THE EVALUATION OF BETA BLOCKER AND CALCIUM ANTAGONIST DRUGS

DEVELOPMENTS IN CARDIOVASCULAR MEDICINE

VOLUME 18

THE EVALUATION OF BETA BLOCKER AND CALCIUM ANTAGONIST DRUGS

Proceedings of the Symposium on How to Evaluate New Beta Blockers and Calcium Antagonist Drugs held in Philadelphia, PA, October 21-22, 1981

Edited by

Joel Morganroth, M.D.,
The Lankenau Medical Research Center,
Jefferson Medical College of The Thomas Jefferson University, Philadelphia, PA

E. Neil Moore, D.V.M., Ph.D.,
School of Veterinary Medicine,
University of Pennsylvania, Philadelphia, PA

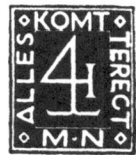

1982

MARTINUS NIJHOFF PUBLISHERS
THE HAGUE / BOSTON / LONDON

Distributors

for the United States and Canada
Kluwer Boston, Inc.
190 Old Derby Street
Hingham, MA 02043
USA

for all other countries
Kluwer Academic Publishers Group
Distribution Center
P.O. Box 322
3300 AH Dordrecht
The Netherlands

Library of Congress Cataloging in Publication Data

Symposium on How to Evaluate New Beta Blockers and
    Calcium Antagonist Drugs (1981 : Philadelphia,
    Pa.)
    The evaluation of beta blocker and calcium
antagonist drugs.

    (Developments in cardiovascular medicine ;
v. 18)
    1. Adrenergic beta receptor blockaders--
Congresses. 2. Calcium--Antagonists--Congresses.
3. Cardiovascular agents--Testing--Congresses.
I. Morganroth, Joel. II. Moore, E. Neil.
III. Title. IV. Series. [DNLM: 1. Adrenergic
beta receptor blockaders--Congresses. 2. Calcium

antagonists, Exogenous--Congresses. 3. Cardiovascular diseases--Drug therapy--Congresses.
4. Cardiovascular agents--Standards--Congresses.
W1 DE997VME v. 18 / QV 150 S9893e 1981]
RM347.S95 1981   616.1'061   82-2267
                                    AACR2

ISBN-13: 978-94-009-7563-7   e-ISBN-13: 978-94-009-7561-3
DOI: 10.1007/978-94-009-7561-3

PREFACE

With the beginning of the 1980's it was becoming increasingly evident that the lack of approval of new cardiovascular agents for use by clinicians in the United States for the treatment of cardiovascular disorders was becoming a problem. Patients requiring medical therapy for hypertension, angina pectoris, arrhythmias, congestive heart failure, and vasospastic disorders of the coronary arteries could receive in the United States only a small number of the drugs available to physicians in the rest of the world. In fact, as the 1980's began, there was only one available beta blocking agent released by The Food and Drug Administration; and even as of this writing, no oral calcium antagonist agent. This lag, in part, has been due to the confusion of proper and expeditious methods to define safety and efficacy of such agents so that the United States regulatory agency (Food and Drug Administration) could approve the use of such agents by clinicians. The vast number of new beta blocker and calcium antagonist agents being developed, as well as the long-term use abroad of many new drugs, has raised important questions as to how relative safety and efficacy of such agents can be determined to facilitate availability in the United States.

The vast array of conditions in cardiovascular medicine that can be treated with either beta blockers or calcium antagonist drugs and the emerging evidence that such treatment cannot only markedly improve lifestyle by eliminating disease morbidity but also decrease the potential of developing sudden cardiac death emphasizes the importance to these classes of drugs.

The following manuscripts represent the collective efforts of physicians and scientists from the United States and abroad as well as members of The Food and Drug Administration and the pharmaceutical industry to address this problem. The contributors have provided state-of-the-art papers which address the important topics in this field. Discussion sections, provided after each segment of the Symposium, allowed participants to express their viewpoints about the important issues and allowed consensus opinions to emerge. While we do not anticipate that this Symposium would evolve a unanimous consensus on means to expedite the proper evaluation of beta blocker and calcium antagonist agents, it was evident that it did identify important research questions yet to be answered and clarified many problems and points of differences between the various components participating in the Symposium.

We hope that this book will be useful as a reference for those individuals who design study protocols and define guidelines to determine the suitability of new beta blockers and calcium antagonist agents.

Joel Morganroth, M.D.

E. Neil Moore, D.V.M., Ph.D.

Philadelphia, Pennsylvania, U.S.A.

CONTENTS

INTRODUCTION

HOW TO EVALUATE NEW BETA BLOCKER AND CALCIUM ANTAGONIST DRUGS: THE CHALLENGE OF THE 1980s

Joel Morganroth, M.D.

In the 1970s it had become clear that overall cardiovascular mortality in the United States of America has been declining. Whether this improvement in longevity was due to alteration in the American diet, better detection of cardiovascular risk factors and their treatment, or to the more wide use of certain classes of new pharmacologic agents remained yet to be demonstrated.

The primary disorders in cardiovascular medicine which afflict the population include hypertension, coronary artery disease and electrical instability of the heart producing arrhythmias. About one dozen drugs account for about two-thirds of all prescriptions written by physicians in the United States for the treatment of cardiovascular disorders. This points to the relatively limited armamentarian available to clinicians in the United States compared to the scope of medical treatment available abroad.

One of the most important developments in the therapy of cardiovascular disorders was the availability of beta blocking agents because of their versatility, potency and relative safety. While beta blocking agents have important differences in terms of their membrane effects, intrinsic stimulating activity (agonist activity) and cardioselectivity, no data exists that one agent appears to be better than another for the treatment of cardiovascular disease. This class of agents can be used to treat patients with hypertension, coronary artery disease

and arrhythmias as well as other non-cardiovascular conditions. As of this
writing, only three beta blockers have been approved in the United States; and
these three agents account for over one-fifth of all cardiovascular prescriptions
and approximately one-quarter of all new increased numbers of prescriptions so
far in 1981.

Possibly the most significant advance in the last 20 years in cardiovascular
medical therapy was the availability of beta adrenergic blocking agents. It is now
felt that the most significant advance in the next 20 years will be in the
evaluation and use of calcium antagonist blocking agents. Beta blocking agents
provided an important insight into underlying physiologic mechanisms that
regulate body systems in both normal and abnormal sates. While calcium
antagonist agents have been used for many years outside the United States for the
treatment of hypertension, coronary artery diseases and arrhythmias, none have
been available for the treatment of patients in the United States until just
recently.

The title of this Symposium is "How to Evaluate New Beta Blocker and
Calcium Antagonist Drugs" and its purpose is to arrive at more precise and helpful
guidelines to determine how to expedite the evaluation of efficacy and safety of
these agents in order to hasten their release by the Food and Drug Administration.

This Symposium was organized by investigators and has no official sanction
or political affiliations; and therefore, the comments herein expressed represent
only those of the individuals involved. The funding of this Symposium was
achieved by educational grants from over two dozen members of the
pharmaceutical and related health care industries.

The organization of this Symposium was in two parts: Part 1 detailed the
important issues in beta blocker agents. These issues included: #1--Whether
there exists important clinically relevant differences between the various beta
blocker agents; #2--What should be considered the recommendations on the most

expeditious means of defining efficacy of beta blocker agents as used in various clinical indications; #3--Comparative safety of beta blocker issues in general and in particular situations in which beta blocking agents are used with caution or are currently considered contraindicated; #4--Problems in study designs to answer these questions; and #5--The question of whether or not beta blockers prevent sudden death in patients post myocardial infarction.

Part 2 of the Symposium addressed the calcium antagonist agents. Topics included: #1--Whether there exists clinically relevant important differences between the various calcium antagonist agents; #2--How to expedite the definition of efficacy in various clinical indications and #3--Issues of safety and problems in the combined use of calcium antagonist and beta blocker agents.

The discussion sections following each of these segments of this Symposium were held to attempt to answer by consensus opinion the important questions raised. Active discussions between the academic investigators in the United States and abroad, scientists and advisors from the Food and Drug Administration and National Institutes of Health and representatives of the pharmaceutical and health care industry addressed these issues. It is our hope that this information can be used to establish new guidelines which will be used as the basis for an efficient and safe means of providing to the American public these new and important cardiovascular agents which we hope will be important contributions to the further decrement in cardiovascular morbidity and mortality.

FACULTY

William B. Abrams, M.D.
Adjunct Professor of Medicine
Jefferson Medical College of The Thomas Jefferson University
Executive Director, Clinical Research
Merck Sharp & Dohme Research Laboratories
West Point, Pennsylvania 19486

Jay N. Cohn, M.D.
Professor of Medicine and Chairman of Cardiology
University of Minnesota Hospital
Box 488, Mayo Clinic
Minneapolis, Minnesota 55455

Leonard S. Dreifus, M.D.
Professor of Medicine and Physiology
Jefferson Medical College of The Thomas Jefferson University
Chief, Division of Cardiology
Lankenau Medical Research Center
Philadelphia, Pennsylvania 19151

Stewart J. Ehrreich, Ph.D.
Deputy Director, Division of Cardio-Renal Drug Products
Food and Drug Administration
Cardio-Renal - HFD-110
5600 Fishers Lane
Rockville, Maryland 20857

Stephen Epstein, M.D.
Chief, Cardiology Branch
National Heart, Lung & Blood Institute
National Institutes of Health
Building 10-7B-10
Bethesda, Maryland 20014

Curt D. Furberg, M.D.
Chief, Clinical Trials Branch
National Heart, Lung & Blood Institute
National Institutes of Health
Federal Building-216
Bethesda, Maryland 20852

Donald C. Harrison, M.D.
William G. Irwin Professor
Chief, Cardiology Division
Stanford University School of Medicine
Stanford, California 94305

Norman Kaplan, M.D.
Professor of Medicine
University of Texas Southwestern Medical School
5323 Harry Hines Boulevard
Dallas, Texas 57235

Robert E. Kates, Ph.D.
Assistant Professor of Medicine
Stanford University Medical Center
Division of Cardiology C-2E
Stanford, California 94305

Eric L. Michelson, M.D.
Assistant Professor of Medicine
Jefferson Medical College of The Thomas Jefferson University
Chief, Clinical Research Unit
Lankenau Medical Research Center
Philadelphia, Pennsylvania 19151

E. Neil Moore, D.V.M., Ph.D.
School of Veterinary Medicine
Professor of Physiology
University of Pennsylvania
3800 Spruce Street--H1
Philadelphia, Pennsylvania 19174

Joel Morganroth, M.D.
Associate Professor of Medicine
Jefferson Medical College of The Thomas Jefferson University
Chief, Cardiac Research and Education
Lankenau Medical Research Center
Philadelphia, Pennsylvania 19151

Robert A. O'Rourke, M.D.
Professor of Medicine
Chief of Cardiology
University of Texas Health Science Center
7703 Floyd Curl Drive
San Antonio, Texas 78284

Alfred F. Parisi, M.D.
Associate Professor of Medicine
Harvard Medical School
Chief, Cardiology Section
West Roxbury VA Medical Center
1400 VFW Parkway
West Roxbury, Massachusetts 02132

Dr. Edward Rowland
Senior Research Fellow
Royal Postgraduate Medical School
Hammersmith Hospital
London W12 OHS England

James A. Schoenberger, M.D.
Professor and Chairman, Department of Preventive Medicine
Professor of Medicine
Rush Presbyterian-St. Luke's Medical Center
1743 West Harrison Street
10th Floor Schweppe-Sprague
Chicago, Illinois 60612

Ludger Seipel, M.D.
Director of Cardiology
University of Tubingen
Med. Klinik II
D-74 Tuebingen, West Germany

Burton E. Sobel, M.D.
Professor of Medicine and Director, Cardiovascular Division
Washington Cardiologist-in-Chief
Barnes Hospital
660 Euclid Avenue
St. Louis, Missouri 63110

Peter Somani, M.D., Ph.D.
Professor of Pharmacology and Medicine
Medical College of Ohio
C.S. 10008
Toledo, Ohio

Robert Temple, M.D.
Director, Division of Cardio-Renal Drug Products Food and Drug Administration
Bureau of Drugs, HFD-110
Parklawn Building
Rockville, Maryland 20857

Jerome Weinstein, M.D.
Consultant, Cardiovascular Pharmacology
The St. Vincent Hospital & Medical Center of New York
Director, Clinical Research, Cardiovascular/Renal
Hoechst-Roussel Pharmaceuticals Inc.
Route 202-206 North
Somerville, New Jersey 08876

Lars Werko, M.D.
Executive Vice President
AB Astra
S-151
85 Sodertalje, Sweden

Alastair J. J. Wood, M.D.
Associate Professor, Pharmacology and Medicine
Vanderbilt University School of Medicine
Department of Clinical Pharmacology
Nashville, Tennessee 37232

Beta-Adrenoceptor Blocking Agents: Historical Perspectives

William B. Abrams, M.D.

Introduction

The availability of beta-adrenoceptor blocking agents has been recognized as a major therapeutic advance of this century. They have proven effective in the control of certain cardiac arrhythmias, provided the first effective therapy for the chronic management of common angina pectoris, contributed importantly to the control of high blood pressure, provided well-tolerated topical treatment for glaucoma and are clearly useful in the management of IHSS, migraine headaches and other disorders. Even more important, evidence is accumulating that beta-blockers preserve life when used acutely and chronically in patients suffering myocardial infarction. It is self-evident that many of the disease states for which beta-blockers have been found effective are serious, disabling, and/or life-threatening. This speaks for their importance in our therapeutic armamentarium. How did they come to be? Their history will be traced through their basic science, therapeutic and regulatory tracks.

Basic Science

Since there is no substantial evidence that these drugs act by a mechanism other than the blockade of beta-adrenergic receptors, the story begins with the understanding of the pharmacology of the sympathetic nervous system. In 1905, Langley suggested that neuro-muscular cells contained both excitatory and inhibitory receptors in explaining the actions of epinephrine.[1] A year later, Dale reported

the antagonism of ergot derivatives for the excitatory, but not the

inhibitory vascular actions of epinephrine -- except for the heart![2]

On the basis of these observations, he proposed the existence of at

least two types of receptors, one of which could be blocked by ergot.[2]

The concept was temporarily sidetracked by Cannon and Rosenbleuth who

proposed the presence of dual neurohumoral mediators: Sympathin I and

Sympathin E.[3] However, in 1946 Van Euler demonstrated that nor-

epinephrine was the single adrenergic neurohumoral transmitter sub-

stance.[4] Two years later, Ahlquist classified adrenergic receptors as

alpha or beta according to the rank orders of potency of six sympatho-

mimetic amines in several physiologic systems.[5] His concept was con-

firmed a decade later when Powell and Slater synthesized dichloro-

isoproterenol and observed its blocking effects on activities now known

to be beta-mediated.[6] DCI was not useful therapeutically because of

its potent intrinsic sympathomimetic activity. The first clinically

useful beta-adrenoceptor blocking agents were pronethalol and propran-

olol, synthesized by Black and Stephenson.[7,8] Pronethalol was dropped

early because of tumorigenic actions in animals. As research expanded

it became clear that more than one beta-receptor existed[9] and this

was confirmed pharmacologically by Furchgott in 1967[10] and clinically

when the cardioselective beta-blocker practolol was introduced.[11]

Studies in animals and man made it clear that beta-adrenoceptor blocking

agents could be classified according to certain pharmacologic activities

in addition to the common property of beta-blockade. By the end of the

1960s, the beta-mediated sympathetic functions were well-defined and

numerous beta-blocking agents were in use or under investigation.

Therapeutics

The potentially adverse effects of catecholamines and inappropriate sympathetic nervous system activity on the heart and circulation were well-known when the beta-blockers arrived on the scene. It is not surprising, therefore, that their use in cardiac arrhythmias, angina pectoris and hypertension was studied early.[12] It is surprising, however, that the cardioprotective effect in myocardial infarction was also studied early,[13]although it took 15 more years to convincingly prove the value.

Cardiac Arrhythmias

A year after the initial publication on pronethalol appeared, Stock and Dale reported on its effects in various cardiac arrhythmias.[14] Their principal finding was that this beta-blocker was useful in slowing the ventricular rate in atrial fibrillation. They also noted utility in suppressing digitalis-induced ectopic beats and tachycardias. On the adverse side, they observed the drug could precipitate or aggravate heart failure when used in this setting. Although much clinical and laboratory research has followed, not much of clinical relevance has changed. Atrial tachyarrhythmias other than fibrillation are considered indications as are arrhythmias associated with sympathetic over-activity.[16] Therapy is more effective because of knowledge gained by pharmacokinetic studies.[17] Propranolol, approved for this purpose in 1967, is the only beta-blocker available for use in arrhythmias in the United States.

Angina Pectoris

As early as 1948, Raab called attention to the potentially dele-terious effects of cardiac sympathetic activity in patients with angina

pectoris.[18] Furthermore, it was known that sympathetic stimulation increased myocardial oxygen consumption more than coronary blood flow.[19]
The suggestion followed that in the presence of coronary artery disease,
augmented sympathetic activity might provoke angina pectoris at an un-
necessarily low level of activity.[20] These notions were confirmed in
1963 when Alleyne and co-workers reported benefit with pronethalol.[21]
A symposium on beta-adrenergic receptor blockade held in England in
November 1965 and reported in the American Journal of Cardiology in
September 1966, included five reports, four involving double-blind
techniques, of the value of propranolol in angina pectoris.[12] Benefits
included reductions in the frequency and severity of anginal attacks,
improvement in the ECG manifestations of ischemia and increased exercise
tolerance. Significant side effects encountered in these early studies
included heart failure, hypotension, bradycardia, heart block, dyspnea
and wheezing, tiredness, drowsiness, lightheadedness, nausea, mild
diarrhea, sleeplessness, visual disturbances, and mental confusion.[22]
A review published six years later listed 28 double-blind trials with
the same basic conclusions.[23] It would appear that the only clinically
important information gained since the early studies is that administration of beta-blockers should be discontinued gradually.[24] This is not
to suggest that a great deal has not been learned about the hemodynamic
consequences of beta-blocker therapy, the role of sympathetic influences
in cardiac events and, as mentioned before, the complex pharmacokinetic
and disposition characteristics of these drugs. Their role in unstable
angina is controversial.[25] All beta-adrenoceptor blocking agents
studied appear to be effective in angina pectoris,[23] including those
with intrinsic sympathomimetic activity.[26] Cardioselective beta-
blockers, at least in low doses, may be preferable in patients with

obstructive pulmonary disease, peripheral vascular disease and
diabetes.[27] Be that as it may, propranolol and nadolol are the
only beta-blockers specifically cleared for use in angina pectoris in
the United States at this time.

Hypertension

In the early 1960s, drug therapy for hypertension comprised diuretics
and agents which inhibited sympathetic nervous system function. As noted
above, hypotension was an occasional side effect of beta blocker administration when given for the treatment of angina pectoris. Prichard
showed first with pronethalol[28] and later with propranolol[29] that
orally administered beta blockers had clear blood pressure lowering
effects in hypertensive patients. Subsequently, a host of studies confirmed these observations for propranolol and all beta-blockers later
investigated for this disorder. When evaluated comparably, all appear
to be equally effective.[30] It is of interest that in the 1965 symposium referred to above, the antihypertensive mechanism of action is
postulated to be a "gradual conditioning" of the baroreceptors.[31]
Fifteen years later this remains a prominant hypothesis among six proposals.[32] The mechanism of action is still unknown. It is also of
interest that in early studies, as at present, beta-blocker therapy
alone did not control all patients and worked well in combination with a
diuretic.[33,34] The beta-blockers are now official members of the
stepped care approach to the treatment of hypertension.[35] Propranolol,
metoprolol, nadolol, and atenolol are available for use in hypertension
in this country and approval for timolol is expected in the near future.

Myocardial Infarction

As noted above, interest in the use of beta-adrenoceptor blocking agents in acute myocardial infarction began in 1965 with the report of Snow[13] that orally administered propranolol reduced mortality when compared to placebo. Although subsequent controlled trials conducted in the 1960s failed to confirm this observation,[36-38] these studies were limited by the use of low and fixed dose regimens. Interest was rekindled in the subsequent decade by experimental and clinical evidence that beta-blockade opposed the patho-physiologic events in acute myocardial infarction, reduced the symptoms and signs of heart attack and had the potential to preserve myocardial tissue.[39-43] For the post-myocardial infarction state, controlled trials with alprenolol[44] and practolol[45] suggested these beta blockers had the potential to reduce death rates, at least in some groups of patients. However, prior to 1981, these studies were the only completed double-blind, randomized trials with reasonably positive findings. Eight multicenter trials are still in progress.[46] Nineteen eighty-one, however, brought the completion of the Norwegian multi-center trial with timolol, which demonstrated a 45% reduction in total mortality and a 28% reduction in the reinfarction rate in patients treated with timolol versus placebo.[47] The patients were treated from the time of clinical stability to a mean of 17 months post-infarction. The mortality findings obtained whether the results were analyzed according to treatment received or original randomization, i.e., "intention to treat." If the survival rates which occurred in this study persist in the general population, it has been suggested such treatment could save 10-15,000 lives annually in this country.

A very recent paper from Sweden reports metoprolol administered I.V., then oral, from early after hospitalization to three months, reduced mortality by 36% versus placebo.[48] This rate is by initial randomization. If the results of this study stand up to the intensive scrutiny applied to all the beta blocker myocardial infarction trials, one would have to conclude that early, as well as chronic, administration of beta-blockers saves lives in this setting. Three decades of animal and human experimental evidence favoring this conclusion is being endorsed. Since this paper is entitled: "Historical Perspectives," one should note that it took 17 years from the development of the first clinically useful beta-blocker, and 16 years from the first report on this use, to the development of substantial evidence that members of this group of drugs can radically improve the prognosis of heart attack, the greatest killer in the Western world.

Glaucoma

Touching briefly on glaucoma, in 1967 it was observed that systemic administration of propranolol for hypertension lowered intraocular pressure in patients with concomitant glaucoma.[49] Topical application was also effective, but use limited by local anesthetic effects.[50] Timolol, which lacks this property, proved to be effective in lowering intraocular pressure with good tolerance and a long duration of action.[51] Clinical trials began in 1975 and the drug was approved for use in the United States in 1978. As in the various cardiovascular applications of beta adrenoceptor blocking agents, the mechanism of action is unknown. It is clear, however, that the production of aqueous humor is reduced.[51]

Regulatory

The 1962 Amendments to the Food, Drug and Cosmetic Act of 1938, directed the Food and Drug Administration not to approve the use of new drugs in the United States unless there is substantial evidence of efficacy, as well as the previous requirement for safety.[52] "Substantial evidence" is interpreted to mean supported by adequate and well-controlled clinical investigations.[52] This requisite, plus expanded animal safety, biopharmaceutical and control and manufacturing regulations, places the Food and Drug Administration squarely into the drug development process. The agency shares with sponsors the joys and hazards of bringing new therapeutic agents to the American people. The beta adrenoceptor blocking agents have been prominantly mentioned in the "drug lag" discussion because of their wide availability overseas and limited availability in this country.[53]Table 1 shows only propranolol has been approved for use in cardiac arrhythmias. Propranolol in 1973 and nadolol in 1979 have been approved for angina pectoris. For hypertension, propranolol was approved in 1976, metoprolol in 1978, nadolol in 1979 and atenolol this year. Of course, this sparse table provides no information on the quality of the data supplied to the FDA in the past in support of claims. One can say, however, that with proof of efficacy, supported by adequate and well-controlled clinical trials, that beta-adrenoceptor blocking agents preserve life. The substantial efforts of the Food and Drug Administration to eliminate the cardiovascular drug lag are coming just in time.

Summary

The availability of beta-adrenoceptor blocking agents has been recognized as a major therapeutic achievement of this century. The development of clinically useful drugs of this class was preceded and accompanied by basic science and clinical research observations which permitted their rapid incorporation into the therapeutic armamentarium. Their use in cardiac arrhythmias, angina pectoris, hypertension, glaucoma and other important disorders is now well-established. Sixteen years of research efforts and numerous multi-center trials have led to credible evidence that members of this class of drugs can save lives after myocardial infarction. Their progress through the regulatory process in the United States has not been as rapid as their value might have warranted. The current efforts of the Food and Drug Administration to proceed more rapidly with these and other life-saving drugs are fully justified.

Table 1

Beta-Adrenoceptor Blocking Agents

Regulatory History

AGENT	IND FILED	NDA FILED	ADVISORY BOARD APPROVAL	NDA APPROVED
Propranolol				
Arrhythmias	5/64	6/66	-	11/67
Angina Pectoris	12/70	4/68	-	9/73
Hypertension	1/73	12/74		6/76
Metoprolol	8/73	11/76	10/77	8/78
Nadolol				
Hypertension	3/73	9/77	3/79	12/79
Angina Pectoris	3/73	9/77	3/79	12/79
Atenolol				
Hypertension	10/73	12/78	11/79	8/81
Timolol				
Glaucoma	12/74	1/78	6/78	8/78

References

1. Langley, J. N. On the reaction of cells and of nerve-endings to certain poisons, chiefly as regards the reaction of striated muscles to nicotine and curare. J. Physiol., 33:374, 1905.

2. Dale, H. H. On some physiological actions of ergot. J. Physiol., London, 34:136, 1906.

3. Cannon, W. B. and Rosenbleuth, A. Autonomic neuro-effector system. Macmillan Co., New York, 1937.

4. Van Euler, U. S. A specific sympathomimetic ergone in adrenergic nerve fibers (sympathin) and its relation to adrenaline and noradrenaline. Acta Physiol. Scand., 12:73, 1946.

5. Ahlquist, R. P. The study of the adrenotropic receptors. Am. J. Physiol., 153:486, 1948.

6. Powell, C. E. and Slater, I. H. Blocking of inhibitory adrenergic receptors by a dichloro analogue of isoproterenol. J. Pharmacol. & Exper. Therap., 122:480, 1958.

7. Black, J. W. and Stevenson, J. S. Pharmacology of a new adrenergic beta-receptor-blocking compound (Nethalide). Lancet, 2:311, 1962.

8. Black, J. W., Crowther, A. F., Shanks, R. G., Smith, L. H. and Dornhorst, A. C. A new adrenergic beta-receptor antagonist. Lancet, 1:1080, 1964.

9. Lands, A. M. and Brown, T. D. A comparison of the cardiac stimulating and bronchodilator actions of selected sympathomimetic amines. Proc. Soc. Exp. Biol., 116:331, 1964.

10. Furchgott, R. F. The pharmacological differentiation of adrenergic receptors. Ann. N. Y. Acad. Sci., 139:553, 1967.

11. Dunlop, D. and Shanks, R. G. Selective blockade of adrenoceptive beta-receptors in the heart. Brit. J. Pharmacol., 32:201, 1968.

12. Braunwald, E.(ed.) "Symposium on Beta Adrenergic Receptor Blockade," Am. J. Cardiol., 18:303, 1966.

13. Snow, P. J. D. Effect of propranolol in myocardial infarction. Lancet, 2:551, 1965.

14. Stock, J. P. P. and Dale, N. Beta-adrenergic receptor blockade in cardiac arrhythmias. Brit. M. J., 2:1230, 1963.

15. Stock, J. P. P. Beta Adrenergic Blocking Drugs in the Clinical Management of Cardiac Arrhythmias. Am. J. Cardiol., 18:444, 1966.

18

16. Mason, D. T., DeMaria, A. N., Amsterdam, E. A., Vismara, L. A., Miller, R. R., Vera, Z., Lee, G., Zelis, R. and Massumi, R. A. Antiarrahythmic agents: mechanisms of action, clinical pharmacology and therapeutic considerations, chap. III, in "Cardiovascular Drugs," G. S. Avery (ed.), Baltimore-London-Tokyo, University Park Press, 1:75, 1978.

17. Shand, D. G. Pharmacokinetic properties of the beta-adrenergic receptor blocking drugs. Drugs, 7:39, 1973.

18. Raab, W. Adreno-sympathogenic heart disease. Ann. Int. Med., 28: 1010, 1948.

19. Eckstein, R. W., Stroud, M., Eckel, R., Dowling, C. V. and Pritchard, W. H. Effects of control of cardiac work upon coronary flow and oxygen consumption after sympathetic nerve stimulation. Am. J. Physiol., 163:539, 1950.

20. Apthorp, G. H., Chamberlain, D. A. and Hayward, G. W. The effects of sympathectomy on the electrocardiogram and effort tolerance in angina pectoris. Brit. Heart J., 26:218, 1964.

21. Alleyne, G. A. O., et al. Effect of pronethalol in angina pectoris. Brit. Med. J., 2:1226, 1963.

22. Stephen, S. A. Unwanted effects of propranolol. Am. J. Cardiol., 18:463, 1966.

23. Alderman, E. L. and Harrison, D. C. Beta-adrenergic blockade in the management of angina pectoris, chap. V, in "Circulatory effects and clinical uses of beta-adrenergic blocking drugs," D. C. Harrison (ed.), Amsterdam, Excerpta Medica, 67, 1971.

24. Miller, R. R., Olson, H. G., Amsterdam, E. A., et al. Propranolol withdrawal rebound phenomenon. N. Engl. J. Med., 293:416, 1975.

25. Gunnar, R. M., Loeb, H. S., Scanlon, P. J., Moran, J. F., Johnson, S. A. and Pifarre, R. Management of acute myocardial infarction and accelerating angina. Prog. Cardiovas. Dis., 22:1, 1979.

26. DiBianco, R., Singh, S., et al. Effects of acebutolol on chronic stable angina pectoris. Circulation, 62:1179, 1980.

27. Parmley, W. W. Beta-blockers in coronary artery disease. Cardiovas. Rev. & Rep., 2:655, 1981.

28. Prichard, B. N. C. Hypotensive action of pronethalol. Brit. Med. J., 1:1227, 1964.

29. Prichard, B. N. C. and Gillam, P. M. S. The use of propranolol in the treatment of hypertension. Brit. Med. J., 2:725, 1964.

30. Prichard, B. N. C. and Boakes, A. J. The use of beta-adrenoceptor blocking drugs in hypertension: a review. Curr. Med. Res. Opin., Suppl. 5, 4:51, 1977.

31. Prichard, B. N. C. and Gillam, P. M. S. Propranolol in hypertension. Am. J. Cardiol., 18:387, 1966.

32. Frishman, W. H. The beta-adrenergic blocking drugs: a perspective, chap. 13, in "Clinical pharmacology of the beta-adrenoceptor blocking drugs," W. H. Frishman (ed.), New York, Appleton-Century-Crofts, 199, 1980.

33. Richardson, D. W., Freund, J., Gear, A. S., Mauck, H. P. and Preston, L. W. Effect of propranolol on elevated blood pressure. Circulation, 37:534, 1968.

34. Paterson, J. W. and Dollery, C. T. Effect of propranolol in mild hypotension. Lancet, 2:148, 1966.

35. Abrams, W. B. Stepped care approach to the treatment of hypertension, in "Pharmacology of antihypertensive drugs," A. Scriabine (ed.), New York, Raven Press, 423, 1980.

36. Balcon, R., Jewitt, D. E., Davies, J. P. H. and Oran, S. A controlled trial of propranolol in acute myocardial infarction. Lancet, 2:917, 1966.

37. Clausen, J., Felsby, M., Jorgensen, F. S., Nielson, B. L., Roin, J. and Strange, G. Absence of prophylactic effect of propranolol in myocardial infarction. Lancet, 2:920, 1966.

38. Kahler, R. L., Brill, S. J. and Perkins, W. E. The role of propranolol in the management of acute myocardial infarction, in "Cardiovascular Beta-Adrenergic Responses," A. A. Kattus, Jr., G. Ross and V. E. Hall (eds.), Berkeley, University of California Press, 213, 1980.

39. Mueller, H. S. and Herron, R. How, when and why to use propranolol in acute myocardial infarction. Cardiovas. Med., 2:321, 1977.

40. Brunner, H. The pharmacological basis for a cardioprotective action of beta-blockers, in "The cardioprotective action of beta-blockers," F. Gross (ed.), Baltimore-London-Tokyo, University Park Press, 11, 1977.

41. Frishman, W. H. Beta-adrenoceptor blockade in myocardial infarction, the continuing controversy, in "Clinical pharmacology of the beta-adrenoceptor blocking drugs." W. H. Frishman (ed.), New York, Appleton-Century-Crofts, 119, 1980.

42. Braunwald, E. and Maroko, P. R. Limitation of infarction size, in "Current problems in cardiology," W. P. Harvey (ed.), Chicago-London, Yearbook Medical Publishers, Inc., 1978.

43. Parmley, W. W. Beta-blockers in coronary artery disease. Cardiovas. Rev. & Rep., 2:655, 1981.

44. Wilhelmsson, C., Vedin, J. A., Wilhelmsen, L., Tibblin, G. and Werko, L. Reduction of sudden deaths after myocardial infarction by treatment with alprenolol. Lancet, 2:1157, 1974.

45. Multicentre International Study: Supplementary Report. Reduction
     in mortality after myocardial infarction with long-term beta-
     adrenoceptor blockade. Brit. Med. J., 2:419, 1977.

46. Hampton, J. R. The use of beta blockers for the reduction of
     mortality after myocardial infarction. European Heart J., 2:259,
     1981.

47. Norwegian Multicenter Study Group: Timolol-induced reduction in
     mortality and reinfarction in patients surviving acute myocardial
     infarction. N. Engl. J. Med., 304:801, 1981.

48. Hjaimarson, A., Herlitz, J., Malek, I., et al. Effect on mortality
     of metoprolol in acute myocardial infarction. Lancet, 2:823, 1981.

49. Phillips, C. I., Howitt, G.,and Rowlands, D. J. Propranolol as
     ocular hypotensive agent. Brit. J. Ophth., 51:222, 1967.

50. Bucci, M. G., Missiroli, A., Giraldi, J. P. and Virno, M. Local
     administration of propranolol in the treatment of glaucoma. Boll.
     Oculist, 47:51, 1968.

51. Katz, I. M. Beta blockers and the eye: an overview. Ann. Ophthl.,
     10:847, 1978.

52. Abrams, W. B. Introducing a new drug into clinical practice.
     Anesthesiology, 35:176, 1971.

53. Wardell, W. M. and Phil.(Oxon), D. Therapeutic implications of the
     drug lag. Clin. Pharm. Ther. 15:73, 1974.

THE CLINICAL RELEVANCE OF BETA-RECEPTOR BLOCKADE, INTRINSIC
SYMPATHOMIMETIC ACTIVITY AND MEMBRANE DEPRESSANT ACTION

P. SOMANI

1. Introduction

Since the original report of Powell & Slater (38) describing the pharmacological properties of dichloroisoproterenol (DCI), a large number of β-adrenoreceptor blocking
drugs have been synthesized in the last two decades (13,17,
34,35,41-44). Although originally developed for a limited
clinical application, their introduction in medical therapeutics has truly revolutionized the treatment of almost all
cardiovascular as well as many other diseases. Success of
these drugs can be easily recognized by continued interest
in synthesis and clinical evaluation of numerous drugs within
this broad group. Although only a limited number of β-blockers
are currently approved by the FDA for general use, a large
number of such agents are under investigation within this
country and many more are freely available in other parts of
the world. Thus, a physician is often baffled as to the drug
of choice from such a large number of agents and such a decision
should be based upon a rational and objective considerations
of pharmacological properties such as receptor specificity,
selectivity and ancillary effects. Drugs are generally useful
for a specified clinical condition, but it is well known in
clinical medicine that all drugs possess a primary effect which
forms the basis of their main therapeutic indication, and
secondary effects which are either the cause of their side
effects or are clinically irrelevant. The β-adrenoreceptor
blocking drugs are no exception to this rule. In this
chapter, the relevance of some of these factors in clinical
therapy with the β-adrenoreceptor blocking drugs will be
reviewed.

2. PHARMACOLOGY OF THE β-BLOCKERS

2.1. <u>Drug receptor-interactions</u>. The concept that a drug
molecule must interact with a specific receptor in the cell
membrane to produce its pharmacological effect, whether
stimulation or blockade of the organ function, is now well
established (Fig. 1). The **fundamental properties** which

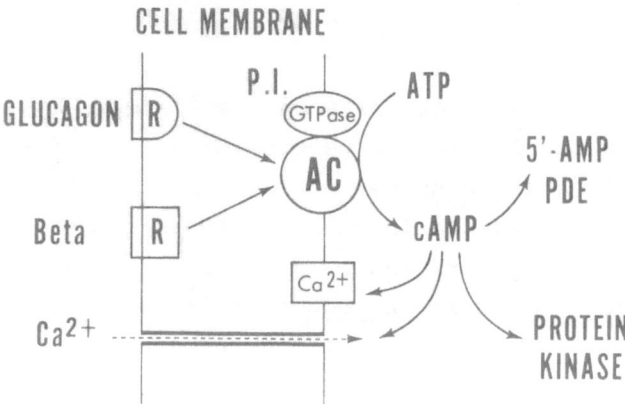

Fig. 1. Schematic diagram to show the concept for specific
drug-receptor interaction in the cardiac tissue. Activation
of the β-receptor stimulates adenyl cyclase (AC), which can
also be stimulated by other drugs such as glucagon. However,
β-blockers inhibit only the response to catecholamines, thereby
suggesting a specific drug-receptor interaction. The drug-
receptor interaction initiates a series of intermediary bio-
chemical reactions which ultimately leads to the observed
pharmacological response.

determine the drug-receptor interactions are affinity,
specificity and intrinsic activity or efficacy. The initial
reaction of recognition of a drug molecule and its binding
to the receptor protein is determined by the *affinity* of the
drug for the receptor. *Specificity* of the binding of the
drug to a given set or subset of pharmacological receptors
determines the selectivity of drug action in the body.
Intrinsic activity of a drug after it forms a drug-receptor
complex determines the intensity of the stimulant effect in
the organism. Drugs which produce a maximal increase in

function are defined as pure agonists or simply as "agonists"; drugs which produce no increase in the organ function but are known to bind with the same receptors, as evidenced by blockade of the response to the specific agonist, are defined as pure antagonists or simply as "antagonists" or "blockers"; there are some drugs which are intermediate between these two extremes they produce less than a maximal stimulant action but block the effects of the agonist - and are defined as "partial agonists". The degree of partial agonism or intrinsic

TABLE 1. Three types of drug-receptor interactions and the pharmacological properties of agonists, partial agonists and a pure antagonist.

DRUG	Specificity Affinity			Intrinsic Activity
AGONIST	+ RECEPTOR ⇌	AR ⟶		RESPONSE
PARTIAL AGONIST	+ RECEPTOR ⇌	AR ⟶		WEAK RESPONSE
ANTAGONIST	+ RECEPTOR ⇌	AR ⊣		NO RESPONSE

activity is usually defined in relation to the maximal (or 100%) response of a pure agonist and therefore may range between < 100 to >1% of the maximum response. Thus, as shown in Fig. 2, it may be seen that when the dose-response curve of a pure agonist is compared to that of a partial agonist, the maximum response of the latter inspite of an increasing concentration is less than that of the agonist. A pure antagonist has no intrinsic activity, but it shifts the dose-response curve of the agonist to the right, indicating its specificity and affinity for the receptors.

2.2. Classification of the adrenergic receptors. Since the original postulate of Ahlquist (1) the receptors in the adrenergic subdivision of the autonomic nervous system are functionally classified into the two broad categories, *alpha* (α) and *beta* (β), each of them being further differentiated into several subtypes (5,6,23,27,28,48). The adrenergic receptor

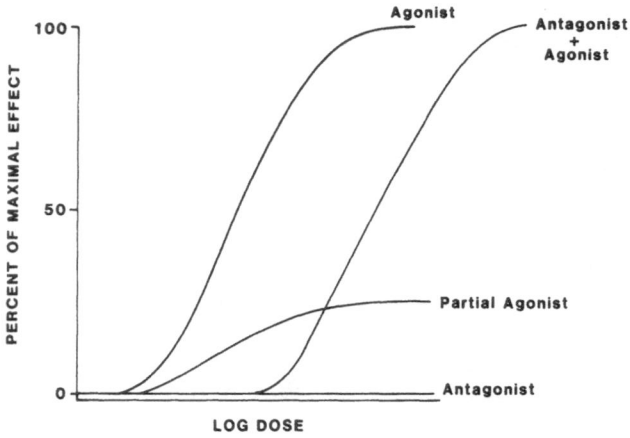

Fig. 2. Three different types of dose-response (D-R) obtained
with a pure *agonist*, a *partial agonist* and a pure *antagonist*
are shown. Note that as the dose of the partial agonist is
increased, a plateau is observed and the maximal response is
less than that of the agonist. A pure antagonist has no
intrinsic activity and therefore elicits no direct response;
however it effectively blocks the effect of the agonist as
evidenced by the shift in the D-R curve to the right.

subtypes may be considered as a family of receptors and while
their differentiation may be very important to the pharmacologist and physiologist, it is equally important to the clinician
because of the opportunity it provides to select either a
receptor-specific agonist or antagonist in an attempt to obtain
the most desirable therapeutic response while minimizing the
potential side effects. Thus, the currently acceptable
receptor classification (Table 2) is supported by the avail-
ability of selective agonists for α_1 or α_2 and β_1 or β_2
receptors in clinical practice and similarly, selective
antagonists for these four subtypes of adrenergic receptors
are currently known. The current list of available receptor-
selective agonists and antagonists is by no means complete
and in future it may be possible to choose from among a series
of organ- and receptor-specific drugs for different subsets
of clinical indications or patient profiles. The extensive
data on the most recent developments in this field are beyond
the scope of this review and in this chapter only the

Table 2. A simplified classification of the adrenoreceptors

Receptor Subtype	Response
Alpha receptors $Alpha_1$	Smooth muscle: Contraction Heart: Prolongation of APD
$Alpha_2$	Presynaptic: Inhibit NE release Renin release:

Beta receptors
    $Beta_1$
	Heart: Increase in heart rate
	        Increase in contractility
	        Cardiac arrhythmias
	        Shortening of APD

$Beta_2$	Smooth muscle: Relaxation Increase in heart rate*

*Carlsson, 1979.

β-adrenergic blocking agents will be considered.

2.3. β-Adrenergic Blocking Agents. Most currently available β-adrenoreceptor blocking drugs are structurally related to the agonist, isoproterenol. These drugs possibly have three sites of attachment to the receptors and the substituent on the aromatic ring determines both the receptor specificity (for β_1 or β_2 subtype) and the intrinsic activity (or lack of it), while the ethanolamine or oxypropanolamine side chain determines their affinity. The clinically useful β-blockers can be classified (Table 3) into either non-selective (i.e., they block both β_1 and β_2 receptors) or cardioselective (i.e., they only block β_1 receptors) groups, although β_2-selective blocking agents have also been synthesized (16,46,55). It should be emphasized that the cardioselectivity of drugs such as metoprolol, atenolol, acebutolol or beventolol is only relative and in large doses, significant blockade of the β_2-adrenoreceptors is indeed possible, and does occur in some patients. Although most of these drugs are highly specific β-receptor blockers, i.e., they do not exert an effect on other types of adrenergic or nonadrenergic (e.g., histamine, serotonin, cholinergic, etc.) receptors, there are at least

the following four pharmacological characteristics of these
agents which must be taken into consideration since these may
prove to be the basis for differences in their clinical activities: potency, receptor selectivity, intrinsic sympathomimetic activity (ISA) and membrane depressant activity (MDA). Thus, potency

TABLE 3. PHARMACOLOGICAL CHARACTERIZATION OF β-ADRENERGIC
RECEPTOR BLOCKING DRUGS.

Group	Drugs
I NONSELECTIVE (β_1, β_2)	
1. Without ISA, without MDA	Bunolol, Nadolol, Sotalol, Timolol
2. With ISA, without MDA	INPEA
3. Without ISA, with MDA	Propranolol
4. With ISA, with MDA	DCI, Alprenolol, Pindolol, Oxprenolol, ICI 72,222
II CARDIOSELECTIVE (β_1) BLOCKERS	
1. Without ISA, without MDA	Atenolol
2. With ISA, without MDA	Practolol
3. Without ISA, with MDA	Metoprolol
4. With ISA, with MDA	CPEP (ICI 89,406)
5. β_1 selective, blocks force > rate	PS-6
6. β_1 selective, blocks rate > force	Mepindolol
III *Beta*$_2$-SELECTIVE BLOCKERS	α-methyl DCI, α-methyl INPEA
IV *Alpha* + *Beta* BLOCKERS	Labetalol

CPEP = 1(2-cyanophenoxy)-3β(3-phenylureido)-ethylamino-2-
propanol; DCI = dichloroisoproterenol; INPEA = n-isopropyl-p-
nitrophenylethanolamine; ISA = intrinsic sympathomimetic activity;
MDA = membrane depressant activity; PS-6 = dl-erythro-1-phenoxy-
3-[(3,4-dimethoxyphenethyl)amino]-butan-2-ol.

describes the mg dose which may exert an effect similar to the
reference compound (propranolol is often used as the reference
compound with potency=1); selectivity defines their relative
affinity for the β_1 or β_2 receptor subtype; ISA describes the
relative intrinsic activity as compared to that of isoproterenol, and MDA is variously described as a direct effect on

the excitable cell membrane. MDA is often equated with the
"local anesthetic like" or "quinidine-like" effect on the
transmembrane potentials or sometimes vaguely described as
"direct" cardiac depressant action.

Potency of a compound is the least important factor in
clinical selection of the drug although a knowledge of relative
drug potencies becomes useful if one is to switch from one
β-blocker to another in a given patient. Cardioselectivity
would be an important consideration in choosing a β-blocker
for a patient suffering from obstructive lung disease,
peripheral vascular disease and possibly for diabetic patients,
but it must be reemphasized that cardioselectivity is only a
relative phenomenon limited to the low therapeutic doses of
presently approved drugs. Other important considerations in
selecting an agent for clinical use are the drug pharmacokinetics, including the bioavailability, extent of the drug
metabolism including the formation of active or toxic
metabolites, plasma half-life, protein binding and renal
handling of the drug and its metabolites and the known
incidence of side effects. These will be discussed in details
by Dr. Wood. The importance of ISA and MDA is discussed below.

2.4. Intrinsic sympathomimetic activity (ISA). The very first
β-blocker ever synthesized, DCI, was found to exert a marked
ISA, and since that time it is known that many other β-blockers
may also possess this property to varying degrees. ISA is
best explained by the direct stimulation of the β-adreno-
receptors as documented in preparations depleted of endogenous
stores of norepinephrine by prior reserpinization (depletion
of the catecholamine stores would exclude release of the amines
as a possible mechanism of ISA). Relative ISA of most β-blockers
has been examined in animal preparations (2,3,4) and I have
grouped them according to their relative ISA in Table 4.
Although ISA of the β-blockers is generally described for
their effect on the heart rate, it is quite likely that a
similar ISA may also be present for cardiac contractile force
and bronchial and arterial smooth muscle for nonselective
β-blockers such as DCI and pindolol (21,38). Thus, on

28

theoretical basis at least, it is possible that a β-blocker
with an appropriate degree of ISA may be superior to propranolol
(or other drugs without ISA) in patients with slow heart rate,
depressed cardiac contractility, A-V conduction delay or block,
bronchospastic condition or peripheral vascular diseases
(Raynaud's phenomenon). For the last two clinical conditions
however, it may be better to use cardioselective β-blockers
instead of the nonselective β-blocker with ISA. Clinical data

TABLE 4. Characterization of β-blockers according to the order
of their intrinsic sympathomimetic activity (ISA)

ISA	DRUGS
100%	Isoproterenol
>50%	DCI, pindolol, ICI 89,406 Carteolol
25-50%	INPEA, practolol, ICI 72,222
10-25%	Alprenolol, Oxprenolol
0-10%	Acebutolol, Atenolol, Beventolo Bunolol, Metoprolol, Nadolol, Propranolol, Sotalol, Timolol

with different ISA in patients with slow heart rate are not
presently available and carefully conducted studies need to
be carried out.

Extensive clinical experience over the last 15 years with
a large number of different β-blockers suggests that all
these drugs, including agents which exert 10-50% ISA in animal
preparations, cause a decrease in resting heart rate in normal
human volunteers, in patients with hypertension or in patients
with angina pectoris (10,17,39,41-44,56). However, pindolol
which has the most pronounced ISA of the currently available
drugs (Table 4) appeared to produce little or no reduction
in resting heart rate in patients with coronary artery
disease (17,51) or hypertension (57). In normal healthy

volunteers, however, Gugler et al. (20) observed a decrease
in resting heart rate with pindolol, metoprolol or propranolol,
although the effect of the latter two drugs appeared to be
slightly more marked (Table 5). All three drugs blocked
equally the increase in heart rate in response to exercise
(20,51). Fisher and coworkers (14) recently showed that the
decrease in heart rate is dependent upon pretreatment heart
rate - patients with heart rate greater than 80 beats/min
showed a significantly greater decrease as compared to those
with basal rate of less than 80 beats/min. Svendsen and co-
workers (51) carried out a very careful comparison of five
different types of β-blockers with propranolol in 37 patients
with ischemic heart disease. Each patient was given six
consecutive doses of a β-blocker intravenously and heart rate,
blood pressure and cardiac output (Swan-Ganz catheter) were
measured before and after each of the six doses of the drug.
These investigators found that so far as the resting hemodynamics were concerned, drugs with no ISA (propranolol and

TABLE 5. Effect of maximal β-blocking doses of propranolol,
metoprolol and pindolol on resting and exercise HR.

Drug Group	Dose (mg)	Resting HR (beats/min)	Exercise HR (beats/min)
Control	—	73 ± 10	163 ± 6
Propranolol	77.7 ± 32.3	61 ± 8	115 ± 8*
Metoprolol	80.5 ± 32.5	58 ± 6*	116 ± 8*
Pindolol	7.5 ± 1.7	71 ± 10	124 ± 4*

*Significantly different from control (data from reference 20)

atenolol) produced a dose-dependent maximum decrease in heart
rate and cardiac output; drugs with intermediate ISA (practolol
and ICI 72,222) produced an intermediate degree of negative
inotropic and chronotropic effect and drugs with pronounced
ISA (pindolol and ICI 89,406) had the least effect. Since a
decrease in heart rate itself may decrease cardiac output,
it is not clear whether or not the decrease in cardiac output
could be an independent phenomenon. Cardioselectivity

apparently was unimportant because each drug pair included a
cardioselective β-blocker (atenolol, practolol or ICI 89,406).
Resting supine blood pressure was not affected by any of the
six drugs. The decrease in exercise-induced tachycardia was
of the same order of magnitude after each of the six β-blockers.
These observations suggest that drugs with marked ISA would
exert less cardiac depressant effect, at least in the absence
of overt CHF. These investigators suggest caution in extrapolating the results form this study to patients with CHF,
since sympathetic tone is markedly increased in such patients
and even β-blockers with marked ISA may reduce heart rate
and cardiac output. However, no definitive clinical data
are currently available, although even pindolol or H87/07,
like other β-blockers, have been reported to produce cardiac
decompensation (7,15,22).

Does marked ISA detract from the antianginal or antihypertensive efficacy of the β-blockers? Several early investigators (8,53) postulated that in patients treated with
β-blockers with marked ISA, the maximal antianginal efficacy
could not be obtained since it appeared that blockage of the
heart rate response to exercise was not as effective after
drugs with ISA as compared to propranolol. McDevitt and co-
workers (36) compared the exercise-induced increase in heart
rate after several doses of six different β-blockers and
showed that while inhibition of exercise-induced tachycardia
after propranolol, sotalol, or atenolol was progressively
increased with a parallel shift in the dose-response curve,
oxprenolol or practolol showed a different type of dose-
response curve with a plateau occurring after an initial
blockade of the positive chronotropic response. These
investigators attributed the plateau effect to the ISA of
the latter two drugs and suggested that very large doses of
β-blockers with ISA are unlikely to be more effective than
smaller doses in treating patients with angina pectoris.
Other investigators (22,25) showed that H87/07, an anolog of
metoprolol but with pronounced ISA, was less effective than
metoprolol in decreasing the frequency of anginal pain,

although no objective difference could be found upon exercise
tolerance test.

Data obtained by several investigators demonstrate that
pindolol is as effective as propranolol in patients with
angina pectoris. Thadani and coworkers (52) recently compared
the antianginal efficacy of five β-blockers with different
degrees of ISA in a randomized, double-blind, placebo-controlled
study. The drugs included propranolol, oxprenolol, practolol,
metoprolol and tolamolol. These investigators found that all
five drugs were equally effective and their hemodynamic
properties were remarkably similar in patients with angina
pectoris. It was concluded that ISA had no appreciable effect
in antianginal efficacy of β-blockers. Frishman et al. (17,18)
showed that 10 mg every 6 hours of pindolol was as effective
as 40 mg every 6 hours of propranolol in reducing the frequency
of anginal attacks, in decreasing the exercise-induced heart
rate, blood pressure or double product (HR X BP), and in the
exercise-tolerance test. Alprenolol and oxprenolol, drugs
with moderate ISA, are also well known to be effective
anti-anginal drugs. It may therefore be concluded that while
drugs with pronounced ISA may or may not decrease resting
heart rate, they are effective antianginal drugs.

Drugs with ISA also are well established to be as effective
as pure β-blockers in treating hypertension (39,41-44,56).

2.5. <u>Membrane-depressant activity (MDA)</u>. There is some confusion in the definition of the MDA in the literature. Early
pharmacology of DCI, pronethalol, INPEA and sotalol clearly
showed that there were distinct differences in their ability
to produce local anesthetic and antiarrhythmic effects against
digitalis glycoside-induced arrhythmias in experimental
preparations (11,31-33,47-49). These antiarrhythmic effects
were shown to be independent of β-adrenergic blocking action
and were believed to be due to a nonspecific quinidine-like
action. Subsequent electrophysiological studies in the canine
Purkinje fibers confirmed that propranolol had a distinct
transmembrane effect (9) similar to that of quinidine and
other antiarrhythmic drugs (Fig. 3). This, in a sense,

should be considered as the MDA of β-blockers, although
sometimes MDA is equated with the direct negative inotropic
action of propranolol (15).

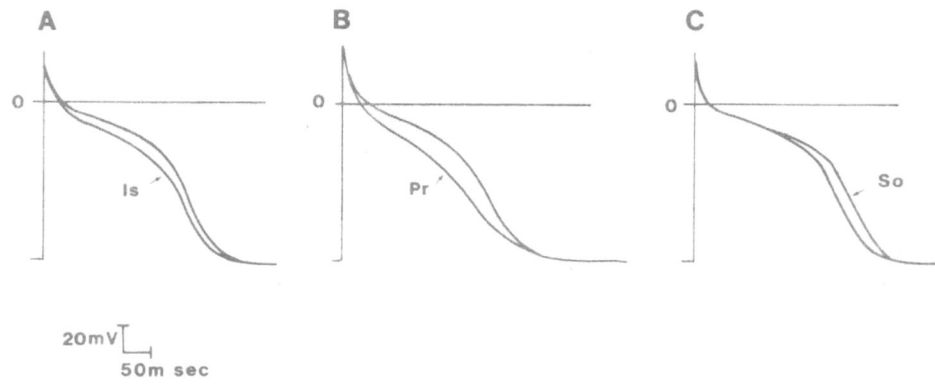

Fig. 3. Schematic diagram showing the differences in the
direct transmembrane effects or propranolol and sotalol on
the electrophysiological properties of the canine Purkinje
fibers. Note that the effect of β-receptor stimulation by
isoproterenol (Is) is to shorten the plateau phase, similar to
that obtained after propranolol (Pr); however, sotalol (So),
a pure β-blocker, prolongs the action potential duration (see
Table 6 for further details).

Early observations showing differences in the antiarrhythmic profile of the β-blockers were confirmed with the
availability of more and more agents, and in experimental
animals it is clearly established that only some of these
drugs are capable of *suppressing* ventricular arrhythmias
induced by toxic doses of ouabain. However, pretreatment of
the animals, especially cats or guinea pigs, may increase the
lethal dose of ouabain. Transmembrane effects of sotalol,
nadolol, INPEA and practolol, β-blockers which fail to
suppress ouabain-induced arrhythmias (12,19,33,47-50) suggest
that their experimental antiarrhythmic profile can be directly
correlated with differences in their transmembrane effects
as compared to those of propranolol (Table 6, Fig. 3). While
propranolol and other β-blockers with MDA reduce phase 0

deplorization and APD (9,26,58,60); sotalol and other drugs lacking MDA prolong the APD (19,45,48,50).

TABLE 6. Comparison of the direct electrophysiological effects of the two groups of β-adrenoreceptor blocking drugs on canine Purkinje fibers[a]

Transmembrane potential	β-Blockers that *fail to suppress* ouabain-induced arrhythmias (sotalol, INPEA, practolol)	β-Blockers that *suppress* ouabain-induced arrhythmias (propranolol, alprenolol, pindolol)
Resting potential	No change	Decreased
Phase 4 depolarization (automaticity)	Slowed	Slowed
Phase 0 depolarization (Vmax)	No change	Decreased
Amplitude of action potential	No change	Decreased
Plateau phase (phase 2)	Prolonged	Shortened
Duration of action potential (APD)	Increased	Reduced
Effective refractory period (ERP)	Increased	Decreased
ADP/ERP ratio	Increased	Increased
Membrane responsiveness	No change	Depressed
Conduction	No change	Depressed

[a]These data are based on the results reported by Davis and Temte (1968), Strauss et al. (1970), Singh and Vaughan Williams (1971), and Kumakura and Somani (1974).

2.6. Relevance of MDA to antiarrhythmic efficacy. The experimental and clinical antiarrhythmic activity of all β-blockers is very well established against cardiac arrhythmias of diverse etiologies. Experimental antiarrhythmic and transmembrane electrophysiological data suggest that the mechanism of their antiarrhythmic action includes not only their β-adrenergic receptor blocking action but also the MDA. However, the direct MDA is seen only in very large concentrations and for those agents which possess MDA, it is associated equally with both dextro- and levo- rotatory isomers, whereas the β-blocking action is associated predominantly with the levo-isomer. Thus, while d-propranolol and l-propranolol exert

an equal MDA, l-propranolol is 100x more potent as a β-blocker
(33).

In clinical practice, drugs such as nadolol, bunolol,
sotalol and practolol, which are entirely devoid of either MDA
or local anesthetic action, are as effective as propranolol,
alprenolol, acebutolol, pindolol and other drugs which possess
these properties (18,44) in the management of cardiac
arrhythmias. In this connection, several points should be
made: (a) in general, β-blockers are highly effective against
arrhythmias which are either caused by or aggravated by the
adrenergic nervous system; (b) these drugs are more effective
in supraventricular arrhythmias rather than in ventricular
arrhythmias due to non-adrenergic etiology (Table 7, Fig. 4);
the dose of β-blockers required for antiarrhythmic efficacy is

TABLE 7. Repeated 24-hour Holter tape analyses in patient C.C.

Holter data	Control	Propranolol 20 mg TID	Propranolol 40 mg TID	Propranolo 20 mg TID + Lorcainid 100 mg BI
Total beats	115,906	93,843	91,756	88,081
PVCs/24 hr	33,079	17,155	19,115	1,087
PVCs/hr	1,378	715	797	45
Isolated PVCs	8,520	8,792	6,520	1,065
Pairs	8,068	1,224	1,478	8
Bigeminal beats	10,515	7,133	11,000	14
VT beats	5,976	6	27	0

quite similar to that required to block β-receptors and clinically
it may not be possible to achieve the same very high plasma
or tissue concentrations necessary to produce the direct
transmembrane changes observed in the tissue bath; (d) drugs
which lack MDA are as effective as drugs which possess MDA.
These data suggest that in clinical application of the
β-blockers as antiarrhythmic drugs, direct electrophysiological
effects are not very important.

35

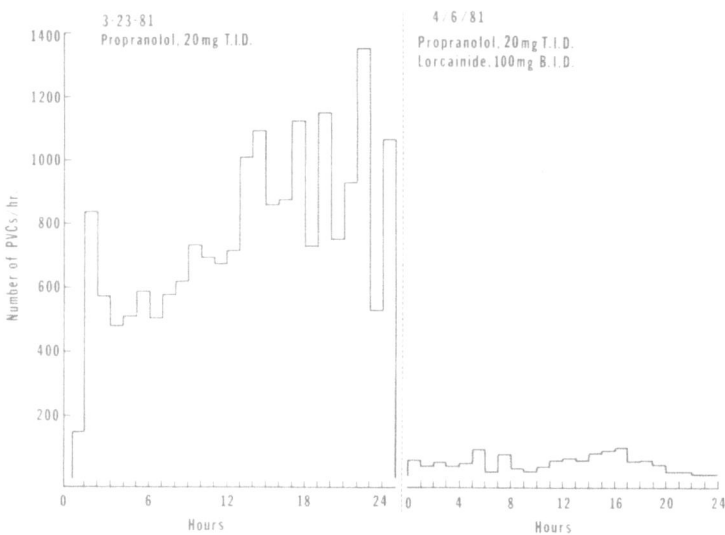

Fig. 4. Histogram showing hourly analysis of the number of
premature ventricular complexes (PVCs/hr) obtained with
24-hour Holter tapes in a 44 year old white female (CC) with
mitral prolapse. During the control two consecutive Holters,
she had an average of 1,378 PVCs/hr; treatment with propranolol
upto a maximum of 20 mg TID reduced the PVCs in a dose-dependent
manner (left panel) and an increase in the dose of propranolol
had no further effect. Addition of lorcainide, an antiarrhythmic
drug, produced further suppression of the arrhythmias (right
panel; Table 7).

2.7. Relevance of MDA to antianginal or antihypertensive efficacy.

Does a lack of MDA make any difference in the choice of
a β-blocker in the treatment of angina pectoris or hypertension?
Perhaps the answer to this question may be provided by comparing the direct hemodynamic actions of propranolol with those
of sotalol, nadolol, bunolol or timolol, drugs which are pure
β-blockers and show no MDA and negative inotropic action in
animals experiments (24,29,44). Clinical data, however, suggest
that the decrease in heart rate and contractile force with
these drugs is quite similar to that observed with propranolol.
Turner et al. (54) and LeWinter et al. (30) recently showed
that both propranolol and nadolol in equal β-receptor blocking
doses produced similar decreases in heart rate or cardiac
contractility (ejection fraction). Thus, a lack of MDA
per se may not offer any special advantage in the choice of the

β-blocker in clinical practice.

3.   CONCLUSIONS.

A large number of β-adrenoreceptor blocking agents have been synthesized over the last 20 years and many of them are clinically available.   There are several important pharmaco- logical properties which should be considered in the clinical selection of an appropriate agent.   β-receptor blocking potency of various drugs differs widely and this is important only in terms of the clinical dose of the drug.   Drugs with some degree of receptor selectivity towards β_1 cardiac receptors may be preferred in patients with obstructive lung diseases.   Intrinsic sympathomimetic activity and membrane depressant actions are ancillary pharmacological properties of β-blockers which may not exert either beneficial or detrimental influence in clinical efficacy of these drugs in patients with angina pectoris, hypertension or cardiac arrhythmias.   Selection of a β-blocker in clinical practice should be dependent upon these considerations and other pharmacokinetic properties.

REFERENCES
1.   Ahlquist, R.P. (1948) A study of the adrenotropic receptors. Amer. J. Physiol. 153:586-599.
2.   Barrett, A.M., Carter, J. (1970) Comparative chronotropic activity of β-adrenoreceptor antagonists. Br. J. Pharmacol. 40:373-381.
3.   Bartsch, W., Dietmann, K., Leinert, H., Sponer, G. (1977) Cardiac action of carazolol and methypranol in comparison with other β-receptor blockers.   Arzneim.-Forsch. 27: 1022-1026.
4.   Bartsch, W., Sponer, G. and Dietmann, K. (1977) Experiments in animals on the pharmacological effects of metipranolol in comparison with propranolol and pindolol. Arzneim.-Forsch. 27:2319-2322.
5.   Berthelsen, S., Pettinger, W.A. (1977) A functional basis for classification of α-adrenergic receptors.   Life Sci. 21:595-605.
6.   Carlsson, E. (1980) On the classification and distribution of β-adrenoceptors.   Acta Pharmacol. Toxicol. 44 (Suppl. II) 17-20.
7.   Collins, I.S., King, I.W. (1972) Pindolol (Visken, LB-46), A new treatment for hypertension: Report of a multicentric open study.   Curr. Ther. Res. 14:185-194.

8. Conolly, M.E., Kersting, F. Dollery, C.T. (1976) The clinical pharmacology of beta-adrenoceptor blocking drugs. Progr. Cardiovas. Dis. 19:203-234.

9. Davis, L.D., Temte, J.V. (1968) Effects of propranolol on the transmembrane potentials of ventricular muscle and Purkinje fibers. Circ. Res. 22:661-667.

10. Dollory, C.T., Paterson, J.W., Conolly, M.E. 1969. Clinical pharmacology of β-receptor blocking drugs. Clin. Pharmacol. Ther. 10:765-799.

11. Dresel, P.E. (1960) Blockade of some cardiac actions of adrenaline by dichloroisoproterenol. Canad. J. Physiol. Pharmacol. 38:375-381.

12. Evans, D.B., Peschka, M.T., Lee, R.J., Laffan, R.J. (1976) Anti-arrhythmic action of nadolol, a beta-adrenergic receptor blocking compound. Eur. J. Pharmacol. 35:17-27.

13. Evans, D.B., Fox, R., Hauck, F.P. (1979) β-Adrenergic receptor blockers as therapeutic agents. Annu. Rep. Med. Chem. 14:81-90.

14. Fisher, M.L., Plotnick, G.D., Hamilton, J.H., Hamilton, B.P., Peters, R.W., Carliner, N.H., Mersey, J.H. (1981) Intrinsic sympathomimetic activity of pindolol: evidence for interation with pretreatment sympathetic tone. Clin. Res. 29:650 A (Abstr).

15. Fitzerald, J.D. (1969) Perspectives in adrenergic beta-receptor blockade. Clin. Pharmacol. Ther. 10:292-306.

16. Fitzerald, J.D., O'Donnell, S.R. (1979) The antagonism by propranolol and α-methyl propranolol (ICI 77,602) of vascular and cardiac responses to isoprenaline in anesthetized dogs. Clin. Exp. Pharmacol. Physiol. 5:579-586.

17. Frishman, W.H. (1980) Clinical Pharmacology of the Beta-Adrenoceptor Blocking Drugs. New York, Appleton.

18. Frishman, W., Kostis, J., Strom, J. et al. (1979) Clinical pharmacology of the new beta-adrenergic blocking drugs. Part 6. A comparison of pindolol and propranolol in treatment of patients with angina pectoris. The role of intrinsic sympathomimetic activity. Am. Heart. J. 98:526-535.

19. Gibson, J.K., Gelband, H., Basset, A.L. (1977) Direct and beta-adrenergic blocking actions of nadolol (SQ 11725) on electrophysiological properties of isolated canine myocardium. J. Pharmacol. Exp. Ther. 202:702-710.

20. Gugler, R., Krist, R., Raczinski, H., Höffgen, K., Bodem, G. (1980) Comparative pharmacodynamics and plasma levels of β-adrenreceptor blocking drugs. Br. J. Clin. Pharmacol. 10: 337-343.

21. Hamilton, T.C., Chapman, V. (1978) Intrinsic sympathomimetic activity of β-adrenoceptor blocking drugs at cardiac and vascular β-adrenoceptors. Life. Sci. 23:813-820.

22. Hedbäch, B., Nordenfelt, I., Svanström, B., Vedin, A. Wilhelmsson, C. Oberg, K. (1977) Effects of a new β₁ selective β-blocker H87/07 in angina pectoris. Ann. Clin. Res. 9:305-310.

23. Hoffman, B.B., Lefkowitz, R.J. (1980) Alpha-adrenergic receptor subtypes. New Engl J. Med. 302:1390-1396.

24. Kaplan, H.R. (1980) Levobunolol, in Pharmacology of Antihypertensive Drugs. Ed. Scriabine, A., Raven Press, New York, pp. 317-323.
25. Keyriläinen, O., Uusitalo, A. (1978) A comparative study of three β_1-adrenoreceptor blocking drugs with different degree of intrinsic stimulating activity (Metoprolol, practolol and H87/07) in patients with angina pectors. Ann. Clin. Res. 10:185-190.
26. Kumakura, S., Somani, P. (1974) The effects of LB-46, a β-adrenoreceptor blocking drug, on isolated normal and ouabain intoxicated Purkinje fibers of the dog. Eur. J. Pharmacol. 25:335-350.
27. Lands, A.M., Arnold, A., McAuliff, J.P., Luduena, F.P., Brown, T.G. (1967) Differentiation of receptor systems activated by sympathomimetic amines. Nature (Lond) 214: 597-598.
28. Langer, S.Z. (1967) Presynaptic receptors and their role in the regulation of transmitter release. Br. J. Pharmacol. 60:481-497.
29. Lee, R.J., Evans, D.B., Baky, S.H., Laffan, R.J. (1975) Pharamcology of nadolol (SQ 11725), A β-adrenergic antagonist lacking direct myocardial depression. Eur. J. Pharmacol. 33:371-382.
30. LeWinter, M.M., Curtis, G.P., Engler, R.L., Shabetai, R., Verba, J. (1979) Effects of equiblocking doses of nadolol and propranolol on left ventricular performance. Clin. Pharmacol. Ther. 26:162-166.
31. Lucchesi, B.R. (1965) The effects of pronethalol and its dextro-isomer upon experimental cardiac arrhythmias. J. Pharmacol. Exp. Ther. 148:94-99.
32. Lucchesi, B.R., Hardman, H.F. (1961) Influence of dichloro-isoproterenol (DCI) and related compounds upon ouabain and acetylstrophanthidin induced cardiac arrhythmias. J. Pharmacol. Exp. Ther. 132:372-381.
33. Lucchesi, B.R., Whitsitt, L.S. (1969) The pharmacology of β-adrenergic blocking drugs. Progr. Cardiovas. Dis. 11: 410-430.
34. Magnani, B. (1974) β-Adrenergic blocking agents in the management of hypertension and angina pectoris. New York: Raven Press.
35. Mäurer, W., Schömig, A., Dietz, R., Lichtlin, P.R. (1977) Beta-Blockade 1977. Stuttgart: Georg Thieme.
36. McDevitt, D.G., Brown, H.C., Carruthers, S.G., Shanks, R.G. 1977. Influence of intrinsic sympathomimetic activity and cardioselectivity on beta-adrenoreceptor blockade. Clin. Pharmacol. Ther. 21:556-566.
37. Moran, N.C., Perkins, M.E. (1958) Adrenergic blockade of mammalian heart by dichloro analogue of isoproterenol. J. Pharmacol. Exp. Ther. 124:223-237.
38. Powell, E.E., Slater, I.H. (1958) Blocking of inhibitory adrenergic receptors by dichloro analog of isoproterenol. J. Pharmacol. Exp. Ther. 122:480-488.
39. Prichard, B.N.C. (1978) β-Adrenergic receptor blockade in hypertension: past, present and future. Brit. J. Clin. Pharmacol. 5:379-399.

40. Pruett, J.K., Walle, T., Walle, U.K. (1980) Propranolol effects of membrane repolarization time in isolated canine Purkinje fibers: Threshold tissue content and the influence of exposure time. J. Pharmacol. Exp. Ther. 215:539-543.
41. Rahn, K.H., Schery, A. (1978) Betablocker. Munich: Urban & Schwarzenberg.
42. Saxena, P.R., Forsyth, R.P. (1976) Beta Adrenoceptor Blocking Agents - The Pharmacological Basis of Clinical Use. New York: North Holland Publishing Co.
43. Schweizer, W. (1974) Beta-Blockers-Present Status and Future Prospects. Bern: Hans Huber.
44. Scriabine, A. (1980) Pharmacology of Antihypertensive Drugs. New York: Raven Press.
45. Singh, B.N., Vaughn, Williams E.M. (1971) Effects on cardiac muscle of the β-adrenoreceptor blocking drugs INPEA and LB-46 in relation to their local anaesthetic action on nerve. Brit. J. Pharmacol. 43:10-22.
46. Somani, P. (1969) Study on some selective beta-adreno-receptor blocking effects of l-(4-nitrophenyl)-1-hydroxy-2-methyl-isopropyl aminoethane (α-methyl-INPEA). Brit. J. Pharmacol. 37:609-617.
47. Somani, P., Fleming, J.G., Chan, G.K., Lum, B.K.B. (1966) Antagonism of epinephrine-induced cardiac arrhythmias by 4-(2-isopropylamino-1-hydroxyethyl)-methanesulfonanilide (MJ 1999). J. Pharmacol. Exp. Ther. 151:32-37.
48. Somani, P., Guse, P., Toscano, P., Bassett, A.L. (1980) Myocardial transmembrane potentials and adrenergic receptors in Advances in Myocardiol. Vol. I. pp. 189-207. Baltimore: Univ. Park Press.
49. Somani, P., Lum, B.K.B. (1965) The antiarrhythmic effects of Beta adrenergic blocking agents. J. Pharmacol. Exp. Ther. 147:194-204.
50. Strauss, H.C., Biggers, J.T., Hoffman, B.F. (1970) Electro-physiological and β-receptor blocking effects of MJ-1999 on dog and rabbit cardiac tissue. Circ. Res. 26:661-678.
51. Svendsen, T.L., Hartling, O.J., Trap-Johnson, J., McNain, A, Bliddal, J. (1981) Adrenergic beta receptor blockade: Hemodynamic importance of intrinsic sympathomimetic activity at rest. Clin. Pharmacol. Ther. 29:711-718.
52. Thadani, J., Davidson, C., Singleton, W., Taylor, S. (1980) Comparison of five beta-adrenoreceptor antagonists with different ancillary properties during sustained twice daily therapy in angina pectoris. Am. J. Med. 68:243-250.
53. Turner, P. (1974) β-adrenergic receptor blocking drugs in hyperthyroidism. Drugs 7:48-54.
54. Turner, G.G., Nelson, R.R., Nordstrom, L.A., Diefenthal, H.C., Gobel, F.L. (1978) Comparative effect of nadolol and propranolol on exercise tolerance in patients with angina pectoris. Brit. Heart J. 40:1361-1370.
55. VanDeripe, D.R., Moran, N.C. (1964) Comparison of cardiac and vasodilator adrenergic blocking activity of DCI and four analogs. Fed. Proc. 24:712.
56. Waal-Manning, H. (1976) Hypertension: Which β-blocker? Drugs 12:412-441.

57. Wessels, F., Heinze, A., Werth, H.W. (1977) Hochdruck-
     therapie mit timolol, einem neunen beta-blocker. Med.
     Klin (Wien) 72:1689-1695.
58. Wit, A.L., Hoffman, B.F., Rosen, M.R. (1975) Electro-
     physiology and pharmacology of cardiac arrhythmias IX.
     Cardiac electrophysiological effects of beta adrenergic
     stimulation and blockade. Part A. Am. Heart J., 90:
     521-533.
59. Wit, A.L., Hoffman, B.F., Rosen, M.R. (1975) Electro-
     physiology and pharmacology of cardiac arrhythmias IX.
     Cardiac electrophysiological effects of beta adrenergic
     stimulation and blockade. Part B. Am. Heart J., 90:
     665-675.
60. Wit, A.L., Hoffman, B.F., Rosen, M.R. (1975) Electro-
     physiology and pharamcology of cardiac arrhythmias IX.
     Cardiac electrophysiological effects of beta adrenergic
     stimulation and blockade. Part C. Am. Heart J., 90:
     795-803.

Pharmacokinetics and Pharmacodynamics of Beta-Blockers

Alastair J.J. Wood

There are now a number of beta adrenoreceptor blocking agents available in the U.S. and it is likely that this number will substantially increase soon. All of the beta blockers have the property of being competitive antagonists of the endogenous β-receptor agonists epinephrine and norepinephrine. There are substantial differences, however, in their pharmacokinetic properties, i.e, in the way in which they are absorbed, metabolized, distributed and excreted. In addition, the various beta blockers currently available differ in their pharmacodynamic properties, such as their ability to block β receptors of different types (selectivity), their ability to stimulate the β receptor, and their cardiac depressant activity, as well as in their membrane-stabilizing, local anesthetic, or "quinidine-like" activity. The purpose of this presentation is to illustrate the differences that exist between the various agents and to stimulate discussion of the importance of these differences.

PHARMACOKINETICS OF β BLOCKERS

The β blockers currently available and those that we expect to become available in the near future can be divided into two distinct groups according to their route of elimination. Some, such as propranolol, metoprolol, and timolol, are extensively metabolized by the liver, whereas others, such as atenolol and nadolol, are excreted largely unchanged by the kidneys (Table 1); the factors controlling the excretion of the drugs in these two groups are quite different. Propranolol, the first of this group of drugs to become available has been studied extensively, partly because of its therapeutic importance but also because of its utility as a model compound.

TABLE 1: PHARMACOKINETIC PROPERTIES OF BETA BLOCKERS

	Absorption (%)	Systemic Availability (%)*	Protein Binding (%)	Partition Coefficient+	Half-life (hr)	Metabolism	Urinary Excretion Unchanged** (%)
Acebutolol	–	20-60	84	1.87	3-6	50-60%	40
Alprenolol	>90	15	85	2.61	2-3	Extensive	>1
Atenolol	46-62	55	>5	0.23	6-7	Minimal	85-100
Metoprolol	>95	50	12	2.15	3-4	Extensive	>5
Nadolol	15-25	20	25-30	0.71	12-24	Minimal	70
Oxprenolol	70-95	20-60	80	2.18	1.3-1.5	Extensive	2-5
Pindolol	>90	>90	46	1.75	2-5	60%	40
Propranolol	100	33	90	3.65	4-6	Extensive	>1
Sotalol	–	>60	54	-0.79	5-13	Minimal	60
Timolol	>90	75	10	2.10	4-5	Extensive	13-20

*Dependent on both absorption and "first pass metabolism"

** % of absorbed dose excreted unchanged in urine

+ Log partition coefficient octanol/water

Extensively metabolized beta-blockers

These drugs which include alprenolol, metoprolol, oxprenolol, propranolol and timolol (Table 1) are well absorbed following an oral dose, and peak concentrations are achieved quickly (1-6). Food appears to enhance the systemic availability of both propranolol and metoprolol (7). Following oral administration and absorption the drug passes to the liver where it is exposed to the liver's drug metabolizing system. In the case of propranolol, and to a lesser extent metoprolol, the liver avidly removes the drug from the blood (8,9,10).

The avid removal of propranolol from the portal blood prior to its entry into the systemic circulation (first-pass elimination) results in a low systemic availability of the drug following oral administration, in spite of the excellent absorption (10,11). An additional complication is the fact that the avid removal of propranolol by the liver following oral dosing appears to be dose-dependent (2,10). This has two important practical consequences. First, at low doses less of the drug enters the systemic circulation than at higher doses, and second, it is impossible to predict the disposition characteristics of the drug at steady state from a single oral dose because the bioavailability is higher during chronic oral dosing than after the first oral dose (11).

Following oral administration the high hepatic extraction of these drugs is dependent on the liver's drug metabolizing ability, which also accounts for the large difference between intravenous (where there is no presystemic elimination) and oral doses. The factors determining the clearance of propranolol, and hence steady state levels, following oral and intravenous dosing are also different. The oral clearance of the drug is dependent solely on the liver's drug metabolizing ability while, at steady state, the intravenous clearance is influenced mainly by liver blood flow in addition to the liver's drug metabolizing ability. Liver blood flow is much less variable between individuals than is liver drug metabolizing ability; thus, it is not surprising that the variability in propranolol concentrations is less following intravenous administration than after oral administration, when variations of up to twentyfold have been found (12,13). In a strictly controlled trial in which 24 normal volunteers aged 21 to 73 years, received 80 mg of propranolol every 8 hours in hospital, a more than tenfold variation in plasma propranolol concentrations was found (Figure 1) (48).

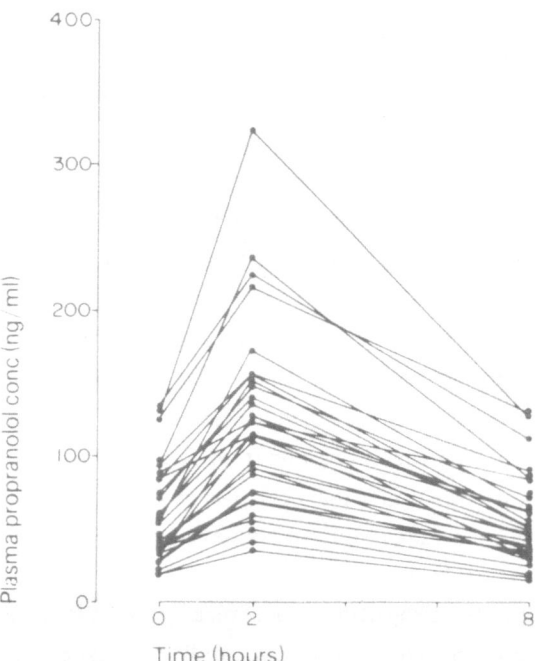

Figure 1:

VARIABILITY IN PROPRANOLOL CONCENTRATION AT STEADY STATE IN A GROUP OF NORMAL HOSPITALIZED VOLUNTEERS RECEIVING 80 mg PROPRANOLOL EVERY 8 HOURS.

From Rutledge, P.A., Shand, D.G. Clin. Pharmacokinet. 4:73-90, 1979.

As pointed out previously, the clearance following oral administration reflects the drug metabolizing ability of the liver. Since this varies widely and is affected by the patients' genetic makeup, the environment to which they have been exposed, their age, and numerous other factors (15), it is not surprising that steady-state drug levels vary so widely. (Some of the factors responsible for this variation will be addressed in more detail later.)

Although most of the studies of the presystemically extracted β blockers have used propranolol, it is likely that these findings can be extrapolated to many of the other β blockers that are avidly removed by the liver.

Renally excreted beta blockers

Atenolol, Nadolol, and Sotalol are mainly excreted by the kidneys as unchanged drug (16,20). Thus, their elimination is impaired in renal disease, but it is not dependent on the vagaries of drug metabolism. It has therefore been suggested that the steady state plasma levels of these drugs will be subject to much less interindividual variation than the highly metabolized beta blockers. While that may well be true, it is important to note (Table 1) that both atenolol and nadolol are poorly absorbed, and although the absorption may be relatively constant (17), it is likely that variability in absorption will result in alterations in steady state levels at least as large as those due to liver metabolism. One must also remember that because of the poor absorption of atenolol and nadolol following oral administration, they too require lower doses intravenously than orally.

EFFECTS OF DISEASE ON THE KINETICS OF β BLOCKERS

Liver Disease

For β blockers such as propranolol and metoprolol and to a lesser extent timolol, all of which are highly metabolized by the liver, liver disease might be expected to have a significant effect on plasma clearance following oral administration. In addition, the alterations in plasma proteins found in cirrhosis may alter the disposition of propranolol, which is highly bound in plasma. Because of the existence of porta-systemic shunts, some of the drug coming from the gut following absorption is able to bypass the liver, resulting in a higher systemic availability of the drug.

The effect of liver disease on the kinetics of propranolol has been carefully investigated using a technique that involves the simultaneous administration of native drug orally and labeled drug intravenously (19). This allows the measurement of all of the parameters controlling elimination including systemic availability, oral or intrinsic clearance (which, as discussed earlier, is dependent on liver drug metabolizing ability), and systemic or intravenous clearance, which is determined at steady state by both drug metabolizing ability (intrinsic clearance) and liver blood flow. In addition, the plasma binding of the drug was measured and used to express the drug concentrations in terms of free or unbound drug in blood. Steady state concentrations of propranolol were markedly higher in cirrhotic patients than in controls (Figure 2). This was due to an increase in systemic availability (38 per cent in the control group as compared to 54 per cent

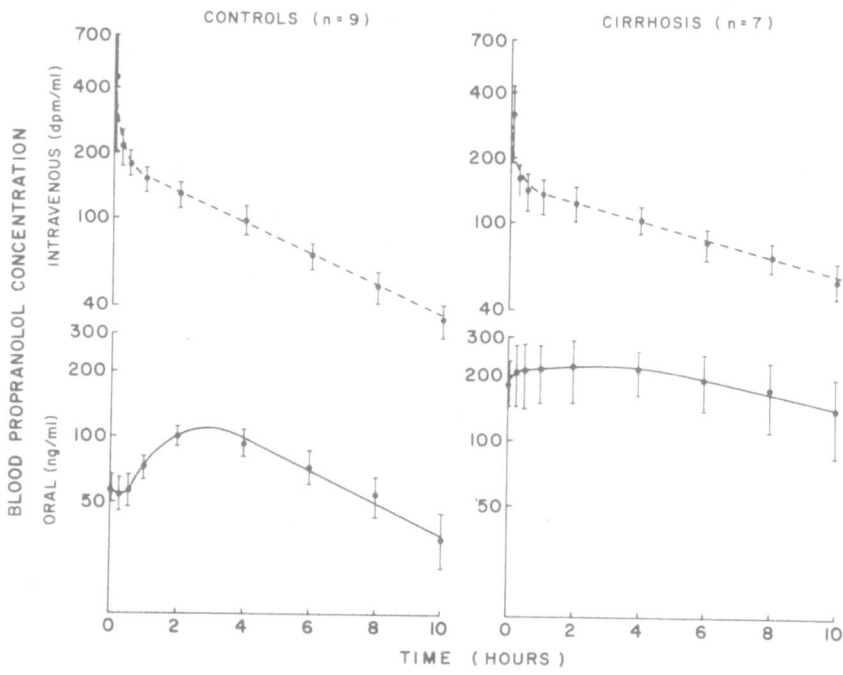

Figure 2

THE CONCENTRATION OF UNLABELED PROPRANOLOL (ng/ml) IN
WHOLE BLOOD AFTER ORAL ADMINISTRATION (●—●) AND THE
CONCENTRATION OF TRITIATED PROPRANOLOL (dpm/ml) AFTER
INTRAVENOUS ADMINISTRATION (●--●) FOLLOWING SIMULTANEOUS
DETERMINATION OF INTRAVENOUS AND ORAL DOSE KINETICS OF
PROPRANOLOL AT THE SEVENTH DOSING INTERVAL IN NINE NORMAL
SUBJECTS AND SEVEN PATIENTS WITH CIRRHOSIS (mean ± SEM)

From Wood, A.J.J., Kornhauser, D.M., Wilkinson, G.R., Shand, D.G. and Branch,
R.A. The influence of cirrhosis on steady-state blood concentrations of unbound
propranolol after oral administration. Clin. Pharmacokinet. 3:478-487, 1978.

in the cirrhotic group) and a decrease in systemic clearance. Because of the increased average total steady state concentrations in blood, coupled with an elevation in the fraction of the drug free in plasma, there was a threefold increase in the average free drug concentration from 7.5 ng/ml to 22.3 ng/ml. It is impossible to predict accurately what the effect of liver disease will be on the steady state levels of other β blockers, but it is likely that drugs such as nadolol and atenolol, which are largely excreted by renal routes, will be little affected, while the drugs that are highly metabolized by the liver will show changes similar to those found with propranolol. However, it should be remembered that changes in protein binding are likely to be less important for drugs such as metoprolol, which is only 12 per cent bound in plasma.

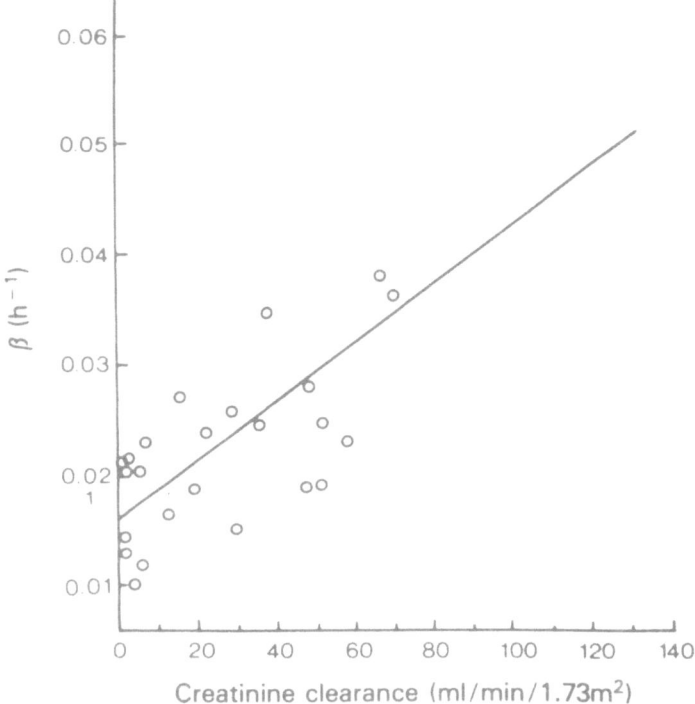

Figure 3

RELATIONSHIP BETWEEN NADOLOL'S RATE OF EXCRETION (β) AND CREATININE CLEARANCE

From Herrera et al. Br. J. Clin. Pharmacol. 8(suppl 2) 227-231, 1979

Renal Disease

It might be anticipated that β blockers that have largely renal routes of elimination might accumulate in patients with impaired renal function; however, it is surprising that there have been suggestions that the excretion of some of the extensively metabolized drugs such as propranolol is also impaired in renal disease. Although a small proportion of timolol (13 per cent) is eliminated unchanged in the urine, the overall clearance of timolol was not prolonged in patients with renal failure (21), and therefore no change in the oral dosage is required.

However, since approximately 70 per cent of nadolol is excreted in the urine (20), its elimination is impaired in patients with renal failure. In fact, the rate of elimination of nadolol correlated well (Figure 3) with creatinine clearance and in patients with the most severe degree of renal failure, the half-life of nadolol was prolonged to 45 hours from the half-life of 14 to 20 hours in patients with normal renal function (20).

The effect of renal disease on the elimination of propranolol has been the source of some confusion with some authors suggesting (3) that the concentrations of propranolol following a single oral dose were higher in patients with renal disease, and absorption appeared to be more rapid. However, others have found impaired absorption and no change in the time to peak levels but did find a reduction in clearance of propranolol in patients with renal failure (22,23). This area has now been clarified following a study of patients with severe renal failure, whether on hemodialysis or not yet on dialysis. No impairment of propranolol elimination, when compared to age matched controls was found (24). Thus, it is unlikely that any adjustment of propranolol dosage is required in patients with renal failure.

Other Factors: age

It is now widely appreciated that the elderly suffer a higher incidence of adverse drug reactions than the young. This higher incidence may be partly due to alteration in their ability to eliminate drugs (25,26).

It has been shown that following 80 mg every 8 hours, blood levels of propranolol were twofold higher in normal subjects over the age of 35 compared to those under 35 (48) (Figure 4). In addition, when the effect of smoking was examined, it was found that the smokers had significantly lower levels of propranolol throughout the dosing interval than nonsmokers (Figure 5). These changes appeared to be due to an age related effect of smoking. The oral or intrinsic clearance of propranolol fell significantly with age only in smokers suggesting that smoking increased the ability to eliminate propranolol only in the young, the elderly being relatively resistant to this effect. Liver blood flow, on the other hand, fell significantly with age in both smokers and nonsmokers and there appeared to be no effect of smoking on the age related fall in liver blood flow. These changes resulted in a significant age related fall in the systemic or intravenous clearance of propranolol in smokers alone (48).

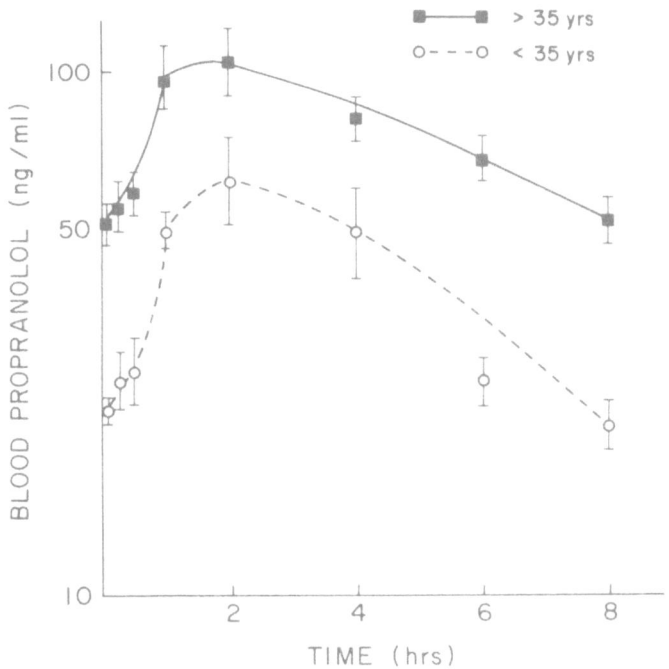

Figure 4:

STEADY STATE BLOOD CONCENTRATIONS OF PROPRANOLOL DURING THE DOSAGE INTERVALS AFTER ORAL ADMINISTRATION OF 80 mg EVERY 8 hr IN NORMAL INDIVIDUALS, ACCORDING TO AGE

From Vestal, R.E., Wood, A.J.J., Branch, R.A., Shand, D.G., and Wilkinson, G.R. Effects of age and cigarette smoking on propranolol disposition. Clin. Pharmacol. Ther. 26:8-15, 1979.

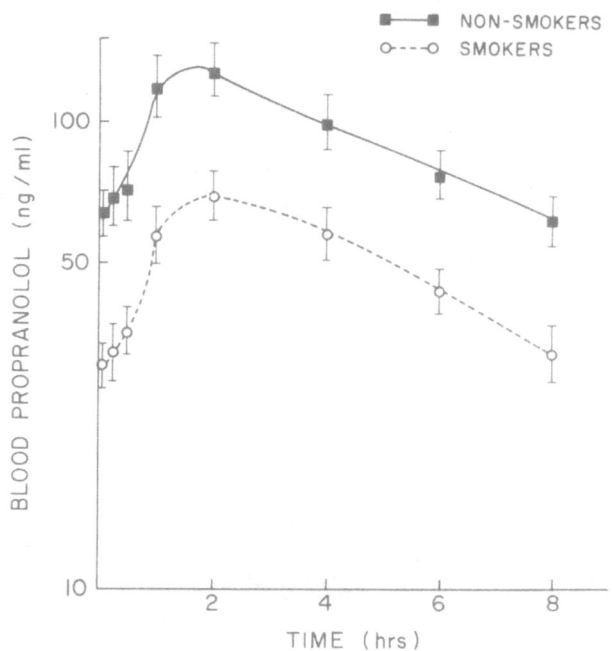

Figure 5:   STEADY STATE BLOOD CONCENTRATIONS OF PROPRANOLOL
DURING THE DOSAGE INTERVALS AFTER ORAL ADMINIS-
TRATION OF 80 mg EVERY 8 hr IN NORMAL INDIVIDUALS -
SMOKERS VS NONSMOKERS

From Vestal, R.E., Wood, A.J.J., Branch, R.A., Shand, D.G., and Wilkinson, G.R.
Effects of age and cigarette smoking on propranolol disposition. Clin. Pharmacol.
Ther. 26:8-15, 1979.

While propranolol is the only β blocker whose kinetics have been studied in detail in aging, the effects of age on the kinetics of some of the others can be predicted. For example, nadolol and atenolol are excreted largely by the kidneys, and as their rate of excretion is known to be closely correlated with creatinine clearance (20), which falls with advancing age, it is likely that their steady state levels will be higher in the elderly, due to poorer renal function in this age group.

From this discussion it is clear that a number of variables affect blood levels of β blockers. As many of the effects of β blockers have a clear relationship to drug concentration in blood, and hence at the β adrenergic receptor site, changes in drug concentration will alter the intensity of the drug's effect.

Liquid Solubility

A feature of beta blockers which is currently receiving more attention is their lipid solubility (lipophilicity). There is considerable variation in the lipid solubility of the available beta blockers (Table 1). As lipid solubility is one of the determinants of drug entry into the brain it is likely that the less lipid soluble agents will enter the brain in smaller amounts resulting in fewer central nervous system side effects.

PHARMACODYNAMIC PROPERTIES OF THE β BLOCKERS

Much has been made of the differences in the actions of the various β blockers. However, all of the β blockers competitively inhibit the effects of both endogenously and exogenously administered catecholamines at the beta-adren-ergic receptors. This means that a larger concentration of agonist is required to produce an effect in the presence of the antagonist, resulting in a parallel shift to the right in the dose response curve.

Assessment of β Blockade

The extent of β blockade can be assessed by a variety of techniques of varying utility. All define the degree of blockade by determining the decrement in a β receptor-mediated response (usually heart rate) to either endogenous or exogenous adrenergic agonist. The sympathetic stimulation produced by standing or exercising can be used as a stimulus for the release of the endogenous agonists epinephrine and norepinephrine. These stimuli will, in the absence of β blockade, increase heart rate. However, the strength of the stimulus for catecholamine-release varies. For example, the degree of catecholamine release following upright posture depends on the subject's previous sodium intake (47). In addition, in the case where the dose-response curve to β agonists is shifted sufficiently to the right by a β blocker (see Figure 6), a given concentration of agonist produced by a constant physiological stimulus may be insufficient to produce any rise in heart rate. Further increase in the degree of β blockade at higher beta-blocker concentrations will then go undetected if this technique is used. This gives rise to the frequent fallacy that two β blockers produce equal degrees of β blockade because they both completely blocked the exercise-induced rise in heart rate.

A better approach to the measurement of the degree of β blockade is to determine the dose of an agent such as isoproterenol which is required to produce a constant response (such as an increase in heart rate of 25 beats per minute) both prior to and following the administration of a β blocker (27). The extent of β blockade can then be expressed as the "dose ratio", or ratio of the dose of isoproterenol required before β blockade to that required after β blockade.

Figure 6 shows the effect of increasing doses of isoproterenol on heart rate. A dose of 1.06 μg of isoproterenol was required to raise the heart rate by 25 beats per minute prior to an infusion of propranolol. Following the propranolol infusion there was a thirty-five-fold increase in the dose of isoproterenol required to produce the same rise in heart rate. This emphasizes a common point of confusion surrounding the effects of β blockers. Since they are competitive antagonists of sympathetic agonists, it is always possible to completely overcome their effects, provided enough β agonist is administered to achieve an adequate concentration at the receptor. There is therefore no such thing as complete β blockade. One can only assess β blockade in terms of the amount of an agonist or the strength of a stimulus required to overcome the blockade.

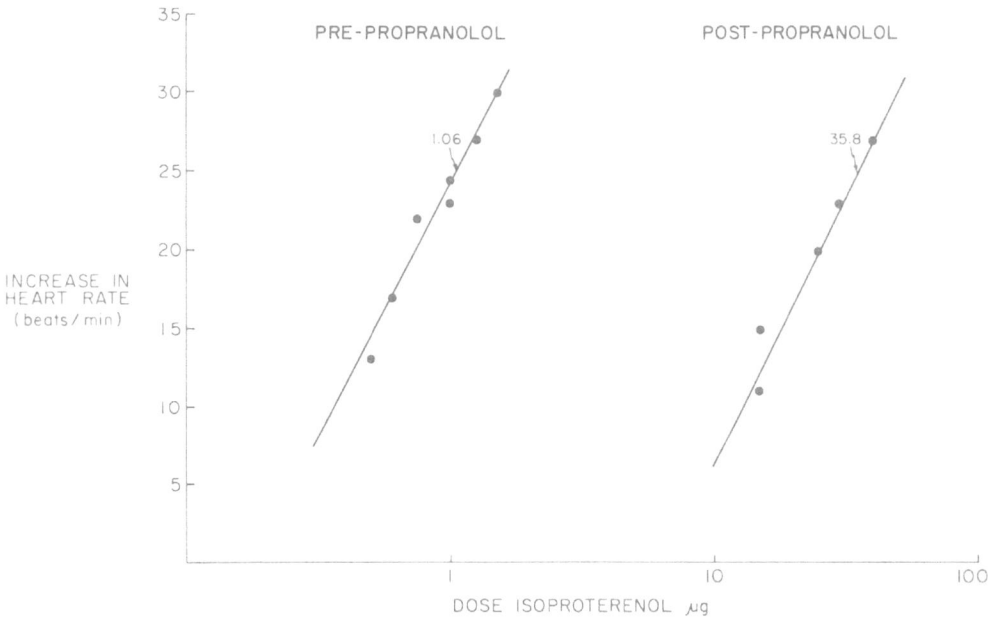

Figure 6:

    INCREASE IN HEART RATE IN RESPONSE TO INCREASING DOSES OF ISOPROTERNOL BEFORE AND FOLLOWING PROPRANOLOL.

Note the parallel shift in the dose response curve.

    This technique has been used to demonstrate (Figure 7) that the dose of agonist required to raise the heart rate by a constant amount (25 beats per minute) increases with advancing age, the elderly requiring around five-fold more isoproterenol than the young (Figure 7) (27).

54

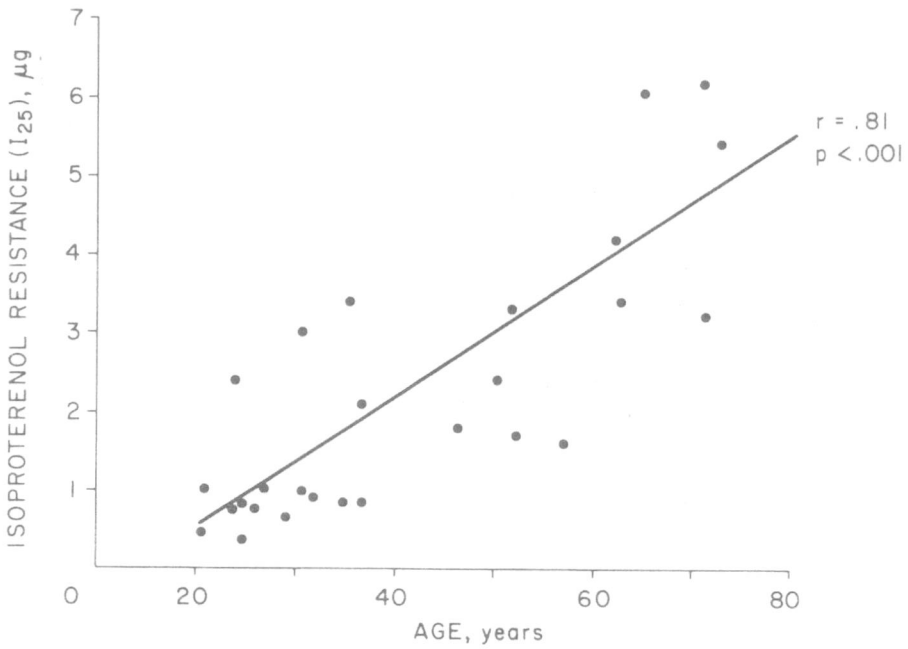

Figure 7:

RELATIONSHIP BETWEEN AGE AND ISOPROTERENOL RESISTANCE AS MEASURED BY THE DOSE (I_{25}) OF ISOPROTERENOL REQUIRED TO RAISE THE HEART RATE BY 25 BEATS PER MINUTE.

From Vestal, R.E., Wood, A.J.J., and Shand, D.G. Reduced beta-adrenoceptor sensitivity in the elderly. Clin. Pharmacol. Ther. 26:181-186, 1979.

Receptor theory would predict that following the administration of an antagonist

$$(DR - 1) = \frac{P}{K_d}$$

where DR is the ratio of the dose of isoproterenol required to raise the heart rate by a given amount (e.g., 25 beats per minute) after propranolol administration to the dose of isoproterenol required before propranolol; P is the unbound propranolol concentration in plasma, that is the concentration available for binding to receptor sites; and K_d is the apparent dissociation constant for propranolol binding to the receptor and hence is a measure of propranolol resistance, since larger values imply less effect. Following the administration of propranolol, it was found that the elderly were four to five times more resistant to propranolol than the young (Figure 8) (27).

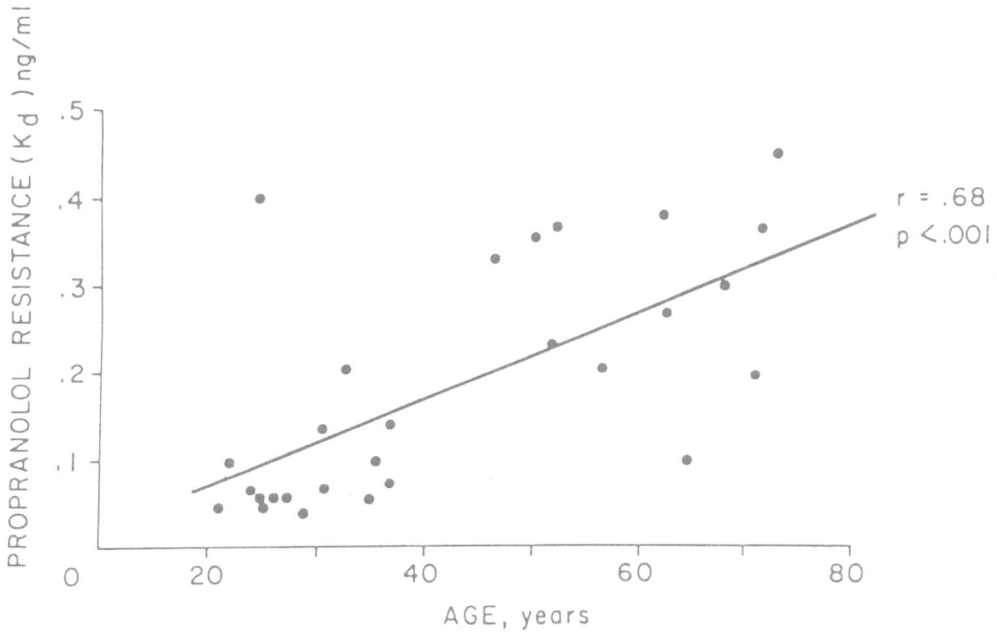

Figure 8

RELATIONSHIP BETWEEN AGE AND THE RESISTANCE TO PRO-
PRANOLOL (k_d - See text). As age advances, greater concentrations of
propranolol are required for beta blockade.

From Vestal, R.E., Wood, A.J.J., and Shand, D.G. Reduced beta-adrenoceptor
sensitivity in the elderly. Clin. Pharmacol. Ther. 26:181-186, 1979.

In addition to their ability to antagonize the effects of β receptor agonists
at the β receptors, some of the β blockers have additional effects that may or
may not be of therapeutic importance (Table 2).

TABLE 2

PHARMACODYNAMIC PROPERTIES OF BETA BLOCKERS

	Potency **	Selectivity for β1 Receptors	Membrane-stabilizing activity	Intrinsic sympathymemetic activity
Acebutolol	0.3	+	+	+
Alprenolol	0.3	0	+	+
Atenolol	1	+	0	0
Metoprolol	1	+	0	0
Nadolol	6	0	0	0
Oxprenolol	0.5-1	0	+	+
Pinodolol	6	0	±	+
Propranolol	1	0	0	0
Sotalol	0.3	0	0	0
Timolol	6	0	0	0

**Relative to propranolol = 1

Membrane Stabilizing or "Quinidine-Like" Activity

Early in the study of β blocking drugs it was found that propranolol had electrophysiological properties that were not related to its antagonism of β adrenergic receptors. Specifically, it was shown that propranolol slowed the rate of rise of the transmembrane cardiac action potential, whereas resting potential and spike duration were unchanged (28,29). It has since been shown that a number of other β blockers possess this effect, including oxprenolol and alprenolol (30). It has been said that this effect has little practical therapeutic importance, since it requires propranolol concentrations as high as 10,000 ng/ml in vitro to produce this effect (31) and inhibition of exercise tachycardia and suppression of arrhythmias occur at levels of only 100 ng/ml (32,33). In addition, D-propranolol, which has much less β blocking activity than L-propranolol while possessing similar membrane-stabilizing effects is devoid of therapeutic efficacy. However, the relevance of some of the in vitro work suggesting that very high concentrations of propranolol are required has now been questioned (34) and recent clinical studies do indeed suggest that propranolol exerts a high dose efect which is independent of beta blockade (35).

Selectivity

Following Ahlquist's original subdivision of adrenoceptors into two types (α and β) according to the relative potency of different sympathomimetic amines (36), almost two decades passed before these receptors were further subdivided into the so-called β_1 and β_2 (37) receptors (Table 3). Stimulation of β_1 receptors produces positive inotropic and chronotropic effects on the heart, whereas β_2 stimulation dilates the bronchi and certain vascular beds. Nonselective β blockers such as propranolol act at both the β_1 and β_2 receptors. However, the so-called selective β_1 receptor antagonists have a relatively greater potency for the β_1 receptor than the β_2 receptor. This means that these drugs will antagonize the effects of agonists on the cardiac receptors at concentrations that have little effect on the β_2 receptors. However, with increasing concentrations of drug, the β_2 receptors will also be blocked. Considerable confusion has surrounded this area; it is important to understand that the drugs are not specific in blocking only β_1 receptors. Rather, they block these receptors at doses that are lower than those required to block β_2 receptors, conveying some degree of selectivity rather than specificity.

TABLE 3

SITE AND EFFECT OF STIMULATING $BETA_1$ AND $BETA_2$ RECEPTORS

$Beta_1$ receptors		$Beta_2$ receptors	
Site	Effect of Stimulation	Site	Effect of Stimulation
Heart	Increased rate	Bronchi	Dilatation
	Increased Contractility	Blood Vessels	Dilatation
		Uterus	Relaxation
		Insulin	Production Increase

In patients with bronchial asthma cardioselectivity may be a useful property, since the selective β blockers are less likely to precipitate bronchospasm in such patients. However, it should be understood that even these selective agents may, in some patients at low doses and probably in many asthmatic patients at high doses, cause bronchial constriction (38). Probably the ideal therapy for such patients, if a β blocker is required, is the concurrent administration of a $β_1$ receptor antagonist along with a selective $β_2$ receptor agonist such as albuterol (salbutamol).

Another situation in which the use of a selective β blocker may be desirable is in the treatment of diabetic patients. Nonselective β blockers may delay the blood glucose recovery from hypoglycemia, whereas selective β blockers such as metoprolol and atenolol do not (39,40). In addition, severe bradycardia and raised diastolic blood pressure have occurred during hypoglycemia while taking propranolol. these effects were milder with a cardioselective β blocker (40). Also the cardioselective beta blockers may not exaggerate the rise in blood pressure during propranolol therapy in response to sysmpathetic stimuli such as the cold pressor test. In conclusion, therefore, cardioselectivity may be of value in some special situations, but these differences are not absolute, and antagonism of $β_2$ receptors does occur, particularly at higher doses.

Intrinsic Sympathomimetic Activity (ISA)

In noradrenaline depleted animal models, it is possible to demonstrate that some of the β blockers (Table 2) have partial agonist activity in addition to their predominant β antagonist properties. The maximum stimulation of the receptors that these drugs can produce is clearly much less than full agonists such as epinephrine or isoproterenol (41-42). It was initially suggested that the β blockers which lacked ISA were more effective in the treatment of hyperthyroidism (43). However, this has now been challenged (44-45). It has also been suggested that drugs with intrinsic agonist activity would be less likely to precipitate cardiac failure in patients prone to this, and that drugs with less myocardial depressant action may be safer in this regard (46). However, it is likely that the principal reason for the precipitation of cardiac failure by β blockers in patients already on the brink of cardiac failure is the removal of the increased sympathetic drive to the heart by β blockade. Patients with compromised cardiac function attempt to maintain adequate cardiac output through increased sympathetic drive to the heart. Removal of this increased drive through the use of a β blocker is likely to precipitate cardiac failure, whatever the drug's effect on the contraction of isolated cardiac tissue in vitro.

Conclusions

There are significant differences between the pharmacokinetics of the various beta blockers. This may be of particular importance in determining the effects of disease states on beta blocker elimination. On the other hand, the pharmacodynamic differences though real, may confer advantages on individual drugs only in special circumstances.

REFERENCES

1. Paterson JW et al. The pharmacodynamics and metabolism of propranolol in man. Pharmacologia Clinica 1970;2:127-133.
2. Shand DG, Rangno RE. The disposition of propranolol. I. Elimination during oral absorption in man. Pharmacology 1972;7:159-168.
3. Lowenthal DT et al. Pharmacokinetics of oral propranolol in chronic renal disease. Clin Pharmacol Ther 1974;16:761-769.
4. Parsons RL et al. Absorption of propranolol and practolol in coeliac disease. Gut 1976;17:129-143.
5. Castleden CM et al. The effect of age on plasma levels of propranolol and practolol in man. Br J Clin Pharmacol 1975;2:303-306.
6. Tocco DJ et al. Physiological disposition and metabolism of timolol in man and laboratory animals. Drug Metab Dispos 1975;3:361-370.
7. Melander A et al. Enhancement of the bioavailability of propranolol and metoprolol by food. Clin Pharmacol Ther 1977;22:108-112.

60

8. Johnsson G et al. Combined pharmacokinetic and pharmacodynamic studies in man of the adrenergic β₁ receptor antagonist metoprolol. Acta Pharmacol Toxicol 1975;36(suppl V):31-44.
9. Shand DG et al. Plasma propranolol levels in adults, with observations in four children. Clin Pharmacol Ther 1970;23:165-174.
10. Kornhauser DM et al. Biological determinants of propranolol disposition in man. Clin Pharmacol Ther 1978;23:165-174.
11. Wood AJJ et al. Direct measurement of propranolol bioavailability during accumulation to steady state. Br J Clin Pharmacol 1978;345-350.
12. Woosley RL, Shand DG. Pharmacokinetics of antiarrhythmic drugs. Am J Cardiol 1978;41:986-995.
13. Chidsey CA et al. Studies of the absorption and removal of propranolol in hypertensive patients during therapy. Circulation 1975;52:313-318.
14. Shand DG. Individualization of propranolol therapy. Med Clin North Am 1974;58: 1063-1069.
15. Vessel ES. Genetic and environmental factors affecting drug disposition in man. Clin Pharmacol Ther 1977;22:659-679.
16. Dreyfuss J et al. Metabolic studies in patients with nadolol oral and intravenous administration. J Clin Pharmacol 1977;17:300-307.
17. Conway FJ et al. Human pharmacokinetic and pharmacodynamic studies on atenolol (ICI 66082)-a new cardioselective adrenoceptor β adrenoceptor blocking drug. Br J Clin Pharmacol 1976;3:267-272.
18. Duchin KL et al. Steady state pharmacokinetics of nadolol and therapeutic efficacy. Clin Pharmacol Ther 1979;25:221-222.
19. Wood AJJ et al. The influence of cirrhosis on steady-state blood concentrations of unbound propranolol after oral administration. Clin Pharmacokinet 1978;3:478-487.
20. Herrera J et al. Elimination of nadolol by patients with renal impairment. Br J Clin Pharmacol 1979;8(suppl 2):227-231.
21. Lowenthal DT et al. Timolol kinetics in chronic renal insufficiency. Clin Pharmacol Ther 1978;23:606-615.
22. Thompson FD et al. Pharmacodynamics of propranolol in renal failure. Br Med J 1972;2:434-436.
23. Bianchetti G et al. Pharmacokinetics and effects of propranolol in terminal uraemic patients and in patients undergoing regular dialysis treatment. Clin Pharmacokinet 1976;1:373-384.
24 Wood, AJJ et al. Propranolol Disposition in Renal Failure. Br. J. Clin. Pharmac. 1980; 10: 561-566.
25. Wood AJJ et al. The effect of aging and cigarette smoking on the elimination of antipyrine and indocyanine green. Clin Pharmacol Ther 1979;26:16-20.
26. Crooks J et al. Pharmacokinetics in the elderly. Clin Pharmacokinet 1976;1:280-296.
27. Vestal RE et al. Reduced β adrenoceptor sensitivity in the elderly. Clin Pharmacol Ther 1979;26:181-186.
28. Vaughan-Williams EM. Mode of action of beta receptor antagonists on cardiac muscle. Am J Cardiol 1966;18:399-405.
29. Morales-Aguilera A, Vaughan-Williams EM. The effects on cardiac muscle of β-receptor antagonists in relation to their activity as local anesthetics. Br J Pharmacol 1965;24:332-338.
30. Singh BM, Vaughan-Williams EM. Local anesthetic and antiarrhythmic actions of alprenolol relative to its effect on intracellular potentials and

other properties of isolated cardiac muscle. Br J Pharmacol 1970;38:749-757.

31. Coltart DJ, Meldrum SJ. The effect of propranolol on the human and canine transmembrane action potential, abstracted. Br J Pharmacol 1970;40:148P.

32. Coltart DJ, Shand DG. Plasma propranolol levels in the quantitative assessment of β-adrenergic blockade in man. Br Med J 1970;3:731-734.

33. Coltart DJ et al. Plasma propranolol levels associated with suppression of ventricular ectopic beats. Br Med J 1971;1:490-491.

34. Pruett JK, Walle T, Walle UK. Propranolol effects on membrane repolarization time in isolated canine Purkinje fibers: Threshold tissue content and the influence of exposure time. J Pharmacol Exp Ther 1980;215:539-543.

35. Woosley RL, Kornhauser D, Smith R, Reele S, Higgins SB, Nies AS, Shand DG, and Oates JA. Suppression of Chronic Ventricular Arrhythmias with Propranalol. Circulation. 60: 819-827, 1979.

36. Ahlquist RP. Study of the adrenotropic receptors. Am J Physiol 1948;153: 586-589.

37. Lands AM et al. Differentiation of receptors responsive to isoproterenol. Life Sci 1967;6:2241-2249.

38. Decalmer PB et al. Beta-blockers and asthma. Br Heart J 1978;40:184-189.

39. Deacon SP et al. Acebutolol, atenolol and propranolol and metabolic responses to acute hypoglycemia in diabetics. Br Med J 1977;2:1255-1257.

40. Lager I et al. Effect of cardioselective and nonselective β blockade on the hypoglycemic response in insulin-dependent diabetics. Lancet 1979;1:458-462.

41. Kaumann AJ and Blinks JR. β adrenoceptor blocking agents as partial agonists in isolated heart muscle: Dissociation of stimulation and blockade. Arch Pharmacol 1980; 311, 237-248.

42. Kaumann AJ, McInerny TK, Gilmour DP, Blinks JR. Comparative assessment of β-adrenoceptor blocking agents as simple competitive antagonists in isolated heart muscle: Similarity of inotropic and chronotropic blocking potencies against isoproterenol. Arch Pharmacol 1980;311:219-236.

43. Turner P. β-adrenergic receptor blocking drugs in hyperthyroidism. Drugs 1974;7:48-54.

44. Carruthers SG et al. The assessment of β-adrenoreceptor blocking drugs in hyperthyroidism. Br J Clin Pharmacol 1974;1:93-98.

45. Nelson JK, McDevitt DG. Comparative trial of propranolol and practolol in hyperthyroidism. Br J Clin Pharmacol 1975;2:411-418.

46. Lee RJ et al. Direct myocardial depressant effects of several β-adrenergic blocking agents in the unanesthetized atherosclerotic rabbit. Proc Soc Exp Biol Med 1978;158:147-150.

47. Fraser J, Nadeau J, Robertson D, Wood, AJJ. Regulation of human leukocyte beta receptors by endogenous catecholamines. J Clin Invest 1981;67:1777-1784.448.Vestal, R.e., Wood, A.J.J., Branch, R.A., Shand, D.G., and Wilkinson, G.R. Effects of age a cigarette smoking on propranolol disposition. Clin. Pharmacol. Ther. 26:8-15,1979.

IMPORTANCE OF ALPHA BLOCKING AND VASODILATOR EFFECTS OF BETA
BLOCKING AGENTS

JAY N. COHN, M.D.

The hemodynamic response to beta adrenergic blockade
includes a number of circulatory effects that might be
viewed as detrimental. The resting heart rate slows, the
cardiac output falls, and maximal exercise capacity is
reduced (1,2). Renal renin secretion is inhibited (3) and
there appears to be an increase in alpha vasoconstrictor
activity. This latter enhancement of vasoconstrictor tone
has been demonstrated in studies utilizing total autonomic
blockade to quantitate the neurohumoral vasoconstrictor tone
before and after beta blockade in hypertensive subjects (4).

Alpha adrenergic receptor blockers and vasodilators have
also been used in the drug treatment of hypertension, but
these theraputic agents when used alone tend also to produce
some adverse circulatory effects. Heart rate is increased,
particularly in the upright position, and the resting cardiac
output tends to rise (5). Renin release is enhanced probably
by virtue of a reflex increase in beta adrenergic activity
(6). Orthostatic hypotension is a problem when alpha blockade
inhibits the reflex vasoconstriction in the upright position
(7).

The cardiac functional effect of beta blockade and alpha
blockade or vasodilation relate not only to the direct effects
of inhibition or stimulation of sympathetic discharge to the
myocardium but also on the peripheral vascular effects of the
drugs. The increase in systemic vascular resistance that
accompanies beta blockade therapy may reduce pump performance
by increasing impedance to left ventricular ejection (8).
Similarly, the decrease in vascular resistance that accompanies

administration of a vasodilator drug may improve pump performance (9). These impedance-related changes in left ventricular performance are counterbalanced in the normal heart by modest changes in left ventricular preload induced by subtle changes in vascular volume or venous capacitance. In the presence of left ventricular dysfunction, however, the preload effects are attenuated and the impedance effects are exaggerated (10). Consequently, in the presence of left ventricular disease the peripheral vascular effects of these drugs can produce rather profound effects on performance of the left ventricle.

These physiologic considerations make it attractive to consider the addition of alpha blocking or vasodilator properties to beta adrenergic blocking drugs. Such an added pharmacologic effect might be expected to enhance the anti-hypertensive action of the beta adrenergic blockers and to counteract some of the deleterious effects of beta blockade, including bradycardia, decreased cardiac output and depressed left ventricular performance. Use of the vasodilators in combination with beta blockers has become standard therapy for the treatment of hypertension (11). Alpha blockers used in conjunction with beta blockers have not provided a good clinical response, possibly because of difficulty in choosing the proper doses of the blocking drugs (12). The development of a pharmacologic agent combining both beta and alpha blocking properties has made it possible to assess the potential usefulness of this dual effect.

Labetalol is a drug that appears to possess both beta and alpha blocking properties. We have studied the receptor blocking properties of the drug, have assessed its antihypertensive efficacy, have evaluated the hemodynamic response in the supine and upright position, have evaluated its effects on blood pressure and heart rate during exercise, and have carried out preliminary studies on the effects of the drug in patients with congestive heart failure.

Receptor blocking properties in man

A group of hypertensive subjects were studied in the
control period, after 4 days of oral therapy with labetalol
at a dose of 800 mg/day and after 4 days of administration
of 1600 mg/day (13). During the lower dose of therapy the
dose response curve relating isoproterenol dose to heart
rate effects was shifted to the right by approximately
eight-fold. After high dose therapy a ten-fold rightward
shift in the response curve to isoproterenol was noted.
Alpha blocking properties of labetalol were studied by
infusion of phenylephrine in a dose of from .02 to 0.2
mg/min. The dose causing an increase in diastolic arterial
pressure was shifted approximately two-fold to the right
during low dose therapy with labetalol and only slightly
more during high dose therapy. Therefore, these studies
indicate that labetalol blocks both beta and alpha adrenergic receptors but that on the basis of this pharmacologic
testing the sensitivity of beta receptors is greater than of
alpha receptors.

A further observation during these receptor studies was
that an infusion of isoproterenol after labetalol blockade
was associated with the patient's awareness of a more force-
ful cardiac contraction with no change in heart rate. This
symptomatic cardiac stimulation was confirmed by measurement
of a progressive increase in stroke volume as the isoproterenol dose was increased with no change in heart rate (14).
In contrast, prior to labetalol therapy the subjects exhibited
a tachycardia at the threshold dose for an increase in stroke
volume. Furthermore, the fall in diastolic pressure that
was observed in the control period during the infusion of
the lower doses of isoproterenol was not noted after
labetalol. Indeed, a slight rise in diastolic pressure
occurred during infusion of isoproterenol in doses that
raised stroke volume without increasing heart rate. These
observations make it unlikely that the stroke volume effects
of isoproterenol could be attributed to peripheral vasodilator

effects of beta-2 stimulation. The most satisfactory
explanation for these observations is that the labetalol is
more effective in blocking beta receptors in the area of the
sinoatrial node than it is beta receptors in the myocardium.
Such a subselectivity of beta receptors might help to account
for the hemodynamic effect of inotropic drugs such as doputa-
mine that have a relatively selective effect on contractility
with relatively little chronotropic effect (15).

Antihypertensive and hemodynamic effects

During eight days of therapy with progressively
increasing doses of labetalol, hypertensive subjects showed
a progressive decline in arterial pressure that rose
promptly when the drug was discontinued (13). This fall in
blood pressure was associated with only a small decrease in
supine heart rate and a slight decrease in standing heart
rate. At doses up to 800 mg/day the standing blood pressure
was affected no more than the supine blood pressure, but at
higher doses a slight accentuation of antihypertensive
effect was noted in the upright position. This finding is
consistent with the additional alpha blocking properties of
the drug and would not be expected in response to a pure
beta blocker. The fall in arterial pressure in both the
supine and standing position during labetalol therapy could
be attributed exclusively to a fall in systemic vascular
resistance, since cardiac output was unchanged by the drug.
Indeed the slight fall in heart rate resulted in a slight
increase in stroke volume during therapy with this drug.

Response to exercise

During therapy with beta blockers the heart rate
response to exercise is usually strikingly attenuated and
there is a modest reduction in the blood pressure rise
during exercise. This pharmacologic effect of beta blockade
leads to a fall in the heart rate-blood pressure product
during exercise and thus a reduction in myocardial oxygen

consumption that probably accounts in large part for the antianginal effect of beta blockers in patients with coronary artery disease.

During labetalol therapy the heart rate response to exercise was attenuated consistent with the expected response to a beta blocker. However, the blood pressure rise during exercise in a group of hypertensive subjects was almost eliminated. This markedly attenuated blood pressure rise during exercise is consistent with a vasodilator or alpha blocking effect of labetalol in addition to its beta blocking property.

Congestive heart failure

Patients with congestive heart failure exhibit heightened sympathetic nervous system activity as manifested by elevated plasma norepinephrine levels (16). The magnitude of the increase in plasma norepinephrine appears to be in part related to the severity of hemodynamic derangement in congestive heart failure (17). Although these elevated plasma norepinephrine levels and heightened sympathetic nervous system activity are often viewed as compensatory mechanisms that help to support left ventricular performance in heart failure, recent concern has been expressed that this sympathetic activity may have a deleterious effect on the heart as well. Increased sympathetic activity may depress left ventricular performance by raising systemic vascular resistance (8). In addition, the heightened adrenergic discharge could play a role in precipitating arrhythmias that are an important cause for mortality in congestive heart failure. Indeed, in recent studies from our laboratory a striking relationship could be observed between shortened survival and elevated plasma norepinephrine levels in patients with congestive heart failure (18). Recent studies from Sweden have suggested that beta adrenergic blockade may be an effective form of therapy for patients with congestive cardiomyopathy (19). The mechanism for this purported

beneficial effect of metoprolol in heart failure has not
been determined.

Acute administration of beta blockers to patients with
heart failure usually results in further depression of left
ventricular performance. Indeed, even in the Swedish studies
that demonstrated long-term beneficial effects of beta blockade,
acute administration of the drug to these patients usually
resulted in some worsening of left ventricular performance (19).
Combining an alpha blocking action with the beta blocking
action might be expected to counteract the negative effects
of beta blockade on pump performance. Therefore we cautiously
administered labetalol to a small series of patients with
congestive heart failure who were in a stable hemodynamic
state while receiving digitalis and diuretics. Oral administration of the drug in these patients produced no striking
change in resting hemodynamics but markedly inhibited the
blood pressure rise that occurs during exercise. In patients
with heart failure blood pressure increases during exercise
are often markedly limited by virtue of poor left ventricular
pump performance. When stroke volume cannot adequately
increase in response to an exercise-induced fall in systemic
vascular resistance, blood pressure will not rise and may
even fall during exercise. Sympathetic stimulation during
exercise has as its peripheral vascular effect vasoconstriction
of nonexercising vascular beds with redistribution of flow
to exercising muscle beds (20). After administration of
labetalol one patient in our series exhibited a striking
fall in blood pressure during exercise and became nearly
syncopal. Although this anecdotal experience with a syncopal
patient cannot be accepted as evidence for a poor response
to this therapy in patients with congestive heart failure,
the likelihood is that in a patient with critical impairment
of left ventricular function that cannot adequately be increased
in response to a vasodilator stimulus, alpha blockade by
blocking the redistribution of blood flow will allow continued
perfusion of nonexercising vascular beds with accentuation

of the fall in systemic vascular resistance.

Although the combination of alpha blocking properties with the beta blocking properties of labetalol should therefore be applied with caution in patients who are normotensive with congestive heart failure, the pharmacologic action of this drug should be particularly beneficial in hypertensive patients who have some left ventricular dysfunction. It is likely that in these patients the use of labetalol would be less hazardous than the use of beta adrenergic blocking drugs which might further impair left ventricular function if the blood pressure is not successfully reduced.

Future directions

It is likely that further modifications of the chemical structure of beta blockers will yield drugs that have numerous additional pharmacologic effects. Varying degrees of vasodilator, beta blocking, and inotropic effects may well be within the capability of pharmaceutical chemists. Study of the interaction of these additional pharmacologic effects with the known pharmacologic action of beta blockers may not only hasten the development of new and more effective antihypertensive drugs that may be useful in monotherapy, but such new compounds may also lead to new insights into the role of adrenergic receptors and vascular tone in the support of circulatory function.

REFERENCES

1. Sowton E, Hamer J. 1966. Hemodynamic changes after beta adrenergic blockade. Am J Cardiol 18: 317-320.
2. Epstein SE, Robinson BF, Kahler RL, Braunwald E. 1965. Effects of beta-adrenergic blockade on the cardiac response to maximal and submaximal exercise in man. J Clin Invest 44: 1745-1753.
3. Johnson JE, Davis JO, Gotshall RW, Lohmeier TE, Davis JL, Braverman B, Temple GE. 1976. Evidence of an intrarenal beta receptor in control of renin release. Am. J. Physiol. 230: 410-418.
4. Khatri IM, Cohn JN. 1970. Mechanism of exercise hypotension after sympathetic blockade. Am J Cardiol 25: 329-338.
5. Richards DA, Woodings EP, Prichard BNC. 1979. Circulatory and α-adrenoceptor blocking effects of phentolamine. Br J Clin Pharmac 5: 507-513.
6. McDonald RH, Corder CN, Leehen FHH. 1977. Alpha and beta blockers: effects on renin release. Prog Brain Res 47: 409-416.
7. Graham RM, Thornell IR, Gain JM, Bagnoli C, Oates H, Strokes GS. 1976. Prazosin: the first-dose phenomenon. Br Med J 2: 1293-1294.
8. Cohn JN. 1973. Blood pressure and cardiac performance. Am J Med 55: 351-361.
9. Cohn JN. 1973. Vasodilator therapy for heart failure: The influence of impedance on left ventricular performance. (Editorial) Circulation 48: 5-8.
10. Cohn JN, Franciosa JA. 1977. Vasodilator therapy of cardiac failure. N Engl J Med 297: 27-31 and 254-258.
11. Zacest R, Gilmore E, Koch-Weser J. 1972. Treatment of essential hypertension with combined vasodilation and β-adrenergic blockade. N Engl J Med 286: 617.
12. Beilin LF, Juel-Jensen BE. 1972. Alpha and beta adrenergic blockade in hypertension. Lancet 1: 979.
13. Mehta J, Cohn JN. 1977. Hemodynamic effects of labetalol, an alpha and beta adrenergic blocking agent, in hypertensive subjects. Circulation 55: 370-374.
14. Mehta JL, Cohn JN. 1976. Dissociation of inotropic from chronotropic effects of isoproterenol during beta blockade with labetalol (SCH 15719W). Clin Res 24: 423a.
15. Akhtar N, Mikulic E, Cohn JN, Chaudhry MH. 1975. Hemodynamic effect of dobutamine in patients with severe heart failure. Am J Cardiol 36: 202-205.
16. Cohn JN, Mashiro I, Levine TB, Mehta J. 1979. Role of vasoconstrictor mechanisms in the control of left ventricular performance of the normal and damaged heart. Am J Cardiol 44: 1019-1022.
17. Levine TB, Francis GS, Goldsmith SR, Simon AB, Cohn JN. Activity of the sympathetic nervous system and renin-angiotensin system assessed by plasma hormone levels and their relationship to hemodynamic abnormalities in congestive heart failure. Am J Cardiol. In press.

18. Cohn JN, Levine R, Levine TB, Gross K, Francis G. 1981.
    Prognostic significance of plasma norepinephrine in
    congestive heart failure. (abstract) Clin Res.
19. Swedberg K, Hjalmarson A, Waagstein F, Wallentin I. 1980.
    Beneficial effects of long-term beta-blockade in
    congestive cardiomyopathy. Br Heart J 44: 117-133.
20. Blair DA, Glover WE, Roddie IC. 1961. Vasomotor responses
    in the human arm during leg exercise. Circ Res 9: 264.

ARE ANIMAL MODELS USEFUL IN DETERMINING IF ALL BETA-BLOCKING AGENTS ARE
THE SAME?

E. Neil Moore and Joseph F. Spear, University of Pennsylvania,
Philadelphia, Pennsylvania.

Sudden cardiac death remains the major cause of death in most western
societies. A number of studies have suggested that administration of beta
blocking drugs can decrease the incidence of sudden cardiac death (1,2,3).
The large Norwegian trial in which timolol was administered 7 to 28 days
following myocardial infarct has provided the strongest evidence to date
that a beta blocking drug can significantly decrease the indicence of
sudden cardiac death following myocardial infarction as well as decrease
the rate of reinfarction (2). The recent studies with metoprolol administered as early as one hour following myocardial infarction also indicates
that beta blocking drugs can significantly decrease the mortality from
heart attack (3).

The exact mechanism by which a beta blocking drug can influence the
incidence of sudden cardiac death remains unknown. A number of possible
mechanisms have been suggested including reduction of life threatening
arrhythmias, slowing of heart rate, decreased myocardial oxygen consumption
or altered metabolism. Since it has been suggested that as many as 85% of
sudden cardiac death victims die from ventricular fibrillation, we undertook
a series of electrophysiological studies to determine the electrophysiological
effects of propranolol, timolol and metoprolol.

The bundle of His technique was employed to help define the precise
locations of conduction delay within the atrioventricular conduction systems
When one records simultaneous electrograms from the atrium, bundle of His,
and ventricles, together with a lead II electrocardiogram it is possible
to define where conduction delays occur in the atrium, AV node, His-Purkinje
system or ventricular myocardium. Figure 1 presents the effects of
increasing doses of timolol (6.25 to 25,100,400, and 800 uq/kg) on conduction
within different regions of the heart in an open chest anesthetized dog.
Conduction times in milliseconds are shown on the Y axis. Following 25 uq/kg
of timolol a delay in AV nodal conduction occurs, but only very small changes

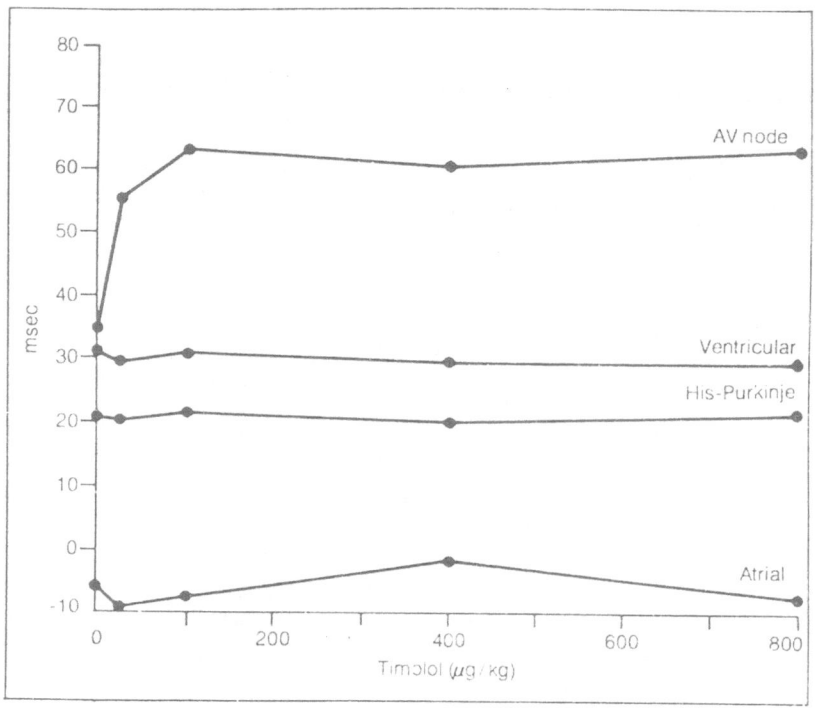

FIGURE 1. The effects in doses of 25,100,400 and 800 ug/kg upon atrial,
AV nodal, His-Purkinje and ventricular conduction are compared in a single
animal whose heart was paced at a constant rate of 200 beats/minute to
prevent the slowing of heart rate produced by timolol. Conduction times
were measured from bipolar electrograms located in the atrium, bundle of
His and ventricles. Only AV nodal conduction was significantly delayed in
this animal. Maximal effects were observed at low doses of timolol, and
further alterations did not occur at higher doses.

in conduction occur within the atrium, His-Purkinje system and ventricular
myocardium. Since timolol has about 10 times the beta blocking potency of
propranolol a similar study on the effects of propranolol on AV conduction
was undertaken using 10 times the amount of propranolol. Figure 2 presents
the averaged results from 5 open chest, anesthetized dog studies. The
intravenous dose of dl-propranolol was increased from 62.5 to 8000 ug/kg.
The percent change from control conduction within the atrium (A-A'), AV node
(A'-H), His-Purkinje system (H-Q) and ventricular muscle (Q-Vs) are shown
as percent change from control. It can be noted that up to 1000 ug/kg
small changes occurred in conduction within the AV node and only a slight
change in ventricular conduction. However, at very high levels of 8000 ug/kg
there was a marked delay in conduction within the AV node and in the His-
Purkinje system. In fact in two of the animals complete AV block occurred.
Thus there does appear to be a difference at these very high doses between
propranolol and timolol; propranolol had a greater tendency to affect
conduction within the His-Purkinje system than did timolol. These doses
exceed those that would be used clinically, but it may suggest that in
the presence of diseased tissue, that timolol may have less depressing
effects on conduction than propranolol.

To further study whether or not propranolol had more depressing effects
upon the His-Purkinje system than timolol we undertook microelectrode
experiments. It had been shown previously by Davis and Tempe that 20 mg/liter
or propranolol significantly depressed resting potential, rate of rise of
the action potential and shortened action potential duration measured both
at 30% repolarization and 100% repolarization (4). In contrast (Figure 3)
200 mg/liter of timolol added to the superfusate does not alter canine Purkinje
fiber action potentials. Microelectrode studies were also completed using
different concentrations of metoprolol added to the Tyrode's solution
superfusing isolated canine Purkinje fibers. At 10 mg/liter of metoprolol
there was no effect on transmembrane action potential characteristics of
canine Purkinje fibers. However, at 100 mg/kg of metoprolol there was a
significant decrease in membrane potential, rate of rise of the action
potential, action potential configuration and an abbreviation of action
potential duration at 30% and 100% of repolarization (5). Thus it
appears that propranolol is more depressant to canine Purkinje fibers
than are equivalent beta blocking doses of timolol and metoprolol.

The ventricular fibrillation threshold (VFT) technique was designed

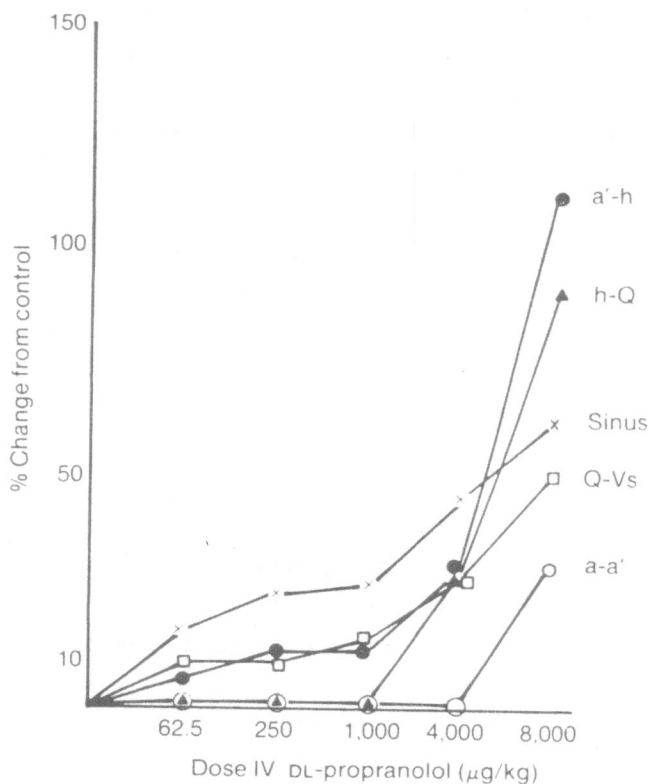

FIGURE 2. Percent change from control values for conduction within the heart are shown for 5 animals paced at a basic cycle length of 300 msec. Doses of dl-propranolol in uq/kq are shown on the x-axis. A-A' = atrial conduction, A-O = His-Purkinje conduction time, sinus = sinus node rate, O-VS = ventricular conduction and A'-H = AV nodal conduction.

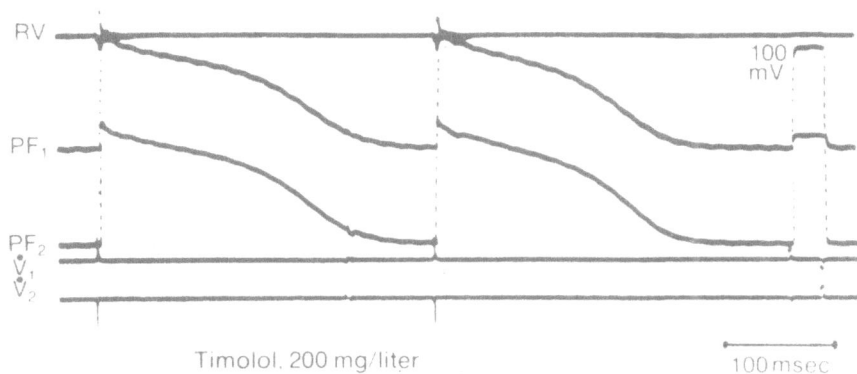

FIGURE 3. A right ventricular bipolar extracellular electrogram was recorded from the right ventricle (RV, top trace) simultaneously with a recording of two transmembrane potentials from two canine Purkinje fibers (PF$_1$ and PF$_2$). The rate of depolarization of the two transmembrane Purkinje action potentials are presented as the electronically derived derivatives in the lower two traces ($\dot{V}_1$ and $\dot{V}_2$). A 100-mV calibration is shown at the far right and the horizontal bar at the lower right of the figure represents a duration of 100 msec. Timolol 200 mg/liter, was added to the Tyrode's solution superfusing this canine Purkinje-papillary muscle preparation.

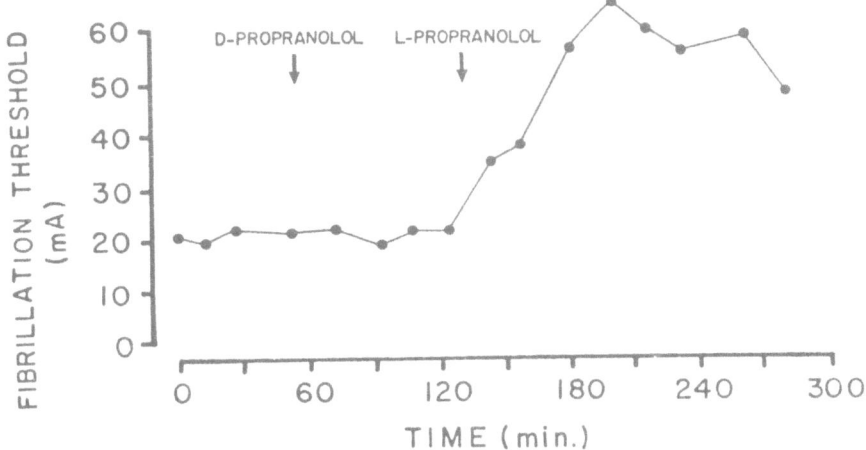

FIGURE 4. Difference between the membrane-stabilizing d-isomer and beta-blocking l-isomer of propranolol upon the ventricular fibrillation threshold (VFT). D-propranolol at a dose of 0.5 mg/kg had very little effect upon the VFT, whereas l-propranolol at the same dose increased the current required to initiate ventricular fibrillation.

to test the electrical stability of the ventricles in order to identify
perturbations that might decrease the likelihood of ventricular fibrillation
developing. We have completed VFT studies in dogs anesthetized with sodium
pentobarbital. The VFT was measured as the minimum current required to initiate ventricular fibrillation. Our techniques have been published previously
(6). Figure 4 is a figure in which the d and l isomers of propranolol were
analyzed as to their effect upon the VFT. Time is shown on the x axis and
ventricular fibrillation threshold in milliamps on the Y axis. It can be
noted that the membrane stablizing isomer of propranolol (d-propranolol)
has very little effect on the VFT. However, following administration of
the beta blocking isomer (l-propranolol) there was an elevation in the
ventricular fibrillation threshold. This strongly suggests that it is the
beta blocking action which has the greatest ability to enhance the electrical
stability of the ventricles as measured by the VFT technique. The effect
of the racemic mixture of dl propranolol on the VFT was measured in 10 dogs
and in all dogs, propranolol increased the ventricular fibrillation
threshold. However, the duration of the effect of propranolol on VFT varied.
Following a 1 mg/kg bolus of dl propranolol an initial elevation of VFT was
followed by the VFT falling back to control levels in some animals in which
beta blockade was still present. (6). The effects of increasing doses of
timolol on the VFT threshold are shown in Figure 5. In three experiments
on male anesthetized dogs doses of timolol increasing from 6.25,25, 100
up to 400 ug/kg timolol were administered. In all 3 experiments there was
an increase in the VFT and timolol caused a more consistent dose related
increase in the VFT than did propranolol. We also have completed a number of
studies with metoprolol as shown in Figure 6. Doses of metoprolol increasing
from 0.1 to 1.0, and 5.0 mg/kg were administered to pentobarbital anesthetized open chest animals. Some animals showed only a modest increase in
the VFT while others exhibited a marked increase in the VFT. With metoprolol we did not observe the VFT threshold falling back to or below control
levels within 100 minutes as we had observed with the racemic mixture of
propranolol. Thus propranolol, timolol and metoprolol all enhance the
electrical stability of the ventricles as measured by the VFT threshold
technique.

One problem in determining whether a given drug is an effective
antiarrhythmic agent has been the lack of appropriate animal test models
exhibiting ventricular tachyarrhythmias similar to those observed during

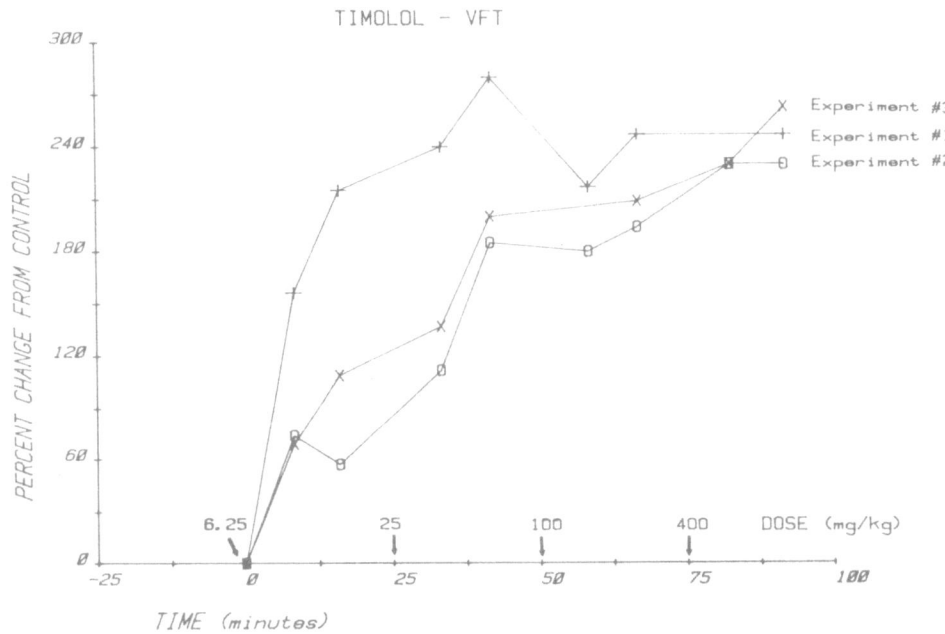

FIGURE 5. The effect of increasing doses of timolol on the VF threshold
are shown for three different experiments. Doses of 6.25 ug/kg timolol
were given at time zero and subsequent doses of 25,100, and 400 ug/kg
timolol were given at 25,50 and 75 minutes respectively. There was a
dose related percent increase from control in the VF threshold after
administration of timolol in all 3 experiments. This suggests that timolol
enhances the electrical stability of the ventricles.

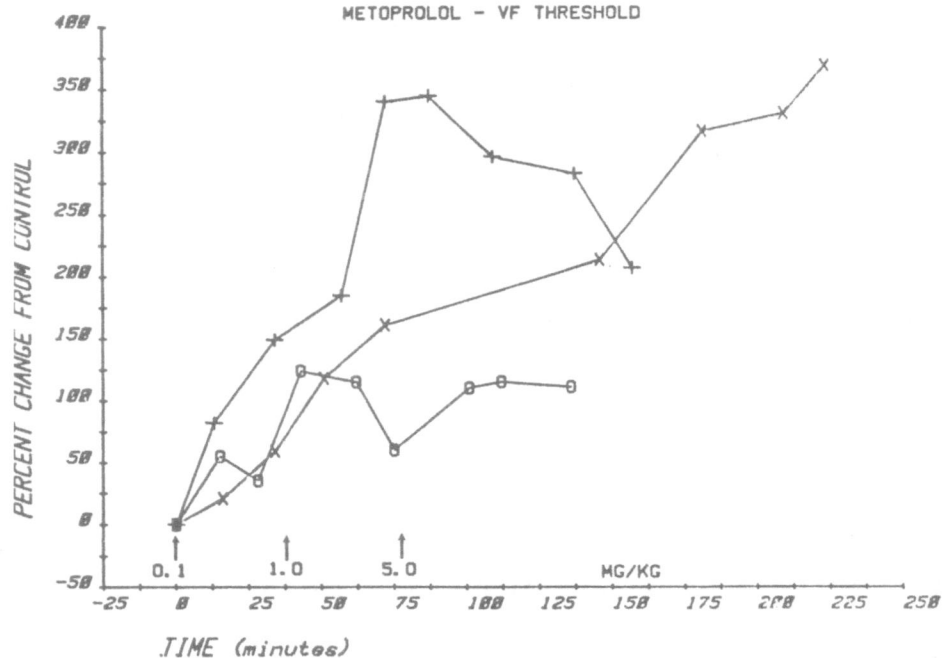

FIGURE 6. The effects of doses of metoprolol of 0.1, 1.0 and 5.0 mg/kg upon the VFT threshold are presented for three different experiments. Time is displayed on the x-axis and percent change from control VFT is shown on the y axis.

myocardial infarction in man. Our laboratory has recently developed
a chronic canine infarct model produced by occlusion and reperfusion of the
left anterior descending coronary artery (7). In this new model, ventricular tachyarrhythmias can be initiated utilizing the same techniques of
programmed electrical stimulation as used in the human clinical catheterization laboratory. Many cardiologists now consider that the most reliable
way to determine appropriate antiarrhythmic therapy in patients at high
risk of sudden cardiac death is to utilize programmed electrical stimulation
to identify effective antiarrhythmic therapy. If an agent prevents the
initiation of a tachyarrhythmia by programmed electrical stimulation after
its administration then that agent is considered an effective therapeutic
agent. We have now studied nine animals in which programmed electrical
stimulation initiated either ventricular fibrillation (VF) or ventricular
tachycardia (VT).

A chronic ventricular tachyarrhythmia infarct animal in which
25 ug/kg of timolol was effective in preventing the re-initiation of
ventricular tachycardia is presented in Figure 7. The lead II electrocardiogram (II) was recorded simultaneously with left (LV) and right (RV)
ventricular electrograms, stimulus artifacts (S), blood pressure (BP),
and 100 msec time marks. The ventricles were paced via bipolar myocardial
plunge electrodes at a basic cycle length of 300 msec and 3 sequential
ventricular extrasystoles were evoked as early as possible. The arrows
at the top of the figure identify the three electrically evoked ventricular
extrasystoles and the arrow in the stimulus artifact trace notes the time
of introduction of the three stimuli. It can be observed in the electrocardiogram that a rapid ventricular tachycardia was initiated. This tachyarrhythmia could be reproducibly initiated at will and was terminated after
several minutes using low-level DC countershock. After demonstrating
that this tachyarrhythmia could be initiated at will, a dose of 25 ug/kg
of timolol was administered. Five minutes after the administration of
timolol the same programmed electrical stimulation sequence was introduced
while recording the same lead II electrocardiogram and electrogram tracings
as in Figure 7. In Figure 8, it can be noted that the three earliest
possible premature extrasystoles only resulted in one non-stimuluated ventricular response occurring. A ventricular tachyarrhythmia (VT) could never
again be initiated despite repeated attempts, i.e., in Figure 8, the triple
extrasystoles were introduced twice and in neither case did a ventricular

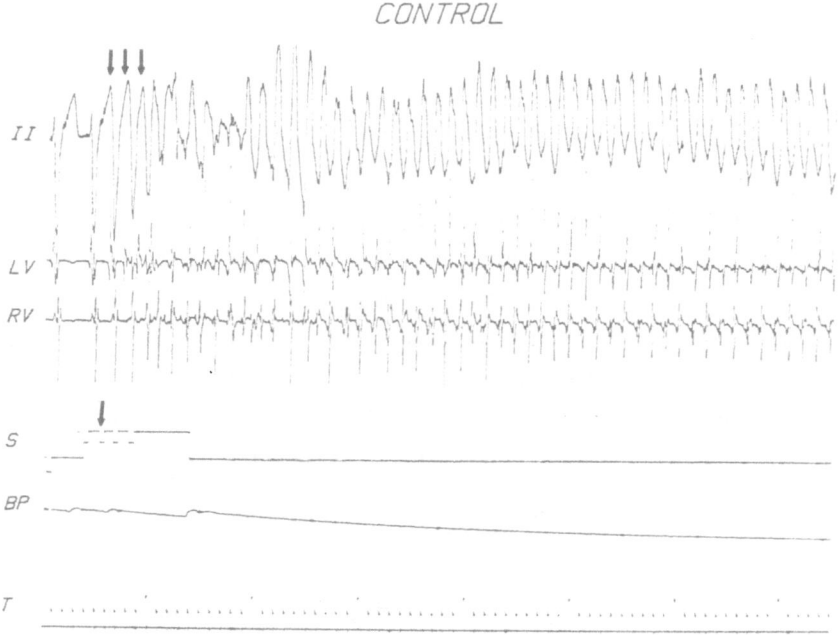

FIGURE 7. The lead II electrocardiogram (II) and right and left ventricular electrograms (RV and LV) were recorded simultaneously with blood pressure (BP), stimulus artifacts (ST) and time marks (100 msec intervals) in a chronic infarct dog. At the time of the 3 arrows above the electrocardiogram, triple ventricular extrasystoles were evoked by programmed electrical pacing. This resulted in a sustained ventricular tachycardia developing in this chronic canine mottled infarct model.

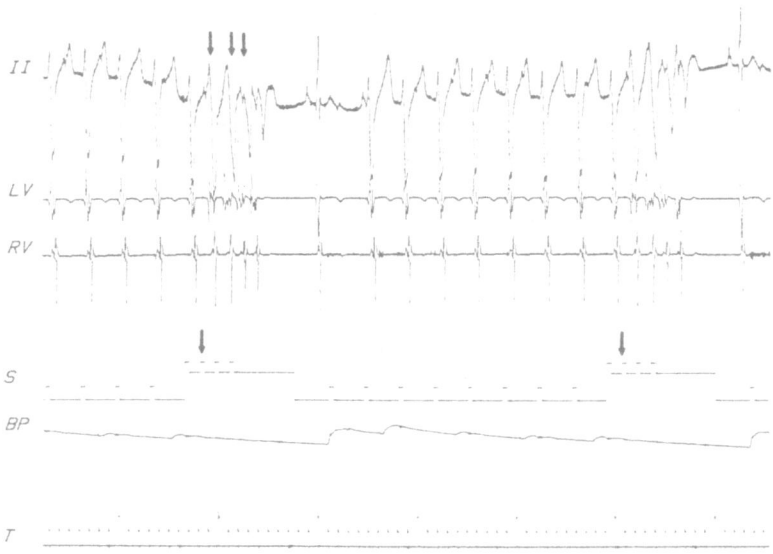

TIMOLOL 25 ug/kg

FIGURE 8. Following the administration of a bolus of 25 ug/kg of timolol the identical electrocardiograms and ventricular electrograms were recorded in the same animal as Figure 7. Five minutes after the administration of this dose of timolol it was not possible to reinitiate any ventricular tachyarrhythmia using the same programmed electrical stimulation sequence as in Figure 7.

tachyarrhythmia develop. In one of the VT chronic animals, ventricular tachycardia was observed to result in ventricular fibrillation following a brief period of rapid VT. In that animal, cumulative doses of timolol up to 0.5 mg/kg failed to prevent the initiation of a ventricular tachycardia, but timolol did result in the tachycardia being markedly slowed and ventricular fibrillation never developed from the slower VT.

In 4 of 5 animals in which ventricular fibrillation was observed following programmed electrical stimulation, it was possible giving doses of ≤ 100 ug/kg of timolol to prevent the reinitiation of ventricular fibrillation. In one of five animals in which programmed electrical stimulation caused ventricular fibrillation, VF still occurred following 100 ug/kg of timolol. Higher doses of timolol than 100 ug/kg were not studied in the one animal in which VF could not be prevented.

Thus, these preliminary studies in our chronic canine mottled infarct model in which ventricular tachyarrhythmias can reproducibly be initiated using programmed electrical stimulation have shown that timolol does have the capability of preventing or altering the ventricular tachyarrhythmias following myocardial infarction. We are undertaking further studies to explore the ability of other beta blocking drugs to prevent lethal arrhythmias in this chronic canine infarct model.

DISCUSSION

The present cardiac electrophysiological experiments in dogs have shown that beta blocking drugs can enhance the electrical stability of the ventricles as shown by the elevation of the amount of current required to initiate ventricular fibrillation and by the studies in which timolol was able to prevent the initiation of ventricular tachyarrhythmias in our canine mottled myocardial infarct model. The recent well controlled studies on timolol (2) and metoprolol (3) suggest that beta blocking drugs can decrease the incidence of sudden cardiac death in man. The precise mechanism of how beta blockade does this is not understood. The action of beta blockade in reducing the incidence of sudden cardiac death may result from their decreasing the incidence of cardiac dysrhythmias by alterations of heart rate, and/or by alteration in the oxygen consumption required by the heart. Our present animal model studies suggest that alterations in cardiac electrophysiology may indeed be important in the mechanism of action of beta blockers. Clearly, these studies are encouraging, but additiona investigations will be required before the precise mechanism as to how beta blockade can influence the incidence of sudden cardiac death will be known.

Acknowledgements

We thank Drs. Stan Nattel and Eric Michelson for assisting in some of these experiments, Ralph Iannuzzi for skilled technical assistance and Bejay Moore for help with illustrative material and manuscript preparation.

References

1. Wilhelmsson, C., Vedin, J.A., Wilhelmsen, L., Tibblin, G., Werko, L. Reduction of sudden deaths after myocardial infarction by treatment with alprenolol: preliminary results. Lancet 2:1157-60, 1974.
2. The Norwegian Multicenter Study Group. Timolol-induced reduction in mortality and reinfarction in patients surviving acute myocardial infarction. New Engl. J. Med. 304-801, 1981.
3. Hjalmarson, A., et al. A double-blind trial of metoprolol in acute myocardial infarction. Effect on mortality. (In Press, Lancet, October 17th, 1981.)
4. Davis, L.D. and Temte, J.V. Effect of propranolol on the transmembrane potential of ventricular muscle and Purkinje fibers in the dog. Circ. Res. 22:66, 1968.
5. Spear, J.F. and Moore, E.N.: The contribution of cellular electrophysiology in the development of antiarrhythmic agents. Pace (In Press, 1981).
6. Spear, J.F., Moore, E.N. and Ricciutti, M. The effects of the d-l-optical isomers of propranolol on the ventricular fibrillation threshold. Europ. J. Cardiol. 7/2-3:117-124, 1978.
7. Michelson, E.L., Spear, J.F. and Moore, E.N. Electrophysiologic and anatomic correlates of sustained ventricular tachyarrhythmias in a model of chronic myocardial infarction. Am. J. Cardiol. 45:583, 1980.

MODERATOR'S COMMENTS ON BETA BLOCKING DRUGS

D. C. HARRISON

I. INTRODUCTION

It has been more than 20 years since the introduction of the first selective beta adrenergic blocking agent. Several agents which block beta receptors have been developed and used in basic research and clinical medicine during this time. In excess of 5,000 publications describing the actions of beta blockers have expanded considerably our knowledge of the role of the adrenergic nervous system in both health and disease. Yet, to date, we have not developed perfect methods for pharmacological or clinical testing of these agents to permit us to compare properties of the drugs or to take advantage of unique characteristics of particular compounds. Therefore, the purpose of this conference is to discuss the important pharmacologic, pharmacokinetic, physiologic and clinical actions of beta blocking agents in order to develop more rational approaches for their evaluation and use.

As an introduction to this session, I want to outline several areas which I hope we can discuss in detail during the next day and a half.

1.1. Pharmacologic concepts

During these past two decades a number of pharmacologic concepts have developed as a direct result of the utilization of beta adrenergic blocking agents in research. These include:

1. Definitions of specific cellular receptors for pharmacologic responses and the definition of the concept of subtypes of receptors.
2. Circulatory and electrophysiologic responses to adrenergic stimulation and blockade.

3. Role of the nervous system in metabolic regulation.
4. Lack of correlation of plasma concentration with effect for most beta blockers.
5. The role of intrinsic sympathetic stimulation of their action.

1.2 Clinical concepts

Experience has shown the importance of the adrenergic nervous system in the etiology of a number of circulatory diseases and in producing their symptoms. The compensation to disease is frequently an appropriate increase in adrenergic stimulation to the altered physiologic state. However, adrenergic compensation can be excessive or inappropriate producing heightened symptoms. The clinical concepts which have been highlighted by beta blockers include:

1. The mechanisms by which they act in hypertension and angina.
2. The role of adrenergic blockage in preventing sudden cardiac death.
3. Mechanisms to palliate and treat obstructive cardio-myopathy.
4. Use in other circulatory disorders such as migraine, dissecting aneurysm, anxiety, etc.
5. The interaction of beta blockers with other drugs.

While many questions remain to be answered, we have made considerable progress in all of these areas. I hope this meeting will lead to better and more effective ways to assess the efficacy and safety of new agents as they are introduced.

GENERAL GROUP DISCUSSION - Are All Beta-Blocking Agents the Same?

Moderator: Dr. Donald Harrison

Dr. Harrison: Several presentations have emphasized the pharmacologic differences in beta blocking drugs, particularly from the laboratory studies, and have outlined the theoretical reasons that there should be some clinical differences. In 1970 it had not been demonstrated clinically that there were great differences in safety and efficiency in the use of these agents in human disease. To be provocative, I would like to say that I am not absolutely certain that has been demonstrated an incorrect concept at this time. Sometimes it is because proper studies have not been performed to try to demonstrate these differences, and in other instances equipotent or equivalent levels of beta blockade have not been demonstrated because the techniques that we have are so limited to demonstrate equipotent beta blockade. For this discussion let us focus on whether or not the laboratory differences that we have talked about, such as membrane properties, ISA cardioselectivity, lipid solubility and protein bonding, can be translated at this point in time to any clinical relevance in terms of differences in the beta blocking drugs. Questions for the panelists should primarily provoke points of discussion.

Dr. Ehrreich: I would like to ask Peter Somani a question and that is related to the effects of these various drugs with intrinsic sympathomimetic activity which you showed had less effects on heart rate since, of course, we do know that they possibly could have somewhat less effects on blood pressure. My question is how can you explain the effects in angina. It may not be possible to answer this; but based on the fact that they have much less effect on the parameter which does indeed waste oxygen, such as tachycardia, what would be the mechanism then to explain the action of these drugs with ISA in angina?

Dr. Somani: This is an interesting question because the mechanism of antianginal action of the beta blockers may include not only a decrease in the heart rate response to exercise but also other factors that may also reduce oxygen requirements. As I showed you this morning, when you compare drugs such as pindolol (which has fairly substantial ISA) and propranolol (which has no ISA), the antianginal efficacy is fairly similar. In the study I mentioned, Frushman and co-workers showed that there was not much difference in the response to exercise with either propranolol or pindolol. The double products were almost identical in this particular study, so that there is fairly good beta blockade in some of these patients. The differences may be in increasing the dose. Some of the earlier studies showed that if one looked at the exercise tolerance and then increased the dose of the beta blockers, those with ISA have a plateau so that there is no further increase in the antianginal property as you increase the dose; whereas,with propranolol-type drugs, as you increase the dose, you may see increased antianginal activity. At the same time from clinical experience, we also know that there are patients who do not respond to a given dose of propranolol, especially if the heart size is increased, and then the efficacy becomes less. This is because now you begin to consume more oxygen. There are other determinants of oxygen requirements in addition to the double product.

Dr. Harrison: I would like to comment on that. Long-term administration of pindolol may not lead during the waking hours to a difference in heart rate for a given level of beta blockade. It has been shown with Holter monitoring that during the night there is less cardiac depression in terms of heart rate, but there are some studies in France in which during the day there was no difference in the resting heart rates. Resting heart rate changes are such a poor mechanism to judge beta blockade, and with prolonged administration of pindolol there are few differences from other beta blockers.

Dr. Wood: I think that the resting heart rate is an almost worthless measure of beta blockade in that there are so many things that determine your resting heart rate, including your parasympathetic tone. The critical data are what happens during sympathetic stimulation, and Dr. Somani showed in the data with exercise that pindolol, which is a partial agonist, is as effective in blocking the exercise-induced rise in heart rate as is propranolol. Secondly, it seems to me that the advantages of an increase in supine heart rate which have been claimed for those drugs that have intrinsic sympathomimetic activity is at the best dubious, and I think very doubtful. It is very seldom that one ever has to stop, if ever, a beta blocker or even reduce the dose because of supine bradycardia. The only indication to that, I think, is when the patient develops hypotension which is a separate issue.

Dr. Orringer: Perhaps one of the most disturbing side effects in most of the patients whom we treat with beta blockers in our clinical practice is the fatigue syndrome. We were hoping that with the advent of nadolol that some of these problems would be resolved primarily because some of the marketing information indicated that its diminished lipid solubility was going to play a substantial role in abating some of these symptoms. Unfortunately, a substantial number of patients we have had on nadolol have also complained of the fatigue syndrome. Is there anything any of you can contribute to the recurrent problems we have had with the beta blocker fatigue syndrome to more than just lipid solubility and is there anything on the horizon, particularly with atenolol, in terms of helping us resolve some of the problems that our patients have been having?

Dr. Somani: I think that with all the beta blockers fatigue is commonly observed in clinical practice. As a pharmacologist, I imagine direct metabolic effects on skeletal muscle and that response or the blockade of the response to catecholamines on skeletal muscle may to some extent contribute to fatigue. The second possibility is the question of the double product, the heart rate times blood pressure in response to exercise. There again, all beta blockers seem to reduce the double product which then translates to the reduced exercise tolerance. I am not sure if other properties contribute to this problem clinically or not.

Dr. Harrison: I think Dr. Wood showed some important data on this question. It is not just the lipid solubility versus the water solubility of the agent. It is protein binding and a number of other factors, and the binding in central nervous system for beta blockers is not well known.

Dr. Wood: There is another study with samples during neurosurgery in brain biopsies. The problem with that study is that they were not all taken at the same time after dosing and they were not all taken in terms of steady states.

Dr. Cohn: I certainly think that what you are talking is a CNS effect. The problem is the measurement of concentrations in the brain including concentrations in fat which doesn't necessarily tell you what the activity is at the receptor site in the brain. I think that most of our experience with these drugs is that patients respond differently to different beta blockers. It is nice to have a series of them available, and for some unknown reason you often can find a patient who will be relieved of the side effects and have equal therapeutic efficacy when you switch from, say, propranolol to atenolol to nadolol. Trial and error is all you can do until we have a better understanding of the mechanism.

Dr. Epstein: I just would like to get back to the question of intrinsic sympathetic activity from a practical clinical point of view. I discussed this previously with Dr. Harrison, where some people are worried about giving a drug like propranolol in individuals who have resting heart rates of 45. A drug like pindolol seems to be attractive, but I wonder if there is any experience on the part of the panelists that would indicate that it is dangerous to give a drug like propranolol to individuals who have slow resting heart rates. From the practical point of view, does the issue arise that you would like to give a drug with intrinsic sympathetic activity to avoid bradycardia in an individual who starts out with a resting bradycardia? Is that a real issue?

Dr. Somani: This is one of the points I raised in comparing the drugs with and without intrinsic sympathomimetic activity. There is no clear cut clinical data to suggest that pindolol with slow heart rates would be better compared to propranolol. We have seen some cases with sick sinus syndrome where propranolol can produce almost complete cardiac standstill. I am not sure whether pindolol would be of any real benefit in these patients or not.

Dr. Harrison: I don't think there is any documented clinical study that shows a difference. If you are dealing with heart rates of 45 in the absence of intrinsic conduction system disorders, then propranolol would be acceptable.

Dr. Epstein: May I ask one other important question that comes up clinically. Is it demonstrated to your satisfaction that a given beta I beta blocker is safer to give to the diabetic patient than is a drug like propranolol? Where do matters stand on that issue?

Dr. Wood: I don't think it is clearly demonstrated. I think one can review the advantages. One of the problems of giving a beta blocker to a diabetic is that it may block the symptoms of hypoglycemia, not the symptom of sweating, which in fact is increased by administration of a beta blocker due to hypoglycemia. The other effects that have been shown to be different are the hypertension associated with hypoglycemia and also the appearance of non-selective beta blockers to prolong the period of hypoglycemia.

Dr. Altman: I just want to address a question to Dr. Moore. I was interested in the animal models that you discussed which is about as close as we can get to an animal model from sudden death. My question is do you have a dog model you have been able to use and reproduce with occlusion and reperfusion? In view of the literature on catecholamine receptors and histamine receptors in various animal species, have you thought about using other types of animal models, say the guinea pig, which may more closely simulate the human condition.

Dr. Moore: We have not used the guinea pig. Actually, the guinea pig has a number of problems to which a lot of people don't seem to pay attention.

Dr. Harrison: The latest animal model that many people are trying to work with is the Japanese quail. The Japanese quail develops atherosclerosis and gets arrhythmias, so it is a model with which you can work.

Temple: The explanation of why a drug with ISA might be satisfactory in angina seems pretty clear; but if resting heart rate is not much affected and if more or less such drugs replace what they are blocking, at least at rest, why do they work in hypertension?

Dr. Cohn: It is not fair for me to answer that, because Bob and I have discussed this together many times.

Dr. Somani: I think we are still searching for the answer for this clinical observation. With all the possible mechanisms that were suggested by Dr. Wood there is a possibility of antihypertensive effect. The latest addition to the list is the interaction with prostoglandins where propranolol has been shown to inhibit the effects of sympathetic stimulation or potentiation of the response to prostoglandins by sympathetic stimulation.

Dr. Harrison: I think that with at least seven antihypertensive possibilities for beta blocking drugs, to try to pick out one and look at it differentially with the others, is very difficult in this point in time.

Temple: You would almost have to assume some differential receptor responsiveness to the stimulatory part also, wouldn't you?

Harrison: Yes.

Dr. Sami: I really came here to try to find out what is an equipotent dose of two beta blockers and how we can use such methods for the pharmacokinetic studies. For example, if isoproterenol stimulation of heart rates in defining equipotent doses of those drugs in the clinical setting of 1) control of angina pectoris (for which you can use exercise testing or something like that to compare drugs, and even then I am not sure that we can define an equipotent dose) but the more important one is if we start using beta blockers for prophylactic means such as prevention of myocardial infarction, then what dose do we give? What is an equipotent dose of one beta blocker with another?

Dr. Harrison: Dr. Wood had some comments about that, and he clearly showed that resting heart rate was not good. Exercise heart rate may be better than the resting heart rate, and he showed the data with the shifts in the isoproterenol dose response curves. Dr. Robin Shanks has written several papers on this, trying to use that method to determine equipotent doses. If you deal with populations, you are going to have difficult problems because there is such variability of at least tenfold in the plasma concentration of drugs which you can't use as any measure for this, and there is the similar individual variability in responsiveness—so it is a very difficult question to answer.

Dr. Sami: There is no answer to that question.

Dr. Wood: Well, no, there is an answer if you want of define relative potency. You have to do it by something such as isoproterenol testing. You can't do it by exercise testing because once you have blocked the effect of exercise, then any further increase in blockade will go undetected so that you could have a drug that was three times as potent as another and completely miss that effect in terms of exercise testing. It is true that there is individual variability and response is less than the variability in pharmacokinetics, probably two to three times within an age group in comparison with the tenfold variability in pharmacokinetics.

Dr. Sami: Let me just follow up on your test for a moment. If I define a population of ten patients and let's say that pindolol is eight times as potent as propranolol dose per dose. Can I use that fact in the clinical setting and say that I can use pindolol in 8 to 1 potency for clinical control of angina; do I have to test each patient individually?

Dr. Wood: I guess the question is can you use it, or may you use it. You certainly can use it. Whether it is valid is a separate question; and, first of all, you should not look at potency in terms of dose but rather in terms of plasma concentrations because at least that gets by some of the pharmacokinetic variability. Secondly, you have to match your group; and I think this is the key and has not been addressed in the past for a variable such as age. You can't do potency determinations in the 20 to 25 age group and then go and do your studies in elderly patients with angina. So that is an important issue. If that is the best you can do, you may have to go with that if you can't or don't want to do isuprel testing.

Dr. Moore: One important thing to look at as far as equal beta blocking ability is whether it depends upon what heart rate you actually start from or as to what effect a given perturbation such as isoproterenol will do.

Dr. Wood: That is not so. People have looked at that; and if you raise the heart rate with something like atropine, you produce the same increment in response with the same dose, so that it doesn't appear to be true in terms of man.

Dr. Fitzgerald: I would like to address myself to two areas. The first one is the question of the dose of a beta blocker. Whilst I agree that Dr. Wood is correct in terms of practical use, I think the panel should in fact give advice to practicing clinicians as to what exactly to do because it is obviously not feasible to do isoprenolol dose response curves. The question of the duration of beta blockade, as long as it is super maximal and there are no additional unwanted effects from having supermaximal blockade, in practical terms, do you believe that that matters? I am talking in terms of a practicing clinician. The second point that I would make about the isoprenaline test is that with a beta I blocker, if you don't have the periphery blocked, you have a problem with the isoprenaline curve because you have a reflex vagal withdrawal due to the unopposed action of isoprenaline on the periphery; and, therefore, an isoprenaline test, it would seem to me and certainly in practical terms, has a limitation for assessing beta I blockers. I would like to make some comments on ISA too; but, perhaps, you would like to respond to that first.

Dr. Wood: Well, certainly, there are snags in the isoprotenerol test. For example, you can't do repeated tests over a period of 1/2 hour which you certainly can do with exercise or standing. In practice, if you have patient in the clinic and the question is whether this patient is adequately beta blocked, there are two ways to go. You can look and see if the patient has a rise in his heart rate on standing; you can exercise test him with some standard test and see if he responds to that; and, thirdly, you can measure his concentration if that is available to you. That has the advantage in that it detects the patients who are either not taking the drug or who have extraordinary low levels of the drug and gives you some feel for what the likely advantage is in increasing the doses relative to the side effects. So I think in practice, which is not necessarily the same thing about which we are talking here, if you are trying to assess whether a patient is going to get added benefit from an increasing dose, then you can use these simple tests, but they are not of value in determining relative potency. In terms of the beta I and beta II effects, I well recognize these problems and would turn it around in that sometimes that can be a strength in that you can actually use interarterial monitoring as a way of demonstrating beta I and beta II differences, but that is not the issue here.

Dr. Fitzgerald: You can't get dose ratio shifts that way; you can't get nice clean shifts that is. I would suggest we need to address three things. The first thing is that there are species differences in the response of tissues to partial agonists which are not seen with full agonists. It has recently been shown, for example, that the response of the isolated guinea pig atrium is quite different from the isolated kitten atrium. I don't think we have studied partial agonist in human tissues sufficiently to really understand precisely what we are talking about, and I think I would make a plea for that. The second point of course is that most of the partial agonists that we have don't have a very wide range in partial agonist activity which does not lower blood pressure in normal volunteers. It has much more partial agonist activity than the other agents, and so I think what one really needs to do is answer the questions that have been raised is to think about two things. First, to think about the difference in tissues on which partial agonists have an influence; and, secondly, the clinical condition because there is a condition which has been recently published in which pindolol has increased cardiac output by about 1 liter per minute in people with autonomic dysfunction. I think if we are going to discuss these things in any depth, we need to talk about the condition in which we are making comments about partial agonism because clearly in thyrotoxicosis there is a marked difference between beta blockers with partial agonists and without; whereas, there isn't in angina pectoris. So I think we have to be much more rigorous in defining what conditions we are talking about when we are making comments about partial agonism.

Dr. Barker: I would like to ask the question, since you skirted the issue to some extent about plasma levels, whether the interindividual variation of fat solubility, exercise, age, smoking, adiposity allows you to use plasma levels to determine when you have achieved your hope of maximum beta blockade; and does it relate to the differences between the drugs?

Dr. Wood: Yes, I think there is a use for plasma levels, provided you start off with limited objectives. If you are talking about using it in the clinic, then the situation in which I use a plasma level is if you draw a plasma propranolol level, for example, because that is the drug with which you have had the most experience in terms of examining plasma concentrations and you find that the patient has a blood concentration just to take one extreme of 200 nannograms per mil, then the chances of getting further therapeutic effect in that patient, if you are looking at antihypertensive effect, the side effects are small. You are not going to get much additional beta blockade from further increases in concentration. On the other hand to take the other extreme if you have levels of down around 40 nannograms per mil, then you know you have a good bit in terms of increasing dose before you are going to get into dose related side effects; but additional beta blocking effects will be picked up.

Dr. Harrison: I would agree, and the other use of plasma concentration of beta blockers is to measure compliance. I think threshold level determinations and compliance are the two reasons for measuring plasma concentration of beta blocking drugs.

Dr. Bayer: In isolated preparations you find a very good correlation between the degree of lipophilia of beta blockers and their membrane depressant activity. That means that with the increasing lipophilia, the side effect increases. My question now is do you mean that the mode of action is unspecific, that is by hydrophobic membrane constituents, the conductances of all channels, sodium, potassium and calcium channels is disturbed? Is there any evidence that the side effects are similar in humans related to lipophilia? Also is there any evidence for steriospecific pathway of metabolism of beta blockers?

Dr. Somani: In response to membrane depression versus lipid solubility in humans, I am not sure there is much correlation shown. The spectrum of side effects with propranolol in one extreme with highly lipid soluble compounds and nadolol and timolol with poor lipophilia, the differences are more in their relation to their pharmacological properties because one can see the spectrum of side effects with each group of drugs. In terms of their effectiveness, if you compare propranolol to nadolol which has no membrane depressant activity and on depression of force of contraction in patients with angina, these two drugs are practically identical in terms of reducing the cardiac output, and heart rate; so they do not translate from animal experiments to human studies. I am not sure whether this can be explained in terms of lipid solubility.

Dr. Abrams: In preparing for this Symposium, I tried to see whether there were any studies that looked at that particular point; and I could find no evidence for this.

Dr. Bayer: Yes, the question is unspecific side effects do not depend on which isomers you use and the question would be if you use the minus isomers, you wouldn't have much side effects.

Dr. Somani: Yes, but they are not active.

Dr. Bayer: The dextro-isomer is not an effective drug in terms of beta blocking activity; only the levo-isomer is effective.

Dr. Harrison: I think the question is not answerable with the evidence we have at hand.

Dr. Anderson: Relative to Dr. Moore's work, I was stimulated by the preliminary results on ventricular fibrillation threshold; and we recently have also been interested in the mechanism of prevention of sudden death and have looked at, I might add, six animals to the two or three that you have studied and our results have been similar. We have looked at a spectrum of beta blockers to see whether or not there would be various effects on elevation of ventricular fibrillation threshold; and what we found was that the relative order or potency was approximately timolol, pindolol, propranolol, metoprolol and finally labetolol approximately in the same order more or less as beta blocking potency. The elevation in VF threshold is approximately fourfold. There wasn't any gross difference in the maximum elevation of VF threshold but the potencies were approximately similar to the beta blocking potency. The other characteristics of the molecule we feel now are probably of relatively minor importance in determining elevation of VF threshold. Unfortunately, we also have seen some variability as you indicated with propranolol, with timolol and some of the other drugs; so there does seem to be a variable response that is difficult to quantitate. I wonder if you would comment on the differences in your model; the relative success with beta blockers as opposed to the relative failure in humans.

Dr. Moore: I really don't know why there would be differences in our model versus man. Propranolol has not been very effective in many other types of animal models of sudden cardiac death.

Dr. Michelson: The reason we studied so few dogs with propranolol in our model was that initially our experience confirmed what we had learned in the cath lab, and I lost interest in studying it further. It was not very successful using doses in animals that were considered to be beta blocking or high beta blocking doses. The drugs were only given intravenously and not with oral long-term dosing, so I can't tell you what might have happened with metabolites and other factors. One thing that bothers me about some of the animal studies that have been done previously and studies done in cells is that they are very often done in normal cells, normal tissue. Presumably patients who are at risk for sudden death and other arrhythmic problems have many abnormal cells, and it is much more important to be studying animal models and cells that are abnormal; and the properties of a beta blocker or the properties of a drug which has membrane stabilizing activities might be very much different if the cells are not normal.

Dr. Harrison: In line with that, Dr. Keef in the laboratory at our hospital has found that using induction techniques in a chronic myocardial infarction model with beta blocking drugs, she can prevent induction arrhythmias now. Whether those are related to spontaneous arrhythmias in the sudden death syndrome again becomes the question, but at least with beta blocking drugs you can prevent the induction of arrhythmia with programmed stimulation in the chronic model.

Dr. Hjalmarson: I would like to bring up the question about the intrinsic stimulatory activity that was discussed by Dr. Fitzgerald. It doesn't seem to be an absolute fact, and to say that pindolol has 40-50% intrinsic activity I think is an incorrect statement. I am quite sure that it could vary from 0 to 40-50%. We have experiences with various partial agonists in man which are in agreement with what has been found in different species and different conditions of the papillary muscle from the same species; that is, there can be a marked difference in the response. So in some patients, even with partial agonists with very high intrinsic activity, there could be almost no stimulatory response at all. So these could act more like blockers in some patients and more like stimulating agents in other patients; and it is not only different from person to person but also from time to time. There might be receptor changes by time. If we believe in regulation or down regulation, there seems to be changes in time; and I think it is a question of the changes in the coupling between receptor activation and effect response.

Dr. Somani: You have raised a very interesting question; and I think that was the major emphasis of my talk, trying to relate the animal data to clinical information. The information about the ISA that I presented is obtained on an average from a number of studies showing that pindolol and others have maximal ISA. Now in preparation for this Symposium I reviewed a lot of data about ISA in man and most studies employing dose response to pindolol in antihypertensive or antianginal studies in man could not show the same degree of ISA in terms of either increasing heart rate or increase of cardiac output. There is distinct species difference, and this is something we ought to keep in mind in extrapolating the information from animal laboratories into clinical pharmacology.

Dr. Cohn: Many of the pharmacologic studies in animals are done with acute dosing, and in the clinic we are using chronic therapy; and I don't know if we can translate so easily the acute effects of these agents in their chronic use because of such things as up and down regulation of receptors which might be quite different if you have a partial agonist as opposed to a blocker. So I think we have a lot more to learn about the differences between acute and chronic responses.

Dr. Parisi: Have any practical differences emerged in switching patients from one to another beta blocker in terms of break-through or symptoms?

Dr. Harrison: I would say that is a very difficult question to answer and very few, if any, studies have been reported that have made that attempt. At this point in time, it is probably difficult to get into that from a clinical viewpoint.

Dr. Somani: In one study in angina patients there was a well-controlled double-blind placebo control where they switched from one beta blocker to another one and there was no difference.

Dr. Harrison: He is talking about the one with failures or the ones with side effects. Not showing that the responsiveness is the same which is the kind of study that needs to be done.

Dr. Woosley: I would like to make a couple of comments. One, regarding the differences you see between propranolol and the various beta blockers in VF threshold, and some of the variability that you see might be explained based on the data of Pruitt and his work with isolated Purkinje fibers that Dr. Wood mentioned. In showing that it takes two hours for tissues in vitro to accumulate concentrations of propranolol that are at steady state, these concentrations of d or dl propranolol have membrane effects. They are not classical antiarrhythmic effects, but they are changes like you described earlier that could be antiarrhythmic and that means that any of the acute IV studies have to consider this time delay effect and a lot of the variability that you may see may be because you are getting beta blockade early. This goes along with some results we had several years ago when we tried to take people who responded to propranolol or during oral therapy; and then do acute I.V. testing to equivalent blood levels; and there is no correlation at all between antiarrhythmic efficacy of propranolol acutely I.V. versus chronic oral dosing, so I think there is an awful lot that we can't explain about the various effects of propranolol; and I think there may be other non-beta-blocking, perhaps some other action. In that same regard, I think Dr. Brahm Singh has shown clearly that the action potential prolongation that Dr. Somani has shown us with sodalol is probably not a beta blocking effect; it is probably a typical Type III antiarrhythmic effect, and something that goes along with that is that other pure beta blockers such as atenolol and timolol don't have this effect on action potential duration. So it is very unlikely that it is a pure beta blocking effect. It again may be some other action. The thing that confuses all these studies is the fact that any tissue or system you look at has some degree of sympathetic stimulation; and whether you are looking at reversal of that sympathetic stimulation or direct effect of the drug is very difficult, to be sure.

Dr. Chelly: The beta blockers decreased the sympathetic tone by the central mechanism. In patients with increased sympathetic tone, as in hypertensive patients, patients with angina pectoris, or patients with congestive heart failure, I would like to know if you have any information concerning the part of the substance on the central mechanisms versus the effect on the heart?

Dr. Harrison: I am afraid that the question you ask can't be answered at this time. We know so little about the central effects of these drugs.

Dr. Somani: It may be true that you cannot answer directly the question you have raised, but I think the animal experiments using direct injection of the drugs into the vertebral artery clearly show that it is possible this central action may be responsible for decrease in blood pressure, because all beta blockers given this way seem to lower the heart rate and blood pressure.

SUMMARY:

Dr. Harrison: I think it is very difficult to summarize this kind of discussion. I believe that the title of the morning session was "Are All Beta Blocking Agents the Same:" I think from the standpoint of isolated tissue studies, animal studies and theoretical considerations clearly are different. There are more than drug differences and specie differences; and while we cannot extrapolate directly from these observations to man, it is likely that appropriate clinical tests, which have not yet either been carried out or may not be possible, will show that there are differences in beta blocking drugs, not just pharmacokinetic differences and difference in mechanisms of action. I think at this juncture, we don't know what those differences are exactly and probably cannot make any practical recommendations at this time.

HOW TO DEFINE BETA-BLOCKER USEFULNESS IN HYPERTENSION: IS AMBULATORY
MONITORING NECESSARY?

Norman M. Kaplan, M.D.

In the past few years, two important findings have been derived from
ambulatory monitoring of the blood pressure: first, the blood pressure
is much more variable than most appreciate and, second, the antihypertensive action of most drugs used to treat hypertension lasts much longer
than most pharmacologists have taught.

Though pioneers such as Sokolow et al. (10) and Bevan et al. (2) described the value of prolonged ambulatory monitoring as long as 15 years
ago, few paid much attention until the English began publishing extensively
on the results obtained with their continuous intra-arterial measurements
and more experience was gained in the US with non-invasive, indirect monitoring equipment. Now, a veritable deluge of data from ambulatory monitoring prompts this analysis of its value in the decision concerning the usefulness of beta-blocker drugs in the treatment of hypertension.

Before addressing that issue, the current status of ambulatory monitoring
will be considered along with a comparison between it and home blood pressure
measurements. Thereafter some of the available data from ambulatory monitoring on beta-blocker therapy of hypertension will be reviewed in order
to answer the question posed by the organizers of this symposium.

THE TECHNIQUES OF AMBULATORY MONITORING

Two techniques are now available to record multiple blood pressures in
ambulatory patients, the direct intra-arterial Oxford device used in England

and the indirect, noninvasive equipment used mainly in the US. There are two models of the latter, the Remler semi-automatic recorder and the Avionics Pressurometer automatic monitor. The Remler requires the patient to pump air into the balloon at his own discretion whereas the Avionics device automatically inflates the balloon and records the pressure at predetermined intervals.

Direct intra-arterial devices

An intra-arterial cannula is placed percutaneously in the brachial artery and attached to an automatic pump which keeps perfusing the cannula with heparinized saline to prevent clotting. The cannula is also connected to a strain gauge transducer which transmits the pressure signal to a miniature tape recorder. The latest model seems to provide reliable recordings (3) and a low cost hybrid preprocessor and minicomputer have been developed to record and convert the individual readings into manageable data (4). With such equipment, multiple recordings for as long as 72 hours can be obtained providing reproducible data (5). With such recordings a circadian variation of the blood pressure has been clearly defined (6) (Figure 1).

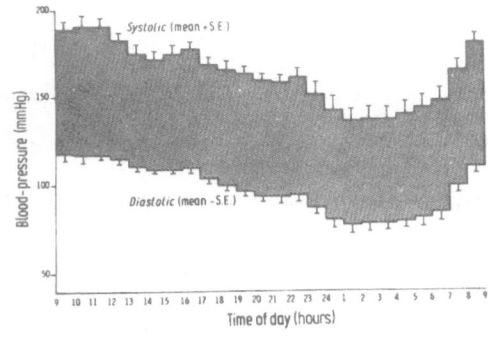

FIGURE 1. The hourly mean systolic and diastolic blood pressures over 24 hours in 20 untreated hypertensive patients (from Millar-Craig et al. Lancet 1:795, 1978).

Though these direct measurements provide precise data that is particularly useful for detailed study of variables affecting physiological control of the blood pressure, they will not be applicable to the large-scale
investigation of drug effects.

Indirect noninvasive devices

The largest and longest experience with such devices has been that of
Sokolow et al. (7) using the Remler recorder (Figure 2).

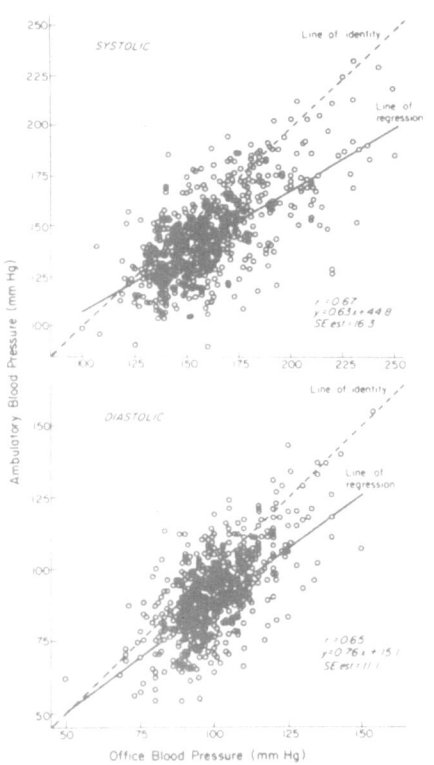

FIGURE 2. A scatterplot of
the average of all ambulatory
blood pressure readings taken
with a Remler recorder over a
24 hour period versus the average
of 3 readings taken in the office
on the same day with a mercury
sphygmomanometer in 675 patients
with essential hypertension
studied off treatment (from
Sokolow et al. Cardiovascular
Reviews & Reports 1:295, 1980)

The two sets of measurements were correlated with an r value around
0.65. However the overall ambulatory readings averaged 15/9 mm Hg lower
than the office readings.

The accuracy of the indirect devices. When compared to simultaneously obtained auscultatory sphygmomanometry, these devices provide comparable blood pressure readings. The recording of the Korotkoff sounds by a microphone sensor as used in both the Remler and Avionics devices has been shown to be accurate (8). Excellent correlations between the Avionics Pressurometer recordings and mercury manometry have been noted with simultaneously taken individual measurements (9) (Figure 3). Similarly close correlations have been noted between Remler and Hawkesley random-zero sphygmomanometry (10).

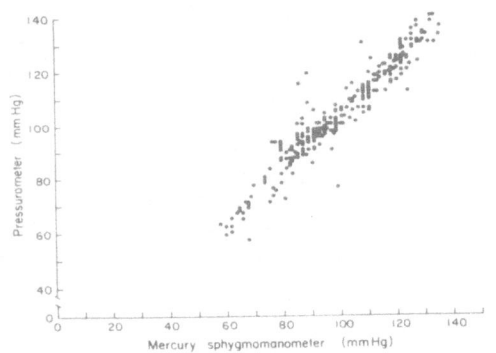

FIGURE 3. The correlation between the Avionics Pressurometer and a mercury sphygmomanometer for 450 readings of the blood pressure in 15 subjects (from Harshfield et al. Ambulatory Electrocardiology 1:7, 1979)

Only one comparison has been published (in an abstract) between an indirect (Remler) and direct intra-arterial device (11). In 15 patients simultaneously measured in the lab, the Remler readings averaged 0.2/8.9 mm Hg higher than the intra-arterial readings; when the measurements were taken at home, the Remler readings were 2.9 mm Hg lower for the systolic and 3.2 mm Hg higher for the diastolic than the direct readings.

The reliability of the indirect devices. Though one group of English investigators could interpret only half of the Remler recordings (12), Sokolow's group estimate that they successfully measure 90 to 95% of the readings (13). A 90% success rate has been claimed for the Pressurometer (14).

From my own experience with the Remler device and from numerous personal communications with owners of Pressurometer equipment, I believe 90% is too high a figure for the routine use of either device. A 75% success rate would be more realistic and maybe still a bit optimistic.

Overall, these results indicate that indirect noninvasive devices for ambulatory monitoring are probably now adequate to provide generally accurate data though some readings will not be interpretable.

THE NEED FOR MULTIPLE BLOOD PRESSURE READINGS

Let us now turn to the question: are multiple readings, such as obtained by ambulatory monitoring, necessary in assessing the usefulness of drugs, specifically beta-blockers, in the treatment of hypertension. My answer is yes, predicated upon two assumptions: 1) the blood pressure is so variable that measurements taken at a single time may not reflect the patient's overall blood pressure status, and 2) the duration of a drug's antihypertensive action can only be assessed by repetitive measurements taken throughout the day.

The variability of the blood pressure

The blood pressure is highly variable and the variability tends to be more prominent, the higher the blood pressure. In one of the first studies of variability under standardized conditions, Armitage and Rose (15) found that repeated readings in the same individuals over a 6 week period varied up to 30 mm Hg, with a significant fall between the first and 20th pairs of readings. Even in normotensives, variability is significant and the degree of variability is not constant over a one year interval (16).

The factors responsible for such variability have not been completely determined but these seem of major importance: the level of the pressure, the intensity of physical activity, the sensitivity of sino-aortic barorecep-

114

tors (for systolic variability) and the level of sympathetic activity as reflected in plasma norepinephrine levels (for diastolic variability) (17). In this study of 26 patients with uncomplicated hypertension, systolic variability was also directly related to the log values of plasma renin activity but not to plasma angiotensin II values. Though the number of subjects was small, variability was noted to increase with obesity but was unrelated to age, sex, and race.

Such variability is obviously of concern in trying to decide if a person is hypertensive and most find that 3 readings at 3 different times is a reasonable, workable compromise in dealing with individual patients. But our concern is whether this inherent variability could obscure the results of relatively short-term studies of the effectiveness of antihypertensive agents. My conclusion is a definite "yes", based upon the usual way that drug trials are now performed. In most, patients have 2 or 3 readings done once weekly, with a 3 to 6 week placebo period followed by a 4 to 8 week period of active drug therapy. Though most of the fall in blood pressure with placebo or just with repeated readings occurs in the first few days (18) (Figure 4), there may be a continued more gradual fall over 12 weeks or longer (19). Obviously part of the drugs' effects may be attributable to the progressive fall in pressure over time.

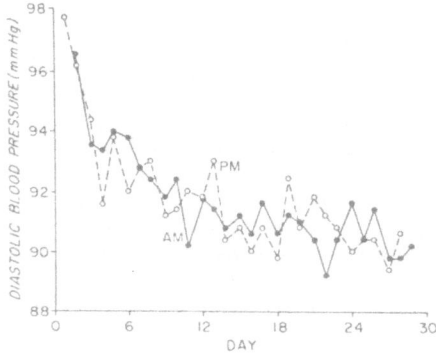

FIGURE 4. The diastolic blood pressures recorded at home twice daily (AM and PM) by 37 hypertensive patients who did not change their medication during the month of study (from Laughlin et al. Am Heart J 98:629, 1979).

The role of ambulatory monitoring in dealing with variability. Though

there are no strong supportive data, it is likely that the potential error

from the obfuscating variability of the blood pressure may be minimized

by obtaining multiple blood pressure readings over entire 24 hour periods.

The reasons include:

1) The anxiety-related higher initial readings should be smothered by

the subsequent readings, as shown in the repeated measurements recorded in

one patient by Perloff and Sokolow (19) (Figure 5).

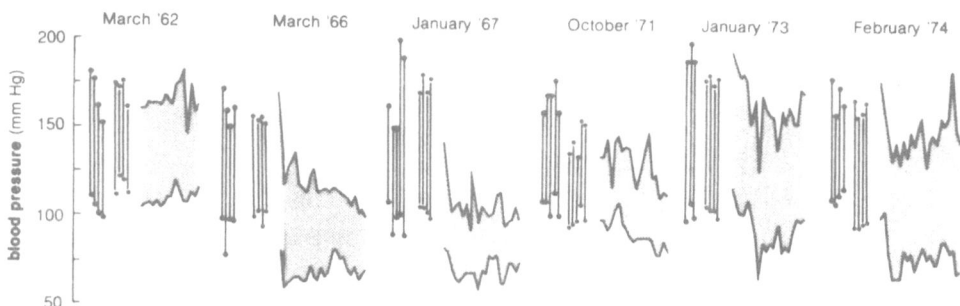

FIGURE 5. Corresponding office (the individual lines) and ambulatory
(the shaded areas) blood pressures measured on six occasions over a 12
year period in a 56 year old woman on various antihypertensive medications.
The degree of control seems better reflected in the ambulatory readings.
Similar data were noted in comparing ambulatory monitoring to readings
taken in the physician's office, at work, at home and asleep in 25 normotensive and 25 hypertensive patients (20). The readings tended to be a
bit higher at work but all were similar except for those taken in the
physician's office, where the hypertensives showed a pressor response.

2) Unless the single sets of readings are taken under carefully control-

led circumstances that are meticulously reproduced at each visit, a variety

of factors that affect the blood pressure may cause errors. These include

ambulation, eating, exercise (21), cigarette smoking (22), and the changing

diurnal pattern (6). The differences introduced by variable degrees of

physical activity are reflected in the direct intra-arterial recordings over two consecutive 24 hour periods taken in five patients (21) (Figure 6). Notice that the two sets of readings are quite similar when the levels of physical activity were similar (periods 1, 2, 4, and 5). But the first set of period 3, when the subjects were active, differs considerably from the second set, when the subjects were inactive.

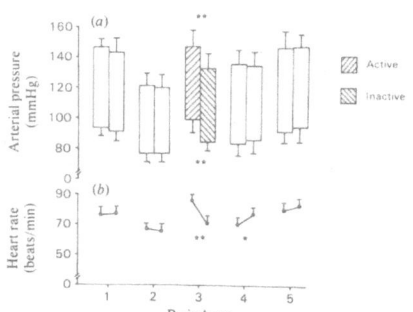

FIGURE 6. Grouped results for 5 patients whose intra-arterial blood pressure and heart rate were recorded for two consecutive 24 hour periods under different levels of physical activity; Period 1, physical activity; Period 2, sleep; Period 3, randomized activity or rest; Period 4, rest in bed; Period 5, physical activity (from Rowlands et al. Clinical Science 58:115, 1980).

Obviously, if repeated ambulatory monitorings are to be compared, the patients should be doing about the same things on the different days.

3) The effects observed at only one time of day may not be an accurate reflection of what happens through the entire 24 hours. Recall that the correlation between the office and ambulatory readings in Sokolow's large experience was only 0.65 and others have observed even lower correlations with smaller groups (23). If what we are trying to show is overall drug potency throughout the day, repetitive readings such as obtained by ambulatory monitoring seem essential.

The efficacy of therapy

This leads to perhaps the most important issue concerning ambulatory monitoring of antihypertensive drug therapy: is the propensity for any given level of blood pressure to cause morbidity and mortality better predicted by the ambulatory readings than by casual readings and, if so, is the effectiveness of antihypertensive therapy in preventing such trouble also better predicted by the effects on ambulatory readings? Once again, proof is not available, but suggestive evidence points to another "yes" answer.

Almost 40 years ago, Alam and Smirk showed that "basal" blood pressures, obtained by repeated measurements over 30 minutes of relaxation, were 10 to 20 mm Hg lower than "casual" readings (24). Smirk used the term "supplemental" pressure for the variable increment between the casual and the basal readings. Smirk subsequently found that the 8 year cumulative mortality, without therapy, was positively correlated with basal blood pressure but not with the supplemental (25).

Sokolow et al. (1) found a higher correlation between the severity of hypertensive complications and blood pressure levels obtained by ambulatory readings than with casual readings. More recently, a group of 32 subjects were found to have office cuff pressures that were more than 10 mm Hg higher than their ambulatory pressures recorded by direct intra-arterial monitoring (26). When compared to 22 subjects with similar office cuff and ambulatory readings, the 32 with significantly lower ambulatory readings had less cardiovascular target organ damage. The investigators therefore suggest that such lower ambulatory readings are indicative of less risk.

The blood pressures of patients included in drug trials are based upon casual readings. The inclusion of many patients whose ambulatory readings are considerably lower than their casual readings and who are therefore at little risk would tend to blunt the apparent effectiveness of any active intervention program.

If, as seems likely but not yet proven, the vascular damage induced by hypertension reflects the usual, overall level of pressure to which the vascular bed is exposed, the use of ambulatory monitoring to obtain the

average level over 24 hours should certainly be more predictive than the
use of casual readings.

The duration of drug effect

Without considering this important issue, ambulatory monitoring seems
necessary just to determine the duration of the antihypertensive action
of a given drug. In the past, most dosage schedules were based upon pharmacokinetic data. A drug such as propranolol with a plasma half-life of 2 hours
was therefore prescribed on a 3 to 4 times a day schedule.

Now that ambulatory monitoring has been done on patients receiving fairly
large doses of propranolol, the duration of its antihypertensive action
is much longer, fully 28 hours in the study by Watson et al. (27) (Figure 7).

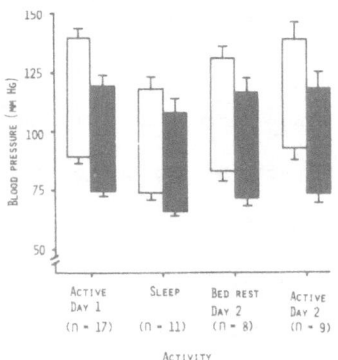

FIGURE 7. The average intra-arterial
blood pressures (± S.E.M.) recorded at
varying times over 28 hours before and
during long-term (mean 11 weeks) therapy
with propranolol (240 mg), metoprolol
(200 mg), or acebutolol (400 mg) given
once daily at 7 AM. On day 2, no drug
was given; bed rest was from 6 to 8:30
AM; the active, ambulatory period from
8:30 to 10 AM (from Watson et al.
Lancet 1:1210, 1979).

Similar results have been noted with virtually every beta-blocker (28)
so that, in the future, these drugs will likely be prescribed on a once a
day schedule which should improve patients' adherence to long-term therapy.

Thus, for multiple reasons, multiple readings seem necessary. But need
these be obtained by ambulatory monitors?

HOME READINGS VERSUS AMBULATORY MONITORING

Long before ambulatory monitoring became technically feasible, Ayman and Goldshine (29) had shown that blood pressures taken by patients at

home were usually lower than those taken in the office. Subsequently, the

degree of this difference has been repeatedly documented (30) (Figure 8).

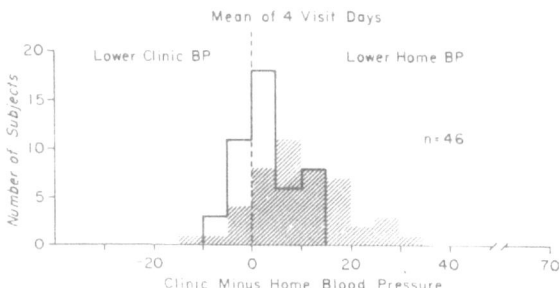

FIGURE 8. The frequency distribution of the differences between weekly clinic and twice a day home blood pressures for the means of four visit days. The diastolic differences are shown in the open figure, the systolic in the shaded. Overall, most of the home readings were lower, averaging 11.3/4.7 mmHg below the clinic readings (from Laughlin, et al. J Chron Dis 33: 197, 1980.)

These differences are similar to what Sokolow observed between ambulatory

monitoring and clinic readings, suggesting that multiple home readings likely

will give the same sort of data as would ambulatory monitoring. Recordings

of blood pressure during sleep are not obtainable by either manual home re-

cording or the Remler device but they are provided by the autonomic Pressuro-

meter. Such night-time recording may be needed in view of such reports as

one that indicates that a long-acting beta-blocker, nadolol, failed to

blunt the early morning rise of pressure (31).

Nonetheless, home blood pressure recordings may be a reasonable substitute

for ambulatory monitoring. In a study comparing the potency of a single

morning dose of a beta-blocker, penbutolol, compared to hydrochlorothiazide

and placebo, the results of the mid-afternoon clinic readings indicated that

the diuretic had a somewhat better effect than the beta-blocker (32). But

the home blood pressure recordings showed that the beta-blocker had a signi-

ficantly better effect (Figure 9).

120

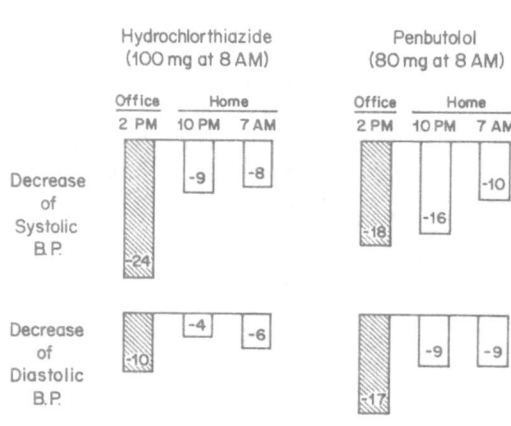

FIGURE 9. The mean decreases
of blood pressure recorded
either by physicians in the
office or by the patients at
home during a double-blind
cross-over controlled trial
of a beta-blocker and a diuretic
(from DePlaen et al. Br J
Clin Pharmacol 12:215, 1981).

When home blood pressures were compared against simultaneous intra-
arterial recordings in 43 hypertensives, the mean differences between them
were 2.0/6.6 mm Hg, the home readings being the lower (33). These differences
were less than those observed between intra-arterial monitors and clinic
blood pressures measured with a random zero sphygmomanometer.

When the cost of ambulatory equipment, currently between $10,000 and
$20,000 for each unit, is compared to that of manual home recording, the
importance of further validation of home recordings becomes apparent. As
they have so often done with other equipment, Japanese electronics manufacturers may offer an excellent alternative to ambulatory monitoring which
will provide most of its benefits at much lower cost. Nielsen and Andersen
have reported their successful use of an indirect, noninvasive Japanese device
that transmits Korotkoff sounds from a microphone to a digital display and
only requires the patient to pump up the balloon and record the numbers
(33). They found a very good correlation between simultaneously recorded
auscultatory measurements with a mercury manometer and offer this device
as an attractive alternative to ambulatory monitoring. Its cost is con-

siderably less than other devices.

CONCLUSION

Much of what I have reviewed is available only in preliminary form as abstracts, reflecting the still unsettled situation concerning the value of ambulatory monitoring in defining the usefulness of beta-blockers in the treatment of hypertension. Nonetheless, recognizing the variability of the blood pressure, the need for repetitive, multiple 24 hour recordings seems essential, if nothing more than to establish the duration of anti-hypertensive drug action. The more important issues concerning the value of such monitoring to establish drug efficacy and long-term benefit remain unanswered. Hopefully, home manual recordings can be substituted for the currently available expensive and cumbersome ambulatory monitors so that we will soon have the answers.

122

REFERENCES

1. Sokolow M, Werdegar D, Kain HK, et al. Relationship between level
    of blood pressure measured casually and by portable recorders and
    severity of complications in essential hypertension. Circulation
    34: 279, 1966.

2. Bevan AT, Honour AJ, Stott FH. Direct arterial pressure recording
    in unrestricted man. Clin Sci 36:329, 1969.

3. Millar-Craig MW, Hawes D, Whittington J. New system for recording
    ambulatory blood pressure in man. Med & Biol Eng & Comput 16:727,
    1978.

4. Cashman PMM, Stott FD, Millar Craig MW. Hybrid system for fast data
    reduction of long-term blood pressure recordings. Med & Biol Eng &
    Comput 17:629, 1979.

5. Mann S, Millar Craig MW, Balasubramanian V, et al. Ambulant blood
    pressure: reproducibility and the assessment of interventions.
    Clin Sci 59:497, 1980.

6. Millar Craig MW, Bishop CN, Raftery EB. Circadian variation of blood
    pressure. Lancet 1:795, 1978.

7. Sokolow M, Perloff D, Cowan R. Contribution of ambulatory blood
    pressure to the assessment of patients with mild to moderate elevation
    of office blood pressure. Cardiovasc Reviews & Reports 1:295, 1980.

8. Wolthuis R, Hull D, McAfoose D, et al. Portable blood pressure mea-
    surements: performance of Korotkov sound analysis techniques.
    Hypertension 3:596, 1981.

9. Harshfield GA, Pickering TG, Laragh JH. A validation study of the Del
    Mar avionics ambulatory blood pressure system. Ambulatory Electro-
    cardiology 1:7, 1979.

10. Fitzgerald J, O'Callaghan WG, O'Malley K, et al. Accuracy of the
    London school of hygiene and Remler M2,000 sphygmomanometers. 8th
    International Society of Hypertension, Milan, June 1-3, 1981.

11. Gould BA, Hornung R, Kieso H, Altman D, et al. A validation of the
    Remler M2000 semi automatic blood pressure recorder with intra-
    arterial and clinic blood pressures. 8th International Society of
    Hypertension, Milan, June 1-3, 1981.

12. Beevers DG, Bloxham CA, Backhouse CI, et al. The Remler M2000 semi-
    automatic blood pressure recorder. Br Heart J 42:366, 1979.

13. Cowan R, Sokolow M, Perloff D. The Remler ambulatory blood pressure
    recording system. Br Heart J 43:715, 1980.

14. Kennedy HL, Padgett NE, Horan MJ. Performance reliability of the Del Mar avionics noninvasive ambulatory blood pressure instrument in clinical use. Ambulatory Electrocardiology 1:13, 1979.

15. Armitage P, Rose GA. The variability of measurements of casual blood pressure. Clin Sci 30:325, 1966.

16. Rosner B, Polk BF.   The instability of blood pressure variability over time. J Chron Dis 34:135, 1981.

17. Watson RDS, Stallard TJ, Flinn RM, et al. Factors determining direct arterial pressure and its variability in hypertensive man. Hypertension 2:333, 1980.

18. Laughlin KD, Fisher L, Sherrard DJ. Blood pressure reductions during self-recording of home blood pressure. Am Heart J 98:629, 1979.

19. Pickering GW, Cranston WI, Pears MH. The treatment of hypertension. Springfield, Ill. CC Thomas, 1961.

20. Pickering TG, Harshfield GA, Kleinert HD, et al. Comparisons of blood pressure and heart rate changes during normal daily activities, sleep, and exercise in normal and untreated hypertensive subjects. 8th International Society of Hypertension, Milan, June 1-3, 1981.

21. Rowlands DB, Stallard TJ, Watson RDS, et al. The influence of physical activity on arterial pressure during ambulatory recordings in man. Clin Sci 58:115, 1980.

22. Houben H, Thien TH, Van'T Laar A. Haemodynamic effects of cigarette smoking during chronic selective and non-selective β-adrenoceptor blockade in patients with hypertension. Br J Clin Pharmac 12:67, 1981.

23. Pickering T, Harshfield G, Kleinert H. Ambulatory blood pressure. Lancet 2:416, 1981.

24. Alam GM, Smirk FH. Casual and basal blood pressures. Br Heart J 5:152, 1943.

25. Smirk FH. Observations on the mortality of 270 treated and 199 untreated retinal grade I and II hypertensive patients followed in all instances for five years. NZ Med J 63:413, 1964.

26. Floras JS, Jones JV, Hassan MO, et al. Cuff and ambulatory blood pressure in subjects with essential hypertension. Lancet 2:107, 1981.

27. Watson RDS, Stallard TJ, Littler WA. Influence of once-daily administration of β-adrenoceptor antagonists on arterial pressure and its variability. Lancet 1:1210, 1979.

28. Mann S, Millar Craig MW, Balasubramanian V, et al. Once daily β-adrenoceptor blockade in hypertension: an ambulatory assessment. Br J Clin Pharmac 12:223, 1981.

124

29. Ayman D, Goldshine AD. Blood pressure determinations by patients with essential hypertension. Am J Med Sci 200:465, 1940.

30. Laughlin KD, Sherrard DJ, Fisher L. Comparison of clinic and home blood pressure levels in essential hypertension and variables associated with clinic-home differences. J Chron Dis 33:197, 1980.

31. Hornung RS, Gould BA, Kieso H, et al. A study of nadolol to determine whether its long serum half life provides reduction in blood pressure over 24 hours. 8th International Society of Hypertension, Milan, June 1-3, 1981.

32. De Plaen JF, Vander Elst E, Van Ypersele De Strihou C. Penbutolol or hydrochlorothiazide once a day in hypertension. A controlled study with home measurements. Br J Clin Pharmac 12:215, 1981.

33. Gould BA, Kieso H, Altman D, et al. Is home blood pressure recording sufficiently accurate to replace intra-arterial ambulatory monitoring? 8th International Society of Hypertension, Milan, June 1-3, 1981.

34. Nielsen PE, Andersen A. Blood pressure device for home-readings. Lancet 2:416, 1981.

EVALUATION OF BETA BLOCKING AGENTS IN THE TREATMENT OF ANGINA PECTORIS DUE TO CORONARY ARTERY DISEASE

STEPHEN E. EPSTEIN, M.D.

I. Traditional randomized double-blind crossover study design
   A. Usually designed with a single-blind run-in placebo period, double-blind periods employing two doses of active agent and one dose of placebo, and finally a single-blind follow-up period. Study duration is usually many months. Although shorter testing periods can be employed, total study duration is necessarily long.

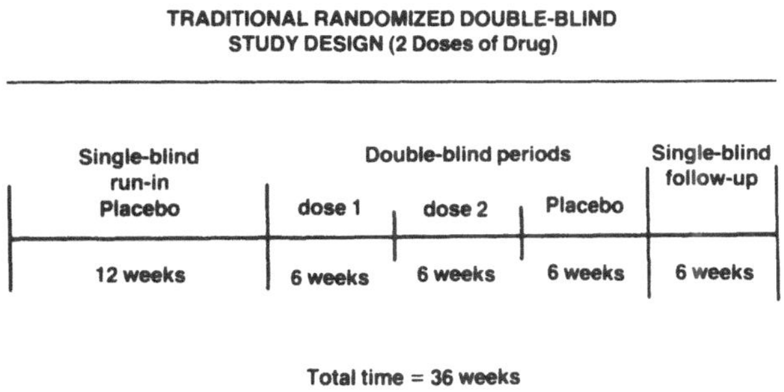

**TRADITIONAL RANDOMIZED DOUBLE-BLIND
STUDY DESIGN (2 Doses of Drug)**

Single-blind run-in Placebo	Double-blind periods			Single-blind follow-up
	dose 1	dose 2	Placebo	
12 weeks	6 weeks	6 weeks	6 weeks	6 weeks

Total time = 36 weeks

Figure 1. Typical design of a traditional randomized double-blind crossover study.

   B. Patient requirements:
      1. Minimal frequency of angina of 5 attacks per week
      2. Stable pattern of angina
   C. Problems with traditional double-blind crossover study
      1. Difficult to find patients with 5 or more episodes per week of stable angina
      2. Long testing period increases possibility of complicating conditions developing that would influence anginal frequency (infection, acute myocardial infarction, unstable angina, concurrent disease, or changes in medication utilization, physical conditioning, exercise patterns, emotional state, body weight, environmental temperature)

126

3. Complicating conditions would increase magnitude of spontaneous
   fluctuations of anginal frequency
   a. Type II error more likely (Failure to detect a significant
      effect when, in fact, such exists)
   b. larger numbers of patients necessary to exclude Type II error
   c. the relation of patient size needed for proving a beneficial
      effect if one exists increases exponentially in relation to
      the coefficient of variation of frequency of spontaneous
      anginal attacks.

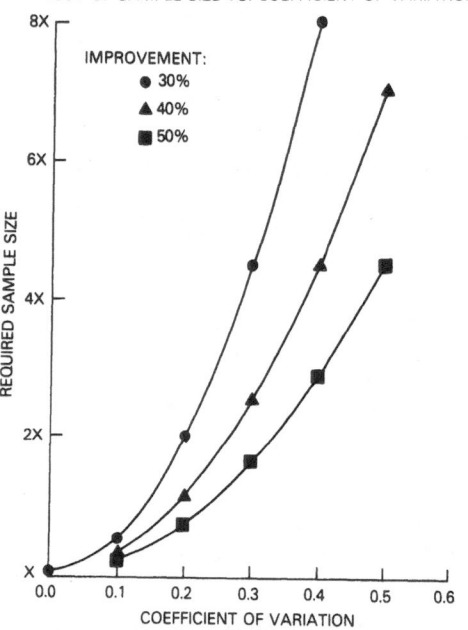

PLOT OF SAMPLE SIZE VS. COEFFICIENT OF VARIATION

Figure 2. Relation between sample size necessary
to detect a significant effect and spontaneous
variability of end point being tested. The three
curves represent relationship for progressively
more powerful interventions.

4. Drop-out rate fairly high (about 25%) due to factors outlined
   in C2. This will further confound statistical analyses.

II. Randomized double-blind exercise testing design
   A. Involves an exercise training and reproducibility period, followed
      by double-blind periods usually employing two doses of active drug
      and placebo period followed by a single blinded period to rule out
      a training effect. Total duration of study can be about 14 days

but might be considerably longer, depending on pharmacokinetics of the drug under investigation. Drugs with longer half lives or prolonged physiological effects will need longer wash-out periods than drugs with shorter durations of action.

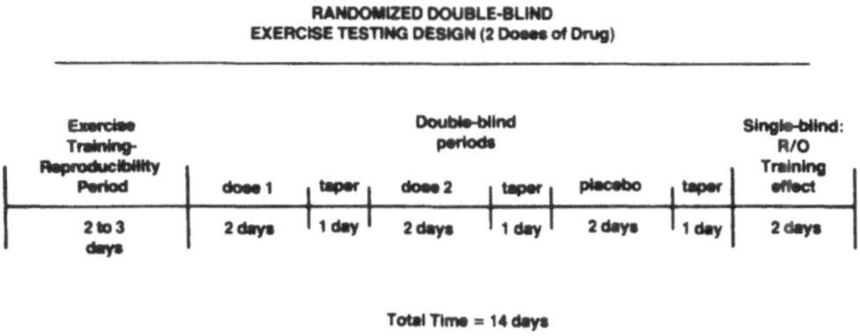

RANDOMIZED DOUBLE-BLIND
EXERCISE TESTING DESIGN (2 Doses of Drug)

Exercise Training- Reproducibility Period	dose 1	taper	dose 2	taper	placebo	taper	Single-blind: R/O Training effect
2 to 3 days	2 days	1 day	2 days	1 day	2 days	1 day	2 days

Total Time = 14 days

Figure 3. Typical design of a randomized double-blind crossover exercise study

B. Patient requirements:
 1. Reproducible exercise-induced angina
 2. Ability to perform bicycle or treadmill exercise
C. Problems with double blind exercise study
 1. Must find patients with reproducible exercise-induced angina
 2. Study is optimally performed in-hospital: hence patient must be able to spend the necessary two or more weeks in hospital
 3. Must determine that no training effect occurred during multiple exercise tests
 4. No assurance that beneficial effects observed over such a short term study will apply to chronic administration (eg - possibility of tolerance developing cannot be excluded).

III. Additional Considerations
A. When comparing relative effects of two or more drugs, arbitrary selection of a single fixed dose will likely lead to erroneous conclusions.
 1. More than one dose of each drug must be tested, or
 2. "Best Dose" testing must be attempted (with best dose determined by prior unblinded empirical testing)
B. If there are multiple factors contributing to determining anginal threshhold:
 1. How can efficacy of a drug that improves a mechanism operative in a minority of patients be demonstrated?

      a. Statistical models must be designed to determine reproducibility of end-point in the group being tested so that if a minority of individuals respond to a drug, the deviation of response of this subgroup from spontaneous variation can be detected. This "searching for subgroups" could lead to "significant" differences when, in fact, none existed. Hence, the subjects so identified must constitute the patient cohort of a second study designed to prospectively test a new hypothesis -- that the therapeutic intervention being tested benefits this specific subgroup of patients.

IV. Are placebo control periods ethical?

    A. Standard double-blind crossover study requires weeks or months of placebo treatment (Fig 1). This can pose some risk to the patient. In one study (1) four of 13 patients (31%) who changed abruptly from 160 mg/day of propranolol to placebo developed unstable angina: one of these four died and one developed an acute myocardial infarction.

    B. Double blind exercise study requires only days of placebo therapy (Fig 3) and patient is observed in-hospital under carefully controlled conditions.

REFERENCES

1. Alderman EL, et al. Dose response effectiveness of propranolol for the treatment of angina pectoris. Circulation 51:964, 1975.

BETA BLOCKING AGENTS IN THE TREATMENT
OF VENTRICULAR ARRHYTHMIAS

Joel Morganroth, M.D.

Sudden cardiac death is due usually to a ventricular arrhythmia such as ventricular fibrillation. An important marker for the development of ventricular tachyarrhythmias has been "premature ventricular beats" which was first recognized in the Coronary Care Unit experience of the 1960's. Epidemiologic studies during the 1970's, particularly in patients post-myocardial infarction or with angina pectoris and more recently with disorders of myocardial function (e.g. cardiomyopathy), have clearly demonstrated that in such groups ventricular premature complexes are potent predictors of the development of sudden cardiac death.[1]

Ventricular arrhythmias occur in two important and different clinical settings. The first is when paroxysmal ventricular tachyarrhythmias occur in patients with manifest cardiac disease; and the occurrence of such ventricular ectopy places the patient in an immediate high-risk for either sudden death or severe disability from congestive heart failure, angina pectoris, or cerebral hypofusion. Such patients must have their ventricular arrhythmias immediately treated to reverse these hemodynamic consequences; and thus, in such patients, placebo periods, noninvasive testing or ambulatory studies are usually not feasible.

The more common setting is when chronic ventricular ectopy is identified in individuals with cardiovascular disease. Ventricular ectopy may occur even to the point of paroxysmal ventricular tachycardia (usually of less than 50 beats in a row) and in such patients symptoms are usually absent or, if present, are merely bothersome palpitations or dizziness. It is in this group of patients in whom it is hoped that antiarrhythmic agents can be used to prevent the apparent high risk of sudden cardiac death. Obviously, placebo periods and ambulatory outpatient studies are feasible as study design methods and noninvasive testing methodology logical for definition of efficacy.

The entire problem of sudden cardiac death is an important challenge to modern day cardiology since in the United States alone approximately one sudden death occurs every minute. This usually interrupts life prematurely and is the leading cause of death in the 20-64 year old age range. The prevention of sudden death by identifying high-risk individuals who are candidates for prophylactic interventions such as antiarrhythmic agents rather than its treatment by resuscitating the victim at its onset it bound to have the most important impact on the elimination of this cause of death.[1]

DEFINITION OF EFFICACY OF ANTIARRHYTHMIC AGENTS IN THE TREATMENT OF CHRONIC VENTRICULAR ARRHYTHMIAS

The definition of antiarrhythmic efficacy depends upon the clinical setting in which the drug is used. We will first discuss the definition of antiarrhythmic efficacy in the more common condition of non-hemodynamically significant chronic ventricular ectopy. In such a setting antiarrhythmic drug efficacy could be simply defined as "the prevention of sudden cardiac death". Unfortunately, such a study endpoint must await the availability of agents in which a high degree of efficacy, compliance and safety exists. Studies to date to attempt to address the issue of sudden cardiac death prevention have either suffered from a high dropout rate due to toxicity of the available antiarrhythmic agent or improper study designs in which sub-therapeutic doses of agents have been used. With the emerging availability of antiarrhythmic agents in which a high degree of potency exists insuring maximal efficacy on ventricular ectopic frequency reduction and in which compliance and safety levels are high, such prospective studies will be possible. To obtain drugs for such evaluation efficacy for now has to be defined on pharmacologic grounds using endpoints relating solely to the frequency and severity of ventricular ectopy under treatment rather than the prevention of sudden death.[2]

Antiarrhythmic drug efficacy should be assessed in individual patients taking into consideration the high degree of spontaneous variability that exists in chronic ventricular ectopic frequency.[3-5] The impact of various statistical methodologies, clinical settings and study protocols,[2,6-7] suggests a definition of efficacy of approximately a 75% reduction in ventricular ectopy frequency when comparing treatment to placebo periods. This should be evaluated in individual patients and thus, the efficacy of the drug will be defined as percent of individual patients so responding to this level of reduction. The practice of pooling placebo and treatment data to define efficacy suffers from the problem of lumping data from patients in which there is marked patient and arrhythmia response heterogeneity. Thus, the percentage responding to the agent will define the relative efficacy for the agent. Of the currently released antiarrhythmic agents in the United States, approximately a 50-75% response rate of tested patients is usually seen. It is also important to remember that antiarrhythmic agents may increase ventricular ectopic frequency as an adverse side effect and this may occur in as many as 5-20% of patients so treated.[8,9]

Recommendations for protocol design based on issues cited above suggest that the minimum ventricular ectopic frequency entrance criteria for patients in this setting should be 30 PVCs/hr for 24 hours. At least 48 hours of Holter monitoring should be obtained on placebo prior to testing the efficacy of the antiarrhythmic agent. At least 24-48 hours of Holter monitoring should be obtained at each dosage level and definition of antiarrhythmic efficacy in general will be approximately 75% reduction as noted above. During the final placebo period one should expect to see at least a 50% return to the initial placebo baseline ventricular ectopic frequency though occasionally, some patients (probably because of high rate of spontaneous variability) do not show this response.

There has been much debate as to the relative advisability of crossover vs parallel designs in these studies, and we believe that the crossover design provides for a more powerful and clinically meaningful study.[10] Study agents should be evaluated for their short-term efficacy which should be defined as several days to a few weeks in order to insure that there is the least possibility of change in underlying cardiovascular condition. Long-term continued efficacy and safety studies should be carried out over months to years with introduction of placebo periods intermittently (e.g. every six months) to insure that ventricular ectopy continues to exist.

BETA ADRENERGIC BLOCKERS IN THE TREATMENT OF VENTRICULAR ECTOPY

Beta adrenergic blocking agents have for many years not been considered one of the first line drugs in the treatment of ventricular ectopy.[11] Electrophysiologic studies have clearly demonstrated that beta adrenergic blocking agents will block the catacholamine induced increased rate of phase 4 depolarization in automatic cells. No change in fibrillation thresholds in the atria or ventricles or change in refractoriness of normal atrial or ventricular tissue is expected. Beta adrenergic blocking agents increase the effective refractory period of the atrioventricular node, thus defining its primary use in patients with supraventricular arrhythmias. Animal studies using large doses of beta blocking

agents have defined a membrane stabilizing effect, "like quinidine" but in the

usual clinical doses, the importance of this membrane effect may be entirely

unimportant.[12]

One of the early and most clearly efficacious uses of beta adrenergic

blocking agents was the intravenous introduction of such agents in patients in

whom volatile anesthetic agents induced catacholamine release and ventricular

arrhythmias during surgery.[13] Additional clinical uses appear to involve the

apparent effectiveness of beta blocking agents in patients with ventricular ectopy

due to actively-induced ischemic episodes, digitalis toxicity, and in the conditions

of mitral valve prolapse and hypertrophic cardiomyopathy. The potential

adjunctive use of beta blocking agents with primary Class I antiarrhythmic agents

has not been precisely studied but there continued use is often seen in clinical

practice. Precisely defined studies in these areas are still wanting.

CLINICAL TRIALS USING BETA BLOCKING AGENTS IN THE TREATMENT OF VENTRICULAR ECTOPY

Table 1 details eight clinical trials that have used a variety of beta

blocking agents to determine their efficacy in the suppression of chronic

ventricular ectopy. These studies were selected because they used ambulatory

monitoring as the means of defining ventricular ectopic frequency and drug effect

and were also oral ambulatory placebo-controlled studies.This table shows that the

efficacy of suppressing ventricular ectopy to a significant level occurs in

approximately 50% of patients with chronic ventricular ectopy either using a

population with mixed cardiac diagnoses or predominantly those with ischemic

heart disease or mitral valve prolapse. The only exception to this appears to be

the study by Woosley and co-workers[17] in which propranolol in doses up to 960 mgs/day were used and 75% of the patients responded. These investigators determined that the plasma concentration of propranolol at the time of ventricular ectopic efficacy was usually greater than that required for beta blockade, thus suggesting that the mechanism for ventricular ectopic suppression may be something other than simple beta blockade. In addition, a biphasic response was seen in five patients in which ventricular ectopic frequency was suppressed at a lower dose of propranolol but at a higher dose ventricular ectopy actually increased. In our study of nadolol[20] using 80 to 640 mgs/day, we determined that in patients in whom ventricular ectopic frequency was suppressed that further suppression could not occur after beta blockade (as measured by heart rate response) occurred. In addition, a biphasic response was not noted in any of our patients, though 10% did have an increase in ventricular ectopy on the agent. Whether these differences reflect observations in different populations or are due to the particular drug remains to be determined.

Other beta blocking agents, such as metropolol, acebutolol, nadalol and atenolol have been studied; and once again, an approximate 50% of patients so treated have demonstrated significant therapeutic efficacy. Side effects in all of these studies have been quite minimal.

Table 2 demonstrates the comparison of the ventricular premature complex response to each of five beta blocking drugs in reference to their pharmacologic properties. One can notice from this table that even though all of these agents appear to be efficacious in an approximate 50% of patients tested, there is no apparent relationship to the degree of cardio-selectivity, agonist activity (intrinsic stimulating activity) or the "quinidine-like" membrane effect. Thus, the mechanism of antiarrhythmic action of beta blocking agents appears to be unclear at the present time.

Later in this Symposium the subject of the use of beta adrenergic blocking drug efficacy in the prevention of sudden cardiac death after in patients with myocardial infarction will be addressed. Whether or not beta adrenergic blocking agents or any type of antiarrhythmic agents will prevent sudden cardiac death when effectively suppressing ventricular ectopic frequency in chronic arrhythmias yet remains to be demonstrated.

USE OF BETA ADRENERGIC BLOCKING AGENTS IN PATIENTS WITH LIFE-THREATENING ARRHYTHMIAS

These patients are characterized by have paroxysmal persistent ventricular tachycardia or paroxysmal ventricular fibrillation. These arrhythmias are of such duration and/or the patient has such severe underlying cardiac disease that hemodynamic symptoms are produced. Such patients are frequently studied by electrophysiologic invasive testing with the attempt at initiating the ventricular tachyarrhythmia so that intravenous (or sometimes oral) therapy may be instituted in order to determine whether or not the dysrhythmia can be re-initiated. To date there are no published controlled studies specifically evaluating beta blocking agents in this setting. Clinical experience, however, suggests that alone these agents are not highly efficacious but may be very useful as adjunct therapy with Class 1 membrane-active antiarrhythmic agents. Studies directed at confirming these anecdotal impressions are needed.

SUMMARY

Beta adrenergic blocking agents using the above-cited study designs and definitions of efficacy appear to be useful as primary antiarrhythmic agents in as many as 50% of general cardiac patients with chronic ventricular ectopy. These agents may also be important as adjunctive therapy with other Class 1 antiarrhythmic agents in patients with severe refractory ventricular tachyarrhythmias. Efficacy of the different beta adrenergic blocking agents does not appear to depend upon their different pharmacologic properties and, thus, a class indication for treatment of ventricular arrhythmias could be considered.

TABLE 1

ORAL BETA BLOCKING AGENTS IN CHRONIC VENTRICULAR ECTOPY

EFFICACY USING HOLTER MONITORING

Reference	Diagnosis	Drug	% Efficacy	Comments [1]; [2]
14	Mixed*	Propranolol	2/16 (50%)	>70%; 240
15	Mitral Valve Prolapse	Propranolol	5/9 (56%)	>75%; 40-320
16	Coronary Artery Disease	Metoprolol	7/13 (54%)	>75%; 100-200
17	Mixed	Propranolol	24/32 (75%)	>70%; up to 960
18	Mixed	Acebutalol	11/20 (55%)	>70%; 300
19	Acute Myocardial Infarction	Propranolol	18/32 (56%)	>70%; 80-480
20	Mixed	Nadolol	7/13 (54%)	>75%; 80-640
21	Mixed	Atenolol	7/12 (58%)	>70%; 50-200

* - several cardiac diseases studied
[1] - percentage reduction required to define drug efficacy
[2] - dose range studied in mgs/day

TABLE 2

COMPARISONS AMONG BETA BLOCKERS IN

VENTRICULAR ECTOPY (VPC) SUPPRESSION

Drug	Cardioselectivity	Agonist Activity	Membrane Effect	VPC Response Rate
Propranolol	-	-	+	About 50%
Metoprolol	+	-	-	About 50%
Nadolol	-	-	-	About 50%
Atenolol	+	-	-	About 50%
Acebutalol	+	+	+	About 50%

+ = present

- = absent

REFERENCES

1. Morganroth J. How to evaluate a new antiarrhythmic drug: The challenge of sudden cardiac death. In: The Evaluation of New Antiarrhythmic Drugs, edited by Morganroth J, Moore, EN, Dreifus LS, Michelson EL. Published by Martinus Nijhoff 1981.

2. Morganroth J. Long-term ambulatory electrocardiographic recording in the determination of efficacy of new antiarrhythmic agents. In: The Evaluation of New Antiarrhythmic Drugs, edited by Morganroth J, Moore, EN, Dreifus LS, Michelson EL. Published by Martinus Nijhoff 1981.

3. Winkle RA. Antiarrhythmic drug effect mimicked by spontaneous variability of venttricular ectopy. Circulation 57:1116, 1978.

4. Morganroth J, Michelson EL, Horowitz LN, Josephson ME, Pearlman AS, Dunkman WB. Limitations of routine long-term electrocardiographic monitoring to assess ventricular ectopic frequency. Circulation 58:408, 1978.

5. Michelson EL, Morganroth J. Spontaneous variability of complex ventricular arrhythmias detected by long-term electrocardiographic recording. Circulation 61:690, 1980.

6. Sami M, Kraemer H, Harrison DC, Houston N, Shimasahi C, DeBusk RF. A new method for evaluating antiarrhythmic drug efficacy in individual patients. Circulation 62:1172, 1980

7. Morganroth J, Michelson EL. Precise determination of antiarrhythmic drug effiacy in individual patients based on individual rather than pooled patient data. Circulation 62:III:305, 1980 (abstract)

8. Winkle RA, Gradman AH, Fitzgerald JW. Antiarrhythmic drug effect assessed from ventricular arrhythmia reduction in the ambulatory electrocardiogram and treadmill test: Comparison of propranolol, procainamide and quinidine. Am J Cardiol 42:473, 1978.

9. Velebit V, Podrid PJ, Graboys TB, Lown B. Aggravation of ventricular arrhythmia by antiarrhythmic drugs. Am J Cardiol 43:359, 1979.

10. Kramer HC. Parallel or crossover designs in evaluation of antiarrhythmic therapy. In: The Evaluation of New Antiarrhythmic Drugs, edited by Morganroth J, Moore, EN, Dreifus LS, Michelson EL. Published by Martinus Nijhoff 1981.

11. Gibson D, Sawton E. The use of beta adrenergic receptor blocking drugs in dysrhythmias. Prog Cardiovasc Dis 12:16, 1969.

12. Coltart DJ, Gibson D, Shand DG. Plasma propranolol levels associated with suppression of ventricular ectopic beats. Br Med J 1:490, 1971.

13. McLish A, Andrew D, Moisan A, Morin Y. Intravenous properties for cardiac disturbance in relationship to halothane anesthesia for cardiovascular surgery. Can Med Assoc J 99:388, 1968.

14. Winkle RA, Gradman AH, Fitzgerald JW, Bell PA. Antiarrhythmic drug effect assessed from ventricular arrhythmic reduction in the ambulatory ECG and treadmill test. Comparison of propranolol, procainamide and quinidine. AJC 42:473, 1978.

15. Winkle RA, Lopes MG, Goodman DJ, Fitzgerald JW, Schroeder JS, Harrison DC. Propranolol for patients with mitral valve prolapse. Am Heart J 93:422, 1977.

16. Pratt CM, Matlack J, Carney S, Waggoner AD, Wichemeyer WW, Martin F, Miller RR. Effect of metroprolol in suppression of ventricular ectopic beats. Circulation 62:III:10, 1980

17. Woosley RL, Kornhause D, Smith R, Reele S, Higgins SB, Nies AS, Shand DG, Oates JA. Suppression of chronic ventricular arrhythmias with propranolol. Circulation 60:819, 1979.

18. DeSoyza N, Kane JJ, Murphy ML, Laddu AR, Doherty JE, Bissett JK. The long-term suppression of ventricular arrhythmias by oral acebutolol in patients with coronary artery disease. Am Heart J 100:631, 1980.

19. Koppes GM, Beckmann CH, Jones FG. Propranolol therapy for ventricular arrhythmias two months post acute myocardial infarction. Am J Cardiol 46:322, 1980.

20. Morganroth J. Evaluation of the efficacy and tolerance of nadolol in patients with chronic ventricular arrhythmias. Data on request and on file at Squibb Medical Research.

21. Morganroth J. Evaluation of the efficacy and tolerance of atenolol in patients with chronic ventricular arrhythmias. Data on request and on file at ICI Americas Inc.

HOW TO DEFINE BETA BLOCKER USEFULNESS IN SUPRAVENTRICULAR
ARRHYTHMIAS.

E. ROWLAND, D.M. KRIKLER.
Division of Cardiovascular Medicine, Royal Postgraduate Medical
School, Hammersmith Hospital, London, W12 OHS, England.

INTRODUCTION.

Although supraventricular arrhythmias usually lack the frequently
malignant implication of rhytnm disturbances arising in the ventricles,
their incidence is considerable and their chronicity often profound.
The young person with paroxysmal supraventricular tachycardia may
not be in grave danger but he may well face years of discomfort in
the absence of effective treatment.   The paroxysmal nature of
many supraventricular arrhythmias, together with their occurrence,
frequently in the absence of organic heart disease, often enables
the afflicted patient to enjoy long spells of normal health which
are interrupted abruptly by disabling and distressing symptoms.
These may be particularly severe when there is associated valvular,
ischemic or myopathic heart disease.   In addition, the presence
of supraventricular arrhytnmia may add its own contribution to tne
prognosis of the associated heart disease and thus contribute
significantly to the patient's outlook.   In rare instances, such
as persistent atrial fibrillation in the presence of mitral stenosis,
embolic complications make the arrhythmia life-threatening and ideal
therapy should achieve the return and persistence of sinus rhythm.

Since the recognition of alpha and beta adrenergic receptors(1)
a specific group of drugs capable of antagonizing competitively the
natural sympathetic transmitters at these receptor sites has been
developed.   These beta-adrenergic blocking drugs have been at the
forefront of treatment for supraventricular arrhythmia.   The basic
action of the beta-adrenergic blockers is to oppose the action of
catecholamines on adenylate cyclase,(2) the enzyme that triggers
the intra-cellular release of a secondary transmitter, cyclic
adenosine monophosphate (cAMP).   The physiological actions are a
reduction in heart rate and depression of atrio-ventricular nodal

conduction (3) due to changes in the cell membrane (4) and via an intra-cellular action, an impairment of myocardial contraction-relaxation (5). All these actions can in some way be traced to an effect on calcium ion transport. At present there are some 12 agents marketed as "beta-blockers" with many claimed to have specific actions. This specificity relates to degrees of cardio-selectivity, partial agonist action and membrane stabilising activity (local anesthetic activity). The latter appears to be an action only seen at doses which are far larger than those seen in the clinical setting. Cardio-selectivity may be relevant in patients with obstructive airways disease; and the presence of partial agonist activity relevant in young people with low resting sympathetic tone. A beta blocker with a unique action is sotalol which has been shown specifically to prolong the action potential to a degree greater than that expected by simple blockade of sympathetic stimulation, an effect which is evident when it is given acutely (6). More recent work with metoprolol appears to suggest that chronic treatment in man, as has been demonstrated with other beta blockers, can prolong repolarisation, an effect not seen when the drug is given acutely (7). With such a wealth of information available on the experimental properties of the many beta blockers available in Europe one must have a clear idea of the desired effects when considering their use in supraventricular arrhythmias. For the purposes of this discussion on possible methods of investigation in the clinical setting we will consider arrhythmias generated in the region of the sinus node, arising in the atrial myocardium, and AV junctional re-entry. Abnormalities in sinus node impulse formation and conduction are clearly important in the context of possible aggravation by antiarrhytnmic drugs and of particular importance in that paroxysmal atrial fibrillation may be the tachycardia component of the bradycardia-tachycardia syndrome. Atrial fibrillation and flutter, whether established or paroxysmal, are frequent rhythm disturbances in all age groups and constitute the commonest supra-ventricular tachycardias requiring treatment. AV junctional re-entry can be broadly classified as being due to an accessory atrio-ventricular patnway (Wolff-Parkinson-White syndrome) or due to dual AH pathways.

Phase 1 and early Phase 2 studies.

Early experimental studies of a new beta blocker will provide
information on the relative beta blocker potency, cardioselectivity
and presence of any partial agonist activity.   Currently available
beta blockers appear to show membrane stabilising activity only
when studied at a dose 10^2-10^3 times greater than that used in the
clinical situation.   Initial clinical studies in addition to
observing drug tolerance should examine the dose-blood level
relationship and examine simple physiological changes such as
heart rate attenuation and pressor effect both at rest and on
exercise.   Experiments with single and chronic dosages will provide
both pharmacokinetic and pharmacodynamic information, the onset
and duration of action being important criteria.   Basic experimental
investigations both in isolated preparation and in intact animals
nowadays provide invaluable information on the electrophysiological
characteristics of new antiarrhythmic drugs.   These are of paramount importance in planning appropriate investigations in the
clinical situation so that tne degree of activity in tne human can
be evaluated without undue risk.   Intracardiac electrophysiological
investigation, by examining the refractory and conductive properties
of cardiac conducting tissues before and after the drug, can
characterize the degree of beta blockade and answer the recurring
question of a membrane stabilising action at clinical doses.   The
onset and duration of action can be incorporated into the triangular
relationship of dose, plasma levels and electrophysiological activity.
These early studies will of course delineate the effect of the beta
blocker on the normal conduction system providing the basis for its
proposed antiarrhythmic spectrum.   The predominant effect is a
depression of AV nodal conduction, the changes in sinus node
recovery time, and atrial and ventricular effective refractory
periods being small or insignificant.   Further investigation
would therefore aim to assess its role in the treatment of supraventricular arrhytnmia where the AV node provides either the
mechanism of initiation and/or pathway of atrioventricular
conduction.

It would be appropriate at tnis point to establish tne
hemodynamic influence following acute administration, and the

fashion in recent years has been to perform angiocardiographic
studies at the same time as the investigation of the basic human
electrophysiological effects. With the growing interest in iso-
tope studies of left ventricular function, especially radionuclide
angiography, an alternative and equally sensitive method of investigation may become feasible.

Acute antiarrhythmic properties.

With this information protocols can be designed to evaluate
the antiarrhythmic actions of the beta blocker in supraventricular
arrhythmias. Appropriate methods of assessment will vary according
to the nature of the arrhythmia and likewise the method of administration. A comparison with either an agent of the same class which
is known to be successful or an effective drug of an alternative
class is desirable to provide a control. Precise and defined end
points to these investigations are also necessary.

Atrioventricular re-entry tachycardia has provided an ideal
substrate for the investigation of antiarrhythmic drugs because of
the classic mechanisms involved and the reliability of initiation
and termination during intracardiac electrophysiological study.
The investigation into the mechanism of re-entry tachycardia in
suitable patients can be combined with an investigation into the
basic electrophysiological behavior as described in the previous
section. Two aspects of the circus movement can be examined when
an antiarrhythmic drug is given intravenously. Termination
requires only that a sufficiently high level of the drug is present,
sufficient to cause second degree block in one or other limb of
the circuit and is most effectively achieved by rapid bolus
administration. Ideally this electrophysiological effect should
appear promptly and before there is significant hemodynamic det-
erioration in an already compromised cardiovascular state. In
the event that termination does not occur the further hypotensive
effect of the drug will stimulate further sympathetic reflex
activity, (9) an influence that will make the AV node even more
resistant to termination. On the other hand evaluation of the
ability of the drug to protect against the initiation of further
attacks requires that an established blood level is maintained

and thus the ideal regime for investigation might be an intravenous bolus followed by an infusion. Again control of inherent patient variability ought to be made by comparing it to a therapeutic regime known to be effective. Such a comparison requires careful planning to select appropriate dosages and intervals between injections.

The other supraventricular arrhythmia that lends itself to investigation of a new beta blocker is atrial fibrillation, or atrial flutter, though in the context of the acute antiarrhythmic properties one needs to examine these arrhythmias once they are established. Intracardiac electrophysiological investigation plays no part in this evaluation, which is more appropriately made by simple methods of electrocardiographic monitoring. Though it has been observed that these agents may produce termination this is uncommon, especially when atrial fibrillation has been established for any period of time, and thus a slower rate of drug infusion is desirable to examine the degree to which the ventricular response is controlled (10). Again concern over possible adverse hemodynamic effects, with the accompanying cardio-accelerator influence on AV nodal behavior, makes slow drug administration desirable. The nature of this method of investigation perhaps makes it suitable for an open titration study in order to obtain further information on the dose-response relationship.

When atrial fibrillation occurs in patients with sinus node disease it is necessary to consider the influence of beta blockade on sinus node function. A similar question is raised in patients with His-Purkinje disease, always a possibility when treating patients with widespread cardiac pathology. While many studies have observed the effects of beta blockers in patients with normal conduction some reports have commented on their influence when the sinus node is diseased (11) or producing HV prolongation when a sufficiently high blood level is achieved (12). Clarification of the safety of chronic beta blockade in patients with His-Purkinje conduction abnormalities is still required, and specific actions of the various beta blockers in these patients evaluated.

Chronic antiarrhythmic properties.

A better understanding of the pharmacodynamics of antiarrhythmic drugs has led to greater interest in examining their influence once the steady state has been achieved. These studies carry the added benefit that they may predict longterm benefit to the patient with greater accuracy. They will also reflect the influence of active metabolites (13) which may not be present when the evaluation is made after intravenous administration. Repeat, but limited, intracardiac electrophysiological study in patients with AV reentry tachycardia provides a suitable mode for demonstrating whether attacks can still be induced. It overcomes the problem that their natural frequency of spontaneous attacks may be low and offers a more objective assessment than patients' symptoms. There are instances when a definitive end point can be established: for instance retrograde atrioventricular block in a patient with an AV nodal re-entry tachycardia shows that the mechanism has effectively been abolished. An additional advantage of repeat electrophysiological study is the ability to study autonomic influences such as tilt testing in order to predict whether the drug is effective under different physiological conditions. This phase of investigation would also be ideally made part of a comparison with an alternative drug for a random cross-over study in a later protocol. Atrial fibrillation or flutter, whether established or paroxysmal, is ideally suited to the investigation of the study of chronic anti-arrhythmic efficacy. Various methods of assessment may be more or less appropriate depending on the precise nature of the arrhythmia and include ambulatory electrocardiographic monitoring when the arrhythmia is established or there are frequent paroxysms, and has the added benefit that atrial extrasystoles may be frequent enough in the paroxysmal forms to offer a further impression of anti-arrhythmic efficacy. Various forms of telemetry or transtelephonic ECG transmission are available which allow longterm arrhythmia monitoring with less discomfort to the patient. However, the diurnal variation and influence of various physiological situations may not be revealed, a deficiency that can to a certain extent be overcome by exercise testing. In the context of paroxysmal atrial fibrillation or flutter the new technique of recording the His

bundle potential by amplifying and signal-averaging the precordial
ECG may be useful for evaluating the long term effect of AV nodal
depressant drugs. Invasive electrophysiological investigation in
paroxysmal atrial fibrillation or flutter has the distinct disadvantage that the arrhythmia may remain inducible despite the
patient being asymptomatic:it can, however, provide a means of
demonstrating that should the arrhythmia return the ventricular
response will be controlled. Objective analyses in this situation
can be made of changes in the ventricular rate, alterations in the
atrial rate in established atrial flutter and prevention of attacks
when these occur frequently enough for statistical analysis. While
the chosen drug regime should ensure that continuous effective
therapy is maintained throughout 24 hours any possible lag effect
due to too great interspersing of dose administration may be
observed with continuous 24 hour ambulatory ECG monitoring.

Phase 3 antiarrhythmic efficacy.

Phase 3 assessment in AV re-entry tachycardia would ideally
be made in a study allocating the new beta blocker randomly in a
comparison with some known effective agent. The infrequent
occurrence of arrhythmia in many of these patients makes the method
of assessment particularly difficult. Electrophysiological
induction has the disadvantage of being invasive and non-physiological:
the substrate for re-entry may still be present but the initiating
factor (eg. atrial extrasystoles occurring in the initiation zone)
may have been abolished. Ambulatory electrocardiographic monitoring
may be inappropriate when attacks occur infrequently. The various
forms of telemetry can cover greater periods of time but require
a greater degree of patient co-operation. Diaries lack the
objectivity of these other methods.

A final protocol for which patients with atrial fibrillation
would ideally be suited is a random non-placebo controlled
comparative study with close monitoring of plasma levels in order
to evaluate the problems of toxicity and side-effects.

148

REFERENCES.

1. Ahlquist RP. 1949. A study of adrenotropic receptors.
   Am. J. Physiol, 153: 586.

2. Sutherland EW, Robinson GA, Butcher RW. 1968. Some aspects
   of the biological role of adenosine 3'5' monophosphate (cyclic
   AMP). Circulation, 37: 279.

3. Smithen CS, Balcon R, Sowton E. 1971. Use of bundle of His
   potentials to assess changes in atrioventricular conduction
   produced by a series of beta-adrenergic blocking agents.
   Br. Heart J. 33: 955.

4. Zipes DP, Mendez C. 1973. Action of manganese ions and
   tetrodotoxin on atrioventricular nodal transmembrane potentials
   in isolated rabbit hearts. Circulation Res. 32: 447.

5. Schneider JA, Sperelakis N. 1974. The demonstration of energy
   dependence of the isoproterenol-induced transcellular ca^{2+}
   current in isolated perfused guinea pig hearts. An explanation
   of mechanical failure of ischaemic myocardium. J. Surg. Res.
   16: 389.

6. Singh BN, Vaughan Williams EM. 1976. A third class of antiarrhythmic action. Effects on atrial and ventricular intracellular potentials, and other pharmacological actions on
   cardiac muscle, of MJ 1999 and AH 3474. Brit. J. Pharmacol.
   39: 675.

7. Edvardsson N, Olsson B. 1981. Effects of acute and chronic
   beta-receptor blockade on ventricular repolarisation in man.
   Brit. Heart J. 45: 628.

8. Härtel G, Hartikainen M. 1976. Comparison of verapamil and
   practolol in paroxysmal supraventricular tachycardia. Eur.
   J. Cardiol. 4: 87.

9. Curry PVL, Rowland E, Fox KM, Krikler DM. 1978. The relationship between posture, blood pressure and electrophysiological
   properties in patients with paroxysmal supraventricular tachycardia. Arch. Mal. Coeur. 71: 293.

10. Singh BN, Jewitt DE. 1974. Beta-adrenergic blocking drugs in
    cardiac arrhythmias. Drugs. 7: 426.

11. Strauss HC et al. 1976. Electrophysiologic effects of propranolol
    on sinus node function in patients with sinus node dysfunction.
    Circulation, 54: 452.

12. Mason JW, Winkle RA, Meffin PJ, Harrison DC. 1978.
    Electrophysiological effects of acebutolol. Brit. Heart.
    J. 40: 35.

13. Cleveland CR, Shand DG. 1972. Effect of route of administration on the relationship between beta-adrenergic blockade and plasma propranolol level. Clin. Pharmac. Ther. 13: 181.

HOW TO DEFINE BETA-BLOCKER USEFULNESS IN HYPERTENSION, ANGINA AND ARRHYTHMIAS: AN OVERVIEW

Eric L. Michelson, M.D.

Beta-blocking drugs have multiple direct and indirect effects on cardiovascular function. Competitive blockade of beta-adrenergic receptors influences heart rate, contractility, stroke volume, MVO_2, vascular tone, renin release, blood pressure, the oxy-hemaglobin dissociation curve, platelet function and even calcium fluxes. Accordingly, beta-blockers have been used successfully as both primary and adjunctive therapy to manage a wide spectrum of cardiovascular disorders including hypertension, angina and arrhythmias. In addition, there has been considerable interest in the potential of beta-blockers to reduce both morbidity (e.g., myocardial reinfarction) and mortality (particularly sudden death) in patients with previous myocardial infarctions. In this session of the Symposium, Drs. Kaplan, Epstein, Morganroth and Rowland detail how to define beta-blocker usefulness in hypertension, angina and arrhythmias, respectively.

Hypertension

The results of recent epidemiological studies provide strong evidence that blood pressure should be controlled at the lowest level compatible with patient acceptance and lack of adverse effects. Multiple pathophysiologic hypertensive mechanisms have been identified which are apparently operative to varying degrees in different subsets of hypertensive patients. Unfortunately, we remain relatively naive in our approach to the treatment of individual patients. This is further complicated by our incomplete understanding of the mechanisms of most antihypertensive drugs. For this reason, algorithms have been suggested (e.g., "step-therapy") by which the majority of patients will get effective therapy.

Beta-blockers as a class are now considered the most useful adjunctive therapy by many hypertension "experts" in this country, with thiazides the initial treatment of choice for most patients. This reflects the large number of "volume" responsive patients in the U.S., including the majority of black hypertensives, as well as the convenience of once daily diuretics and the relative expense of beta-blockers. In addition, it is also known that some patients will not respond at all to beta-blockers and a minority of volume responsive patients may even have a "paradoxical" increase in blood pressure. Furthermore, there is concern that hypertensive rebound or "overshoot" may be a more frequent problem with some beta-blockers than with thiazides, particularly since many hypertensives tend to comply only intermittently with their medical regimens.

However, two developments may alter further the usage pattern of beta-blockers in this country, which has already evolved quickly over the last five years. First, the availability of effective well-tolerated beta-blockers with longer half-lives as well as other advantageous, ancillary properties, such as direct vasodilating effects. Second, the availability of ambulatory, long-term blood pressure monitoring devices. Undoubtedly, blood pressures are quite variable throughout the day in many patients. Presumably, these devices should provide a more rational basis for blood pressure control. At present, most antihypertensive regimens are designed on the basis of isolated resting-supine or relaxed-standing blood pressures, usually measured to coincide with the expected time of peak or trough medication effect. Unfortunately, most hypertensives are abnormal not only at rest, but also have greatly exaggerated blood pressure increases in response to both exertion and "stress". As a class of drugs, beta-blockers therefore offer a potential advantage for many patients in that both their static as well as dynamic blood pressure may be more effectively controlled. However, this needs to be evaluated critically for both beta-blockers as well as other therapies. Ideally, blood pressure should be controlled 24 hours a day and the level of control confirmed. At present these recorders are in still in a developmental stage and controlled studies using these devices have been limited. Their potential roll in clinical investigation is addressed by Dr. Norman Kaplan.

Angina

The use of beta-blockers in the treatment of angina pectoris is well established, and the ability of beta-blockers to decrease MVO_2 in patients with obstructive coronary disease is their major mode of efficacy. Although beta-blockers represent a major advance in the treatment of angina, the available agents, either alone or in combination with nitrates, are often not sufficient in a large number of patients. In evidence, the number of coronary artery bypass grafting procedures continues to increase in this country despite the relative costs, immediate morbidity and mortality, and long-term failure of many patients to resume full activities and gainful employment. Consequently, there is continued commitment to the development of additional drugs to prevent both angina as well as the morbid and fatal consequences of ischemic heart disease. These drugs include the calcium channel influx blockers,discussed elsewhere in this Symposium, whose salutory properties include coronary artery vasodilatation.

Alternatively, a variety of beta-blockers are also becoming available which vary in their ancillary properties, including intrinsic sympathomimetic activity, beta receptor antagonist-selectivity, vasodilating, alpha-blocking and other properties. In addition, structural differences may confer other functional properties unique to specific agents. In addition, the treatment of angina and ischemic heart disease may soon include the use of agents affecting vascular tone,(via blockade of calcium channels, inhibition or activation of prostaglandins, kinins, etc.), vascular endothelium, platelet function and/or ventricular diastolic function as either primary or adjunctive therapy.

The design of angina studies is a challenging problem. First, there are multiple subsets of patients with respect to clinical presentations: stable, exertional angina, (with low, moderate or high workloads); new onset exertional angina; previously stable angina, recently changed in pattern; exertional plus rest angina; non-exertional angina; and angina in patients with recent myocardial infarctions. Second, there are anatomical subsets with respect to coronary angiographic findings. Third, there are ethical considerations: Are there subsets of patients for whom surgery rather than medical therapy should be mandated on the basis of either clinical presentation or angiographic findings? Are placebo-controlled studies ethical? Are there alternative study designs to best determine either the potential efficacy or lack of efficacy (or even deleterious effects) of various agents, either alone or in combination. What subjective criteria of response (e.g., via patient diaries) or objective criteria (e.g., via formal exercise testing) are acceptable? These issues are addressed by Dr. Stephen Epstein.

Ventricular Arrhythmias

In various studies, beta-blockers have been shown to reduce significantly the frequency and/or grade of ventricular arrhythmias in 30-70% of patients, although their mechanisms of action have not been fully elucidated. Anti-adrenergic effects presumably predominate, but anti-ischemic effects may also play a role in some patients. In addition, some beta-blockers (e.g., propranolol) have "membrane-stabilizing" and other direct electrophysiologic properties which become evident at high doses. As with other antiarrhythmic drugs, the response to beta-blockers may be quite variable depending on the dosage, and the therapeutic window may be relatively narrow in an individual patient.

In general, beta-blockers have not been found to be adequate primary antiarrhythmic therapy for the prevention of recurrent sustained ventricular tachycardia, except in those patients with catecholamine hypersensitivity, others with long QT syndromes, and some with recurrent ischemia. However, the potential role of beta-blocking drugs in preventing sudden death, particularly in patients with a recent myocardial infarction is an important subject which is considered later in this Symposium. Dr. Morganroth addresses some of these issues in the chapter on "How to Define Beta-Blocker Usefulness in Ventricular Arrhythmias".

Supraventricular Arrhythmias

The management of supraventricular arrhythmias must be considered in the context of several specific rhythm disorders. In general, supraventricular arrhythmias are not life-threatening, but may precipitate pulmonary edema, angina or hypotension in susceptible individuals. Control of the ventricular rate is often sufficient to limit the incapacity of atrial arrhythmias, although conversion to sinus rhythm is preferred when feasible.

Beta-blockers play an important role in decreasing sympathetic tone, thereby decreasing the sinus rate, the frequency of atrial extrasystoles and the rate of AV nodal conduction. Thus, they can be effective primary or adjunctive therapy for a variety of paroxysmal and chronic supraventricular arrhythmias with varying mechanisms. They can also be used effectively to increase exercise tolerance in some patients with chronic atrial fibrillation whose rates accelarate too rapidly on digoxin. However, they must be used with caution in patients with the"sick sinus syndrome" manifesting as paroxysmal atrial fibrillation, in patients receiving calcium "antagonists", and in patients with underlying bronchospastic pulmonary disease. Dr. Rowland discusses some of these considerations in the chapter on "How to Define Beta-Blocker Usefulness in Supraventricular Arrhythmias". A Panel and Discussion follow this presentation.

Acknowledgment

The assistance of Ann Hagan with manuscript preparation is gratefully acknowledged. Dr. Michelson is recipient of Clinical Investigatorship Award 5 K08 HL00709-02 from the NHLBI, NIH, Bethesda, Maryland.

GENERAL GROUP DISCUSSION - How to Define Beta-Blocker Usefulness In:

Moderator: Dr. Eric Michelson

Dr. Morganroth: I will take the liberty to ask Dr. Epstein a question. Is it practical to do controlled anginal studies in light of the apparent free use of coronary surgery? The lay population particularly seems to be aware of the alternatives to therapy that you use a proper consent that informs them of these proper alternatives to justify placebo outpatient trials, to justify experimental beta blocker or other type of antianginal agents, calcium channel blockers in light of the alternatives. Do you think these studies are actually practical to do in the 1980's?

Dr. Epstein: Yes, I think so. The major problem that you allude to is the availability of the coronary bypass operation; and I think that does pose an alternative form of therapy which, if the patient is a candidate, would preclude for that particular patient inclusion in a protocol. Let's just look at the issue for a moment. The indications for a coronary bypass operation that everyone would agree on would be the patient who already is a therapeutic failure on medical management, but that leaves patients who are under some type of control. Let's just stop at that point. If you do coronary angiography, some of those patients will have left main disease and triple-vessel disease; and probably most people would want to operate on such patients because they are fearful that sudden death may come into play. And one could argue that delay over several weeks or months conceivably in the isolated patient may have a deleterious impact. That is, the patient may die while he is in a protocol. There are a fair number of patients who have single or double-vessel disease, in which case it has not been demonstrated that operation prolongs life. I think that those individuals, ethically speaking, would be ideal candidates for additional trials of pharmacologic therapy to see if their symptoms could be controlled. A not insubstantial number of patients are beginning to come back to us, as cardiologists, who have already had their bypass operation; either patients in whom all of the grafts are closed, or patients who have developed progressive disease in their other native coronary vessels, and are at the threshold for re-operation. I think those patients would be excellent candidates for pharmacologic therapy and new drugs to see if their symptoms could be effectively controlled.

Dr. Kostis: I have a question to Dr. Kaplan and Dr. Epstein. Dr. Kaplan told us that propranolol and others with short half-lives may be used once daily in the treatment of hypertension. The question is what were the blood levels when they were still effective; were they zero or were they detectable? If it was zero, what was the mechanism? For Dr. Epstein, can we use beta blockers with short half-lives in the treatment of angina once a day or twice a day? Is it effective?

Dr. Kaplan: I can't give you the exact levels; but first of all, with higher doses there are obviously much higher blood levels at the peak effects and it does take a good deal longer, than say a half-life of propranolol of two hours, for it to reach a very low level; but I think it should be obvious that it is not in the plasma that these drugs are doing their thing, that they are working within the brain, within receptors in various and sundry places; and I don't think that depending upon blood levels is really going to give us the answers that we want to know. Therefore, monitoring the end result seems to be much more logical.

Dr. Michelson: This is a very important issue. Presumably, under steady state conditions, blood levels do reflect something. The problem is that we are talking about tissue effects of drugs, and this problem is not just a problem in angina or hypertension; it is also the problem that has been alluded to here in looking at disparities of antiarrhythmic effects and dosages given. It is a problem in every field. It is definitely a cardiovascular problem; it is not just limited to one manifestation of cardiovascular disease. Tissue levels and plasma levels may or may not mean something depending upon how the drug is given; it depends upon whether you are in steady state and upon whether or not there are active metabolites. We know there are many drugs that are going to be very tissue active whether or not we detect anything in the blood stream; and, therefore, this is a very complex issue. I don't think we can address here all the pharmacologic aspects. But, perhaps, Dr. Woosley or one of the Vanderbilt group would like to address some aspect of that.

Dr. Epstein: I was just going to say I can't answer the second part of that question, but with respect to the antianginal effects of beta blocking agents and those short half-lives, is a single dose effective? We have not done such studies. I think Dr. Harrison and his group have actually studied that. Don, I think, could shed some light on that issue.

Dr. Harrison: We showed effects for propranolol in angina in terms of physiologic effects going out to about 12 hours, but not after that; whereas, with drugs with longer half-lives we were able to show persistent effects on heart rate responses in double product going out to 24 hours. In hypertension, it is very clear, as Dr. Kaplan pointed out, that even though you may have essentially zero blood levels, you still may have persistent antihypertensive effects; and I don't think anyone knows the mechanisms of that and whether it goes back to resetting of the baro-receptor mechanisms, because this doesn't occur with acute therapy; this occurs with chronic therapy over some period of time. I don't think anyone knows the mechanism for that.

Dr. Epstein: Did you look in your study at the antianginal duration of these drugs or just the physiologic effects? In other words does the antianginal effect of propranolol persist for 12 hours?

Dr. Harrison: In our original crossover study with multi-dose levels, we did find that there was reduction in angina out to about 12 hours as well. It went along with the physiologic effect. It wasn't a perfect correlation but nearly so.

Dr. Temple: Dr. Kaplan, do you think that instead of trying to get blood pressures throughout the day, which could be very difficult, you could sort of surround the problem by measuring them at the approximate peak of the blood level and then just prior to dosing which is a somewhat simpler thing to do.

Dr. Kaplan: I maybe overstated the need for total ambulatory 24 hours around the clock monitoring every 5 minutes. I don't think that is ever going to be necessary or practical. But the idea of looking for duration I really think is two separate issues. One is how long do these drugs last, and I think that can really only be determined by getting repeated measurements for long periods of time. As far as knowing if, say a b.i.d. schedule, if that is what everybody decides to try is effective, I agree, one at say 2 hours if Inderal was the drug to be chosen and another one at the end of a 12-hour period before the next dosing would be given—that would probably serve the purpose very well.

Dr. Michelson: Dr. Temple, let me ask you, based upon what you have seen would you accept the results of ambulatory blood pressure monitoring if that were presented to F.D.A., and someone had designed a study and used that as their means of showing that they had duration of effect.

Dr. Temple: Well I think you have to show that the group does its ambulatory blood pressure measuring well. What we like to see is an in-clinic measurement just before the next dose which is a pretty good way of showing in comparison with placebo or another drug group at the same time that you have persistent effect. For single daily dosing it is not that hard, because you can give the dose at a time such that it is convenient to come to the clinic before the dose. If the dosing is twice a day, it could get harder.

Dr. Morganroth: For accurate efficacy, wouldn't you also want to see by long-term monitoring whether environmental phenomena could change blood pressure on a medication? Wouldn't this be an important aspect of efficacy in addition to a single spot morning reading?

Dr. Temple: I have no information about that. How do we know that antihypertensive therapy prolongs life? We have data on thiazides and reserpine and whatsoever has been used in the HDFP, but its mostly thiazides, reserpine and maybe a little propranolol; and I don't think one can say whether it is important to lower the blood pressure. The evidence that we have is that if the blood pressure is lowered at the time to come to clinic that is good. We don't know what your night-time blood pressure is and so forth.

Dr. Michelson: Cardiovascular physiologists like objective endpoints. For example, an exercise test is very nice because it gives you a double product, and it may be that certain drugs such as beta blockers are very effective in blunting the exaggerated response many hypertensives have to certain types of activitites; and it may be that beta blockers will turn out to be very effective drugs based on that type of testing. Perhaps Dr. Kaplan could address this as well as Dr. Temple. Is there a role for exercise testing for more formal stress-related blood pressure measurements in chronic blood pressure management? Are you satisfied with a recumbant and a relaxed standing blood pressure taken times 3, five minutes apart, five minutes before the next dose?

Dr. Temple: That is a good question. I would just emphasize again, that all of our information comes from measurements made under certain conditions so that it is hard to answer the question you ask. Along the same lines, I remember a presentation a while back of, I think, single daily dosing acebutolol which, when compared to some other drug, the nocturnal control was not as good with acebutolol as it was something else, but the investigator said that it didn't really matter because the pressure was below 120/80. Nobody was measuring blood pressure at night in any studies in which a drug therapy has been shown to lower mortality, and the drugs that were used were very long acting so there is every reason to think that blood pressure was low all the time.

Dr. Michelson: Right, but considering the usual diurnal curves, the kind that Dr. Kaplan has demonstrated so well here using the 24-hour ambulatory monitors, I would not want to use a 1 A.M. pre-dosing blood pressure as my baseline. It might make a difference when that one daily dose was give.

Dr. Kaplan: Well, surely it might. What we obviously don't know, we have very little inferential evidence, mainly from Sokoloff's papers some years ago, that you may be better off if your ambulatory blood pressure is lower throughout the 24 hours than if only your casual blood pressure is lowered. But we really don't have the data that would be mandatory to make the assessment as to whether full 24-hour control is essential or maybe, if your blood pressure is lower for the next 6 or 8 hours, that is enough after you have taken a medication. Another point, you mention about exercise. I think we may make it impossible to ever say a drug works if we put so many stringent requirements on it that it has to keep the blood pressure down under all circumstances. I mean, then you would get yourself into sort of a vicious cycle to say that you never control all exercise or stress or other kinds of blood pressure responses. Again, maybe that is important for the long haul as far as morbidity and mortality is concerned; but I think that may be asking to much.

Dr. Michelson: It does strike me that as we get closer to being more objective we are getting closer to counting PVC's and arrhythmias and that analogy with its advantages and disadvantages, unfortunately.

Dr. Epstein: I think I can't agree more strongly with what Dr. Temple and Dr. Kaplan said. I think you get into a very dangerous situation. You are lucky and you have data showing that controlling blood pressure in certain subgroups of patients reduces mortality and those data were obtained under certain specific conditions, under resting conditions in the clinic and so on. You could develop a drug like propranolol or a drug that doesn't control resting blood pressure very well but it controls the exercise response beautifully. To say that drug should be approved in the control of hypertension because you have a sophisticated measurement of control is doing a disservice to the key data that we have. We know that if you lower blood pressure under specific circumstances in specific subgroups that it prolongs life and until you can come up with data showing that you can prolong life if you just knock the top off the exercise pressure, or if you lower sleeping blood pressure, you just don't have those data. The other thing is if you strive to lower blood pressure as Dr. Kaplan indicated throughout the 24 hours because you think empirically it might be good, just think of the side effects you are going to get into giving higher doses. Until someone shows that it is necessary, I think that you should put yourself in the position of forcing physicians to give such medicines to patients because there is always the issue of side effects.

Dr. Temple: Actually, I would argue that you should probably try for 24-hour control, because in all probability in the one study that showed reduction in mortality, you had it. You are dealing with the longest acting antihypertensive drug known, reserpine, principally along with a diuretic given several times a day at the time. You almost surely did have 24-hour control in those people. To me, the best presumption is that is what you need; and it is someone else's job to show that you don't. So that assessing control 24 hours seem crucial to me.

Dr. Michelson: You would accept the 24-hour ambulatory monitor as data, then.

Dr. Temple: Evidence of 24-hour control is fine.

Dr. Scriabine: I would like to ask Dr. Epstein and also members of the F.D.A. staff present here whether the type of exercise tolerance data which you described to us are acceptable evidence of antianginal activity of a drug for regulatory agencies; and if it is not, what role, if any, such studies would play in the decision to approve or not approve the drug by F.D.A.?

Dr. Epstein: I defer to the F.D.A. As an investigator, its quite clear to me that if you have a well-designed study looking at exercise capacity and you show that a given drug improves exercise capacity then you have demonstrated efficacy at least for the short-term effect and that I think would go into the equation that would be used to decide whether or not the drug is effective and safe; and not being part of the F.D.A. process, I would think that would be an important bit of evidence demonstrating that the drug is effective.

166

Dr. Temple: We've never had to face the issue, I should tell you because we have always had both evidence of reduction in angina attacks in one or more studies and improved exercise tolerance. I think everybody's bias is that exercise tolerance is a fair measure of exercise tolerance in regular life and that if it becomes impossible or difficult to find people with enough angina attacks to show a reduction, we probably would accept that data alone. Obviously, in vasospastic angina you really have to resort to angina attack rate since we're not at the point quite yet of accepting ergonovine testing; maybe we should be, and you don't have exercise testing to help you probably.

Dr. Epstein: I would like to make clear, in case I was misinterpreted, when I put the two protocols up, that is, the traditional long-term, randomized, crossover study, I was not belittling that. I think that is probably the most effective way, the most definitive way, to get at the antianginal properties of a drug. I merely indicated, by the contrast, that there are other ways to make it so you could look at fewer number of patients over a shorter duration of time that might be more practical in this day and age to determine if a given drug had some antianginal effectiveness. But certainly, the traditional way of looking at it would be very important; and if you had both, it would make the case even stronger.

Dr. Temple: Let me add that I think some evidence of persisting effect, say beyond two days, is important. There are clearly drugs around that have a change in their effect after a short early phase.

Dr. Sami: I still would like to pin Dr. Epstein down on the question of crossover design with respect to the washout periods necessary when comparing two beta blockers. I think there are some data that show with some beta blockers, there is a washout effect as long as eight days after stopping chronic oral dosing of a drug;

and I don't know how you can reconcile this with your short 14-day scheme for comparing two drugs.

Dr. Epstein: I think that is a very good point. I didn't mean, and I think I said, that when I put that slide up that this is the way every antianginal drug has to be tested. Clearly, depending on the specific characteristics, the pharmacodynamics of each drug, you are going to have to modify that protocol. If you take a drug with an extraordinarily long half-life, then you are going to have to adjust the protocol. Knowledge of the pharmacodynamics of the agent is essential in designing an efficient, concise protocol; and there may be some drugs that it is going to take a very long time to insure that you have got a proper washout period.

Dr. Sami: I don't think you can even define that with half-life because there are drugs like pindolol with a very short half-life and a very long action after the half-life. So even the half-life is not helpful. I think in designing studies you really have to allow for enough safety time for washout before you test your other drug.

Dr. Epstein: I think you are right. I think what you have to do really is see what the physiologic effects of the duration of effects are and then design your protocol around that. You are absolutely right.

Dr. Fitzgerald: I'd like to address some comment to the relationship between blood level and response in angina on the one hand and hypertension on the other. I think you can get some illumination about the relationship between beta blockade and the hypotensive response by examining in detail the onset and the offset of effect. I have done studies with intravenous atenolol and interestingly you get an immediate onset of beta blockade in terms of the fall in systolic pressure and heart rate. And if you watch them over six hours, the heart rate and the systolic pressure come back. Between four and five hours the diastolic pressure begins to fall and it stays down for 24 hours after a single intravenous dose. Clearly you can interpret these results as saying there's an adaptive response and leave it at that, as everybody else doesn't quite know what the adaptive response is. And then if you look at patients when you stop their oral atenolol and if you look at the rate of return of pressure and the rate of return of heart rate, you will find that the heart rate will return very nearly towards normal, about 36 hours, but the blood pressure will perhaps take up to five days. So I think it is very important to separate the discussion of blood level in relation to hypotensive response from blood level in relationship to antianginal response; and I have no doubt at all, but Dr. Epstein may correct me, that you need persisting beta blockade for an antianginal effect and that as the beta blockade wears off, the antianginal effect wears off, so that would be my comment. I would, if I may, ask Dr. Epstein for a little more detail on his verapamil study which I found very interesting in terms of the mode of action. As I recollect, there was a recent paper in the British Medical Journal comparing propranolol and verapamil in adequate doses, which is only just beginning to happen now; and as I recollect, verapamil had relatively little effect on heart rate response to exercise in this study. It lowered pressure a little bit; it had much less effect on ST segments than did propranolol, but it had a much more profound effect on the duration of exercise to pain. I wonder if he noticed any differences between propranolol and verapamil in his particular study in relationship to those four particular parameters. That is to say ST segment change, time-to-pain, heart rate and blood pressure.

Dr. Epstein: That is an interesting question. We did notice differences. For example, the double product at onset of angina and also at the new exercise intensity achieved. Clearly propranolol has a profound effect on double product. It lowers exercising heart rate and to some extent exercising blood pressure and presumably a major portion, not all, but a major portion of the beneficial effect of propranolol on the increase in exercise capacity is lowering the work demands of the myocardium. Now verapamil, using our particular subgroup of patients who were refractory clinically to propranolol, had a better effect on exercise capacity than propranolol. Despite that, however, its effects on double product were much less. There was a minor effect on heart rate and a minor effect on blood pressure. So even though exercise capacity was considerably better than on propranolol, the effect on double product was much less; so clearly there is another mechanism operative in verapamil, not just the one on at least that parameter of myocardial oxygen demands. Now we have done, and some other people have done, studies showing that verapamil does have an effect on diastolic filling, perhaps compliance, and it may be that the effect that it probably has on the rate of myocardial relaxation, which is impaired in the majority of patients with coronary artery disease, may be another mechanism operative and as is being speculated about, presently. Also, there are dynamic changes that occur even in diseased vessels which may be amenable to a vasodilator like verapamil, and it is possible that this is yet another mechanism whereby verapamil may produce a beneficial effect.

Dr. Wenger: I would like to make a few statements about the relationship of dose to duration of effect because it seemed to be somewhat muddled, and I don't see any pharmacologist leaping up to support anything; so I thought I would. The half-life is not necessarily dose dependent, obviously; but one would expect that the duration of effect is dose dependent in a drug that has a half-life that is not dose dependent. So the half-time of effect is expected to be dose dependent and that can be mathematically modeled, so that is one aspect of this question. This is really a comment that relates to all drugs anyway. A second factor would be the interaction, the kinetics between the site of action and the plasma drug pools, and that would have an effect on the duration of effect. And finally, very importantly, there are some exceptions that don't let the mathematical work unless you include them and that would involve the parameter you are measuring, which may have its own duration of return; and apparently, that seems to be so in hypertension. There are a variety of factors involved here in the duration of effect, many of which can't be modeled really. The half-life is important; and for example, if you use a beta I selective drug in a patient who has asthma and you want to get a long duration of effect, but that drug has a short half-life, you have to use a much larger dose of the drug to get the long duration of effect and then you lose a certain amount of the beta I selectivity. So I don't think that the half-life is relevant in these drugs, depending on what you are looking for. It's one piece of a lot of different pieces in the picture.

Dr. Michelson: It is much more dynamic than even that. Unfortunately, these drugs affect the system and the system is then affecting the drugs differently than it would have had it not seen the drug. It becomes very complex. As a pharmacologist yourself, do you have a suggestion to make to us?

Dr. Wenger: No, I'm going to call myself a cardiologist and pass to Ray Woosley.

Dr. Woosley: I'm really glad I'm here to defend pharmacology. I don't know the name of the pharmacologist who said that drugs can only work for one half-life, but let's find out who it is and stomp him out and realize the the duration of acton, as Dr. Wenger just pointed out very nicely, is the bottom line. Pharmacokinetic studies, as he also said though, are very important in new drug development; and I don't want people to fail to realize at some phase in a drug's development, even if it is an anti-hypertensive, where the clinical input is more important, that there is an awful lot that can be learned from pharmacokinetic studies. You can prevent the undue accumulation of drug by knowing its half-life, its clearance; you can use that to make dosage adjustments in disease states. Also, by finding a discrepancy between blood level and effect, you can, perhaps, identify potentially active metabolites. So pharmacokinetics play a major role in drug development. I think we all realize this, but when they are taken out of context and people say that you have to measure blood levels and you can't do clinical monitoring, I think they are overstating the situation and actually misinterpreting the pharmacokinetic data.

Dr. Michelson: Let me ask this. Based on what we have heard in this session about the beta blockers, we realize that there are differences in certain ancillary properties and certain differences especially in pharmacokinetic and dynamic properties. However, once it has been demonstrated that a beta blocker has a certain effect, for example, whether it is on migraines or antihypertensive, the point that Dr. Morganroth brought up in the discussion of ventricular arrhythmias, once it has been identified, what the class does. Is there enough similarity so that once someone has proven that the drug is safe, and still enjoys the class properties, should that drug then have an easy access to the market place?

Dr. Woosley: My advice is no. I think that the price that you are going to pay by doing that is missing a lot of drug actions that you would pick up by doing controlled systematic trials. I think you may put a lot of other drugs on the market that may have toxicities we don't know about, may have other effects that you are going to miss by not having systematic trials. So it is my bias that you should not give blanket approval for any new indication just because a drug is a beta blocker. I think there are still plenty of questions open about these other actions that need to be answered.

Dr. Michelson: Let me ask Dr. Morganroth. What do you think. You made that statement; are you going to ask for a "class action suit" here?

Dr. Morganroth: I am puzzled by the problem, because on the one hand, I agree with what Ray Woosley said, that one has to be careful about giving any blanket approvals for any reason, just from a scientific and a medical-legal point of view. On the other hand, to do the studies repetitively, because of their high cost and delay, in agents that are quite similar, there really is no clear scientific pharmacologic reason that; for example, atenolol could not be used in arrhythmias today with far less number of studies in depth than one had to do in order to get propranolol aproved. I think this is a complex problem because one has to consider the cost and benefit to the public compared to what one would learn scientifically from doing an extensive degree of studies. I would be curious to see what Dr. Temple's reaction to this dilemma is.

Dr. Michelson: There are two aspects to this. One is a drug which is being newly developed and not approved for any indication for which there has not been a sense of post-marketing experience, and then there is the drug that is already approved for one indication but there is every reason to believe that it should have all the other beta blocking properties. It could then be marketed with much less expensive and detailed studies for an additional indication; and the advantage might be, for example, that the drug might be suitable to once-a-day dosing as opposed to four times a day.

Dr. Morganroth: It is to that latter group that my comments are really addressed.

<u>Dr. Temple</u>: I was planning to talk about that question to some extent this afternoon, so I don't want to say too much. I assume there wouldn't be a total amount of safety data available. You are just wondering whether you should run through each indication. I'll explain it more later. There are enough surprises that come along in the course of looking at what happens when a study is actually done, that my own bias is that we are probably not ready to that. I will try to illustrate that a little bit in a presentation later in the Symposium. It may well be that most of the time you would be right. I am almost certain of that if you assume that a well-documented beta blocker was going to lower blood pressure; but every once in a while I think you probably would be wrong, or you would fail to find out something important like one drug is not as good as another or does something surprising or had some funny interaction; and those things are worth finding out, I think.

<u>Dr. Epstein</u>: I would just like to elaborate. I don't know what you are going to say later on, but I have rather strong feelings about that because we have already seen this morning that each one of these beta blockers has very different effects. They metabolize differently, they have different lipid versus water solubility, some have membrane actions, and some have intrinsic stimulating activities. Take the calcium antagonists. I mean using calcium antagonists as a group, each one has very different effects, and I don't think if verapamil was shown to increase survival in a given situation, I don't think you would be justified in saying that diltiazem and nifedipine would. I think the beta blockers are analogous. It would be nice if you could generalize; but these drugs have so many actions that we know differ, and we have been talking this morning about actions that we don't know anything about, so I think it is dangerous to extrapolate from the beneficial effects of one drug, and then say let's put everybody on another drug, because it is probably the same thing. It may not be dangerous in one sense, but you may be

depriving the individual of a well-demonstrated beneficial effect of another drug. I would feel rather strongly that that type of class decision is not appropriate.

Dr. Michelson: We should appreciate, though, that in the real world clinicians do just that. When beta blockers are released, they pick their indications.

Dr. Epstein: But that doesn't make it right.

Dr Michelson: Of course not, but we should be aware of the responsibility we have then when a drug is released.

Dr. Furberg: I want to bring up a methodological issue. Dr. Epstein was talking about subgrouping and that makes me a little bit nervous, because subgrouping can be good and it can be bad. I think the good thing is that it is intellectually very stimulating, and it is very good to develop new hypotheses to test in new trials; but you shouldn't forget that subgrouping can be used to identify subgroups where the drug has no effect or has a negative effect or is harmful. The danger is if we use the information in the subgroups, the post hoc subgroups, to document the efficacy of the intervention of that subgroup. In particular in a condition like angina pectoris, as you pointed out, placebo has been documented to be efficacious where the heterogeneity has been enormous; and we have a number of known and probably unknown cofounders. So what I am saying, I guess, is in some ways subgrouping is just the first of two steps. We ought to do it to define subgroups. We shouldn't forget that the important step is the next one, where we in a prospective trial study the efficacy of intervention in that particular subgroup. That is the only way to document subgroup.

Dr. Epstein: I am glad you brought that up. Obviously, in the short time available to me I couldn't go into that in detail; but that is a point that deserves re-emphasis. What I was suggesting is that we have to be aware of the subgroups-- that we should have our eyes open and perhaps identify those patients who may look like they are behaving favorably, but that, as you have indicated quite properly, does not mean that they responded favorably to the drug, but to use that information to identify your subgroup of patients, who then undergo a proper study to see if they, in fact, do respond in a favorable way. You are absolutely right about that.

Dr. Wood: I would like to endorse the comments that Dr. Woosley made earlier and to extrapolate them just a little bit further. First of all, when we are trying to relate concentration to effect, I think all pharmacologists believe that there must be some relationship between concentration and effect. The problem is when we are looking at the treatment of high blood pressure, we don't know first of all where we should be measuring the concentration; and, secondly, we don't even know what the effect is we should be looking at. We are measuring the reduction in blood pressure, which is a composite result of who knows what, and a number of different effects which may be exerted at a number of different sites. In taking that point a little further, our group and others have shown that changes in receptor density themselves can be produced by these drugs, such that the administration of beta blockers may increase receptor density; and this may be true for other drugs, such as alpha blockers and so on. There has been a suggestion that a beta blocker with intrinsic sympathetic activity may have different effects on receptor density. So it is probably not fair to imagine that necessarily we are going to find a simple relationship to the plasma concentration effect. Not only are we looking at the effect of the drug, but we are looking at the secondary effects of the drugs on the receptors, such that if you change receptor density, then suddenly remove the drug, you are looking at the half-time for changes to return to normal in receptor density. So there are very complex inter-relationships there that have to be taken into account before we make the simplistic relationship between the plasma concentration and effect, particulary in hypertension, I think.

Dr. Michelson: Yes, absolutely. this interaction I am sure exists, and in angina and probably arrhythmias as well. Host-drug interaction has been alluded to a couple times, but I want to bring this point up again in terms of acute drug testing; we have not spoken too much about that aspect of things in terms of arrhythmias, and we have not yet spoken about supraventricular arrhythmias. As an investigator who does clinical electrophysiologic studies, the limitations of these studies are most elegantly seen in the setting of studies of patients with paroxysmal supraventricular arrhythmias, because autonomic tone is such an important factor. For example, in a patient who is recumbant, quiet, supine in a cath lab in whom you perform a study, especially with a drug which mediates its effects in large part through its effects on autonomic tone, such as a blocker, it may be an excellent drug on the table; and the patient gets off the table and two minutes later is in the same arrhythmia which you indicated by your study the patient was now protected from. Dr. Rowland, would like to comment on that?

Dr. Rowland: Our experience is probably more appropriate to verapamil which we have had a great deal of experience with in supraventricular tachycardias, where we have been very interested in how much you can counteract the influence of verapamil on AV nodal conduction by the simple process of tilting patients up. We have done a limited amount of work with beta blockers and the same thing appears to be true, that if you try to give a drug to terminate their reentry tachycardia in a postion of head up tilt, even a small degree, the drug is far less successful than if you give it in a supine position. That doesn't answer the question. The far more important question is, if the drug works intravenously, does it work automatically when given orally. I alluded to the problem that the mechanism of termination of tachycardia can be different from the mechanism of prevention, and that is why I tried to elaborate on this point that we need to have ways of assessing the antiarrhythmic efficacy in the chronic situation. Probably it may not even include electrophysiologic retesting for the reasons that Dr. Michelson has referred to. Although we can simulate gross changes in autonomic balance, withdrawal of parasympathetic tone and increase in sympathetic tone, we probably can't mimic all the changes the patient will have over 24 hours from day-to-day. It is only by ambulatory monitoring, telemetry and diaries that we are going to be able to answer that question.

Dr. Michelson: I would like to make a plea though, to those of you who are entertaining studies of new antiarrhythmic agents. Although I think there is very valuable information to be gained about these drugs, studying them in the electrophysiologic cath lab, you should not rely only on the results of acute electrophysiologic testing. It must be complemented by retesting during ambulatory oral dosing under chronic maintenance conditions. You should not just depend on acute drug testing, and it should be complemented by other clinical parameters. It should not be just an end in itself at this point.

Dr. Rowland: I didn't mean to decry the electrophysiological retesting, because I think it can tell us very important questions about the way in which the tachycardia may be terminated and the way in which you can protect against it. But I think so far, a lot of the electrophysiological retesting that is being done has already been done too early after chronic administration; and we need to wait, for instance, probably with a beta blocker, for two to three weeks to see the sort of morphometric and electrophysiologic changes that are probably very important to the prevention of both supraventricular and ventricular arrhythmias.

Dr. Michelson: And with drugs like amiodorone, it may not ever be appropriate to evaluate; and it probably takes two-to-five months before you can retest the patient on oral therapy, and maybe never.

Dr. Goldstein: I would like to direct a question to Dr. Morganroth. You talked about the frequency of PVC's as an indicator. I wonder if you would like to comment about complexity of PVC's which in many epidemiologic studies have been the strongest predictor, exclusive of PVC frequency. How do you deal with that question in a trial?

Dr. Morganroth: I think that there is no question that complex arrhythmias are in my mind more important than simple ventricular arrhythmias in terms of the potential endpoint of sudden cardiac death. I think this is reasonably well documented now, not only in the post infarction group from the Ruberman study, but also from Moss' data, which did show a difference between simple PVC's and complex PVC's. A number of studies have clearly demonstrated that it is only the complex ventricular arrhythmias that seem to correlate with sudden cardiac death. Thus, there is no question that complex arrhythmias are important. How to deal with that form from a methodologic statistical point of view is difficult because these seem to be more random as an event. A high degree of reduction as a minimum is usually what has been accepted in most of the studies that have been launched to date. My only bias is that I am most comfortable with a drug that eliminates the complex arrhythmias entirely, or almost entirely. I would, in fact, from a statistical point of view like to see total complex arrhythmia reduction. I think we have antiarrhythmic drugs now than can do that. In terms of defining whether or not such reduction actually prevents sudden death of course is the major issue.

Dr. Epstein: But don't your statistics change dramatically because of the increased random nature of the complex event; a 75% reduction may not be statistically significant. I know in our experience with hypertrophic cardiomyopathy it is not unusual to see ventricular tachycardia on one day, not on another, and present on a third day. What does it do to your statistics?

Dr. Morganroth: We have actually looked at that and published that in Circulation. It turns out that from the ANOVA analysis of variance model we used, slightly less reduction was required than for simple PVC's. I have not yet really understood why that occurred, because my bias would be the same as yours, that you would have to have at least as much reduction, if not more so. Again, I think we are talking a numbers game anyway when we ask how much percent reduction is needed. I think for pharmacologic effect for simple PVC's it is 75%, if you will, for complex PVC's. It is probably at least that; and, preferably, I would like to see for sudden death trials the total abolishment of complex arrhythmias, eliminating arrhythmias. We are trying to prevent sudden death, so we should try to eliminate arrhythmias in clinical studies.

Dr. Michelson: I know Dr. Kostis wants to say something about the statistical analysis of complex arrhythmias.

Dr. Kostis: I don't even have to ask the question.

Dr. Michelson: He is going to tell you that it is very difficult to analyze the frequency of complex PVC's and depending upon what method you use, it could require less or more than a 65% reduction to show statistically significant drug effect, because the analysis is non-parametric.

Dr. Kostis: You have non-parametric methods, and you are using methods assuming normal distribution.

Dr. Morganroth: I wish such methods existed.

Dr. Michelson: The methods that we used were completely wrong; but they were the only methods available. That is the problem.

Dr. Wenger: I would like to comment on the same topic. Most of the studies that have looked at complex PVC's don't look at the frequency separately, so that you are looking at frequency as well as complexity. There is a paper I believe that Dr. Bigger has published recently in the British Heart Journal that relates to that topic, and I would refer whoever started this off, to read that article as an interesting place to start looking at relationships.

Dr. Levitt: I wanted to comment on that philosophical question about approval of drugs by class, and I think there is a misconception involved. I think that when propranolol did its thing as an antiarrhythmic, antianginal, antihypertensive drug there was a great big clinical fishing expedition going on which lasted for years to try to define exactly what the clinical properties of the drug were. When one comes to new beta-adrenergic blocking drugs, one has a distinct advantage; one knows what the target is precisely. One also has a distinct advantage. One knows what the successful study designs were; and I think for those people in the audience who are in industry, I think they would be well advised to be more selective about the targets they are shooting for with drugs of a similar class to other drugs which have proved efficacy. I think one of the problems that industry gets into is they try to get an antiarrhythmic drug approved like quinidine for all possible arrhythmias in all possible circumstances with the implication, of course, of prolonging life. And I think if one is selective in terms of study design and one uses the benefits that one has derived from the previously demonstrated protocols and approved efficacy with the other drugs of the class, I don't think one is dealing with an overwhelming task for the remaining drugs in the class. And if indeed there are differences, then the additional work certainly should be done. If it turns out that the very simple protocols to prove drug A effective don't work with drug B, then drug B certainly should be studied anew; so I really don't think there is an argument. I think drug B can be approved with much less to do than drug A if the proper protocols are used. I think the academic community has an obligation to guide the pharmaceutical industry into the most effective protocols to prove the limited points that need to be proved.

Dr. Morganroth: The definition of "useful" is not clear. If you are giving antiarrhythmic treatment of a chronic VPC patient who doesn't even know they have VPCs who happens to have a cardiomyopathy or is post-infarction, and the reason the physician is giving that agent is to prevent sudden cardiac death, then obviously the endpoint should be sudden cardiac death. How to do such studies is more difficult than to simply find that an agent isn't inert and decreases VPCs. If we jump to the next step and assume that VPC reduction prevents sudden death, an analysis we had for years with hypertension and as we are doing now for cholesterol and sugar etc, then to do so is useful; but we don't have the data to jump to that step. In addition, we have to find out whether we need to eliminate all complex VPC's or just reduce VPC's to prevent sudden death. The only way to answer these questions is to do a sudden death trial using antiarrhythmic therapy.

182

Dr. Michelson: There is nothing magic about 75%. It is taken from the analysis of a group of patients; and if you had a more sophisticated analysis available and could look at individual patients, your results might be somewhat different. For example, if someone had approximately 500 PVCs every hour of their life and you gave a drug and then the next day they had 400 PVCs every hour, although that is only 20% decrease, there would be so little variability, that this small decrease would still be significant. The requirement for a 75% reduction is based on taking a large number of patients and saying what number can we routinely apply in looking at this group of people; but if you really are capable of doing a more sophisticated analysis, patient-by-patient, in some patients even 100% reduction would not be significant; whereas, in other patients even 10% would be sufficient.

Dr. Temple: I just wanted to be sure of the distinction between activity and usefulness.

Dr. Michelson: A 75% percent reduction in PVCs is not a measure of clinical usefulness. It is merely a guideline for statistical significance; that is, it suggests a drug is different from placebo, has antiarrhythmic activity, and is not inert.

SUMMARY:

Dr. Michelson: I think that the only way to summarize this session is to say that it looks like there are no short cuts in the near future to getting new drugs aproved, but at least we have gotten some useful guidelines on better ways of doing these studies. Presumably, the implementation of simple, well-designed studies with clear endpoints and careful scientific methods will facilitate new drug evaluations and subsequent approval as indicated.

COMPARATIVE SAFETY OF BETA BLOCKING DRUGS

D.C. HARRISON, M.D.

1. INTRODUCTION

The relative safety of one beta blocking drug as compared to another has been the subject of considerable debate. However, confusion has resulted since few studies have documented that equivalent levels of beta blockade had been achieved in the reported studies which suggest there is differential safety for one agent when compared to another. Therefore, it is difficult to demonstrate with certainty that there are significantly less circulatory, electrophysiologic or metabolic consequences produced by any given beta blocker unless it possesses a different pharmacologic spectrum of action.

On the other hand, certain pharmacologic properties of beta blocking agents would tend to reduce specific side effects and thereby result in a safer drug under certain pathological conditions.[1] The three pharmacologic properties most often studied are cardioselectivity, intrinsic sympathetic activity, and membrane stabilizing properties. These properties appear to provide a margin of greater safety for some agents in a few disease processes.

2. CARDIOSELECTIVITY

The cardioselectivity of beta blocking agents is not an "all or none" finding.[1] It is the relative ability to block sympathetic stimulation of the beta or cardiac receptors while not influencing stimulation of the $beta_2$ or peripheral, respiratory and other receptors.

Table 1. Physiologic and pharmacologic effects of β_1 vs β_2 agents.

I. β_1 adrenoceptor block

    1. Heart - hemodynamics and electrophysiology

    2. Small coronary arteries

    3. FFA production

II. β_2 adrenoceptor block

    1. Bronchial muscle

    2. Large coronary arteries

    3. Peripheral blood vessels

    4. Uterine muscle

    5. Lactate, glucagon, and insulin production

    6. Gastrointestinal tract

III. Unspecified

    1. Plasma renin

    2. Glycogenolysis

    3. Platelet production

The pharmacologic consequences of $beta_1$ and $beta_2$ receptor stimulation are outlined in Table 1. Thus, agents which are cardioselective would be less likely to aggravate hypoglycemia, produce hypertensive crises during hypoglycemia, and compromise the peripheral circulation.[2,3] Cardioselective agents would also have less effect on airway resistance in patients with asthma and chronic obstructive lung disease than nonselective agents. However, at higher doses even cardioselective agents such as atenolol and metoprolol reduce airway function in asthmatic patients and those with lung disease.

A major problem with evaluating cardioselectivity is the lack of standardized methods for studying the phenomenon. For example, studies on resting respiratory function do not establish cardioselectivity and the use of isoproterenol to produce marked sympathetic stimulation is artificial and does not always permit a distinction of cardioselectivity. Classification of existing beta blockers into cardioselective and nonselective agents has been made from isolated organ or animal studies (Table 2).

185

Table 2. Classification of beta blocking drugs.
A. Non-selective
   Propranolol   Timolol
   Oxprenolol   Alprenolol
   Pindolol
B. Cardioselective
   Practolol   Metoprolol
   Atenolol   Acebutolol (partial)

2.1 Cardioselectivity and respiratory function

Several published reports[4] utilizing single dose administration in patients with lung disease have demonstrated that selective agents have lesser effects on airway resistance than nonselective agents. However, cardioselective agents decreased airway function when given at higher doses.[1] Nevertheless, when given in roughly ten times the equipotent doses, atenolol produces an average of 17% decrease in specific airway conductance versus a 54% decrease for propranolol. When compared with a series of beta blockers,

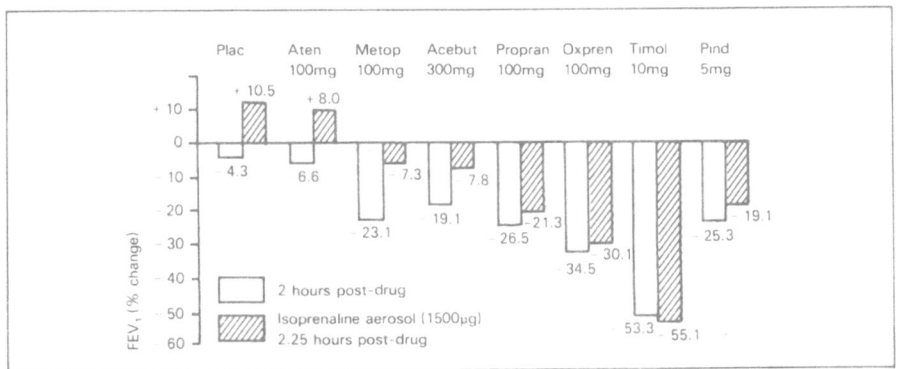

FIGURE 1. Effect of a placebo (plac; n = 10), atenolol (aten; n = 10), metoprolol (metop; n = 9), acebutolol (acebut; n = 5), propranolol (propran; n = 10), oxprenolol (oxpren; n = 8), timolol (timol; n = 4), and pindolol (pind; n = 5) on forced expiratory volume in 1 second in asthmatic patients.[5] Wheezing occurred with metoprolol (4 of 9 patients), acebutolol (1 of 5), propranolol (5 of 10), oxprenolol (6 of 8), timolol (4 of 4) and pindolol (1 of 5), but not with atenolol.*

*Reprinted with permission of the journal, Drugs

atenolol produced the smallest decrease in forced expiratory volumes in one second (FEV$_1$) and did not inhibit this broncho-dilation response to isoproterenol as usually occurs with the nonselective beta blockers. In comparable studies I.V. atenolol (3 mg) only partially blocked the bronchodilator response to inhaled salbutamol and orally administered atenolol (50 and 100 mg) produced less shift in specific airway conductance dose response curves to salbutamol than acebutolol.[4]

In patients with both asthma and hypertension, atenolol reduced blood pressures without causing specific changes in lung function tests.[6,7] In approximately 75% of patients with ob-structive airway disease, atenolol was tolerated well on a long-term basis.[7]

In summary, several studies demonstrate that cardioselectivity is an important pharmacologic characteristic of beta blocking agents for safety when they are to be used in patients with respiratory disease. Although at higher doses the cardioselec-tive properties may be lessened, the agents are generally safe in patients with obstructive airway disease.

2.2 Cardioselectivity and metabolic effects

In comparative studies none of the beta blocking agents have important effects on resting plasma insulin levels. All beta adrenergic agents antagonize the isoproterenol-stimulated increase in plasma insulin levels, but the cardioselective agents, metropolol and atenolol, had less activity than the non-selective agents, propranolol and pindolol.[8] A number of studies[9,10,11] showed that cardioselective agents did not delay recovery from insulin-induced hypoglycemia while nonselective agents prolonged recovery. Similar observations have been made in insulin-treated diabetic patients, and in patients treated with oral hypoglycemic agents.[12]

2.3. Central nervous system effects

Fewer depressive side effects and greater feeling of well being have been reported with atenolol as compared with pro-pranolol, but the significance of this is uncertain.

2.4. Intrinsic sympathetic activity (ISA)

While the pharmacologic significance of ISA is now known, beta blocking drugs which have this property may produce less circulatory depression when given intravenously than agents which lack ISA. No such effect has been documented for oral administration. In 1970, I stated, "For equivalent levels of beta blockade there is no difference in circulatory effects of available beta blockers." To date that pronouncement is true!

Physiologically, agents which raise peripheral vascular resistance, as does propranolol given acutely, should produce greater heart failure in patients with markedly reduced ventricular function; practically this has not proven true. My assessment is that there are no intrinsic safety factors for one agent over the other when equivalent beta blockade is produced.

3. MEMBRANE STABILIZING PROPERTIES

Several agents have been characterized as having membrane stabilizing properties, but no physiologic significance has been documented. The dextro isomer of propranolol gives this agent membrane stabilizing or "quinidine-like" properties, but they are very weak and μg/ml amounts are required to have anti-arrhythmic actions. Thus, in doses given in man these characteristics are unlikely to have pharmacologic effects.

4. INDIVIDUAL RESPONSES TO BETA BLOCKADE

The response to acute beta blockade depends upon the degree of adrenergic tone present in a patient at the time of administration. Since this cannot generally be quantitated, reports of acute comparisons of the effect of agents is likely to be misleading. Moreover, subjective responses of patients to the administration of drugs is highly variable and unless placebo controlled studies are performed, it is difficult to judge relative safety of one agent as compared to another.

5. SUMMARY

Cardioselectivity, intrinsic sympathetic activity, and membrane stabilizing activity may be important factors in

188

determining the relative safety of beta adrenergic blocking
agents. When given in higher doses and for long duration, these
factors are less important clinically.

REFERENCES

1. Heel RC, Brogden RN, Speight TM, Avery GS: Atenolol: A
   review of its pharmacological properties and therapeutic
   efficacy in angina pectoris and hypertension. Drugs 17: 425-
   512, 1979.
2. Waal-Manning HJ: Can β-blockers be used in diabetic patients?
   Drugs 17: 157, 1979.
3. Waal-Manning HJ: Atenolol and 3 nonselective β-blockers in
   hypertension. Clin Pharmacol Therap 25: 8, 1979.
4. Astrom H: Comparison of the effects on airway conductance
   of a new selective beta-adrenergic blocking drug, atenolol,
   and propranolol in asthmatic subjects. Scandinavian Journal
   of Respir Dis 56: 292, 1975.
5. Delcalmer PBS, Chatterjee SS, Cruickshank JM, Benson JK,
   Sterling GM: Beta-blockers and asthma. Brit Heart J 40: 184,
   1978.
6. Boye NP, Vale JR: Effect in bronchial asthma of a new beta-
   adrenergic blocking drug atenolol (ICI 66,082). European
   J Clin Pharmacol 11: 11, 1977.
7. Henningsen NC, Mattiasson I, Ohlsson O, Arborelius M, Bulow
   K: Long-term treatment of asthmatic and resistant hypertensive patients with selective beta-blockade (atenolol).
   8th World Cong. of Cardiol. Tokyo, Sept. 1978, p. 353.
8. Hansson L, Aberg H, Karlberg BE, Henningsen NC, Jameson S,
   Gudbrandsson T: Five years experience with atenolol in
   hypertension. 8th World Cong. of Cardiol. Tokyo, Sept.
   1978, p. 352.
9. Harms HH, Gooren L, Spoelstra AJG, Hesse C, Verschoor L:
   Blockade of isoprenaline-induced changes in plasma renin
   activity in healthy human subjects by propranolol, pindolol,
   practolol, atenolol, metoprolol, and acebutolol. Brit J
   Clin Pharmacol 5:19, 1978.
10. Deacon SP: Effect of atenolol and other beta-blockers on
    insulin-induced hypoglycaemia. Proc. Royal Society of
    Medicine 70 (Suppl. 5): 50, 1977.
11. Deacon SP, Barnett D: Comparison of atenolol and propranolol
    during insulin-induced hypoglycaemia. Brit Med J 2: 272,
    1976.
12. Deacon SP, Karuwanayake A, Barnett D: Acebutolol, atenolol
    and propranolol and metabolic responses to acute hypo-
    glycaemia in diabetes. Brit Med J 2: 1225, 1977.

Current Problems in the Evaluation of New Beta-Blocking Agents

Robert Temple, M.D.

Evaluating a new beta-blocker is certainly no harder than it ever was, and there really are no major problems in carrying out the basic evaluation of effectiveness and safety. There is, if anything, more guidance from the errors and successes of the past. But there are a number of regulatory and scientific questions that remain, and some relate to the question posed for the first panel today: "Are all beta-blockers the same?"

They are not exactly the same, as Dr. Somani and others have described in detail, but the real questions are:

1. To what extent may conclusions about one beta-blocker be carried over to another without an actual human study to confirm the conclusion?

2. What are the truly useful differences among beta-blockers?

At present our operating policy is that effectiveness conclusions reached about one beta-blocker cannot be applied to another without confirmation, however tempting it may be to do so. Not only that, because we believe physicians will assume, not without some reason, beta-blockers all have the same effectiveness, we require that this assumption be tested, at least partially. Beta-blockers are approved on the basis of effectiveness in at least one of three "major" indications, angina, hypertension, and arrhythmia, but on condition that the other indications be studied after marketing. We have not asked that some of the "minor" indications -- migraine or IHSS -- be studied, although of course manufacturers may choose to study them. Studying all three indications is plainly a lot of work and it could reasonably be asked whether it is really necessary. Could some pharmacodynamic response, such as change in exercise rate-pressure product, substitute for full-fledged effectiveness trials?

Perhaps it could but a difficulty is that because we are not quite sure how beta-blockers work, it is not easy to say in most cases what pharmacologic endpoint will correlate with clinical effectiveness. Moreover, in a number of cases, the logical or predicted result of a trial has not occurred when studies were carried out.

1. One of the most obvious instances of redundant effort, I would have said 6 months ago, was our requirement that a combination of beta-blocker and thiazide diuretic had to be studied formally to show the contribution of each component to the blood pressure lowering effect. But since then I have seen well-controlled trials with 2 cardioselective beta-blockers that give me pause. The changes from baseline in the 4 trials were:

Drug	Trial	T	B	C	Thiazide Contribution
		Change in Blood Pressure (no. of subjects)			
Atenolol	1	12/6 (17)	20/11 (17)	20/13 (17)	0/2
	2	14/10 (24)	21/19 (24)	38/22 (24)	17/3
Metoprolol	3	26/12 (20)	23/15 (24)	33/20 (24)	10/5
	4		24/17 (34)	23/17 (36)	-1/0

T = thiazide   B = beta-blocker   C = Combination

In studies 2 and 3 the thiazide did seem to contribute to the effect on systolic pressure but there was no significant effect on diastolic pressure in any of the studies. In contrast to these very modest, at best, diuretic contributions, studies of propranolol and a thiazide have usually shown a larger thiazide effect, generally about equal to the effect of a thiazide alone.

Obviously, these few studies do not provide enough data for a conclusion that cardioselective beta-blockers behave differently from non-selective blockers when used with a thiazide. The major limitation is that none of the studies compared a selective and a non-selective beta-blocker, so we cannot tell how these populations would have responded to a non-selective agent. There are therefore possible explanations for the minimal added effect of the thiazide in these studies that would not indicate a real difference from other beta-blockers. For example, the studies of cardioselective agents may in some cases have been carried out in relatively low salt intake patients, who might have a relatively small effect of thiazides in any circumstance, although in several of the studies a separate thiazide group seemed to have a typical response. In some cases the blood pressure on beta-blocker alone was fairly low, perhaps leaving relatively little room for improvement. Finally, the two impressively negative studies (Nos. 1 and 4) may represent nothing more than a chance occurrence. It is possible, however, that there really is a difference between the beta-blockers. Perhaps, for example, the selective agents have somewhat less effect on plasma renin and do not correct the thiazide-induced elevation of renin as well as the non-selective agents. Alternatively, if they tend less than other beta-blockers to unmask peripheral alpha-receptors, perhaps there is less room for a favorable effect of the direct dilating effects of the thiazides.

Whatever the ultimate explanation, if the interaction of beta-blocker and diuretics is not predictable for the class, it is not easy to say what is.

2. It seems logical to predict that a drug with a lot of intrinsic sympathomimetic activity (ISA) would have relatively little effect on hemodymanics at rest. One might therefore deduce that such an agent would not be a very good antihypertensive agent (blood pressure is usually assessed at rest), but would be effective in exercise-induced angina, where it would block the high levels of adrenergic activity resulting from exercise. So far, however, and noting that the conclusion is based on fairly small studies, it appears that pindolol, with the most ISA of any of the well-studied beta-blockers, is an effective antihypertensive agent, about as effective as propranolol, despite minimal effects on resting heart rate and, according to a recent report, little effect on cardiac output. On the other hand, oxprenolol, with less ISA than pindolol, appears to be a less effective antihypertensive agent than propranolol, at least when each is added to a diuretic (based on results from two large controlled comparative studies), and a less effective anti-anginal drug as well, which one would probably not have predicted. The latter conclusion is based on results of a single comparative study by Frishman.

The reason for these surprises may be simply that we do not entirely understand the mechanism of action of beta-blockers, especially the possible interplay of several mechanisms. If, for example, the effects of a beta-blocker are a summation of effects on cardiac, vascular, kidney and central nervous system receptors, each of which could be differently affected by the beta-selectivity of the drug, its degree of ISA, and the extent of its lipid solubility, it is no wonder we cannot always predict what will happen. Apart from this, the drugs can have properties not related to beta-blockade at all, such as local anesthetic activity, alpha-adrenergic blocking activity, or direct vasodilating activity, to complicate matters further.

The examples above may prove exceptional and, thus far, most beta-blockers have had generally similar effectiveness, at least insofar as this has been studied. But the total comparative data are relatively limited, and most of the controlled studies we have seen have been in hypertension, with a much smaller number in angina, and fewer still in arrhythmias. Moreover, few of the studies include sizable comparisons with other beta-blockers, which would be needed to detect anything but quite large differences.

At this time, therefore, it still seems necessary to ask that the major indications for beta-blockers be studied formally, rather than accepted based on pharmacologic observations. It seems especially important to carry out more adequate comparisons of one agent with another.

Perhaps the best reason to believe beta-blockers are likely to prove similar in effectiveness is the very small number of clinically important differences that have been discovered among them, even though one might have thought there is a very great commercial and therapeutic incentive to discover such differences. This is not very reassuring, however, because, despite the perceived incentives, the search for clinically important differences between beta-blockers has been desultory at best. The pharmacologic differences among the drugs have often been studied carefully in animals, and sometimes in man as well, but the hints of differences, even exciting differences, offered by pharmacologic data have rarely been pursued by adequate human trials.

Consider, for example, the question of adverse effects. It is recognized that beta-blockers cause a few serious, and many less serious but quite annoying, adverse effects. There seem to be reasons to suspect that drugs with cardioselectivity, with ISA, with alpha-blocking properties, or with decreased concentration in the brain might have less tendency to cause some of these effects, e.g., unpleasant dreams, fatigue, listlessness, cold extremeties, Raynaud's phenomenon, impotence, depression, heart failure, respiratory distress, heart block, or extreme bradycardia. Nevertheless, virtually no controlled trials to find out whether the suspicion is correct have been conducted.

Two straightforward trial designs could be used to look for such differences. The more conventional approach would be to compare the frequency of such effects with two of the agents, but it might be hard to succeed with this design as the side effects are, in most cases, not very common and a very large number of patients could be needed to show a difference. An approach more likely to be successful would be to identify patients with a particular adverse effect, e.g., dreaming or cold extremities on propranolol, and randomize them to propranolol or to another beta-blocker. Any substantial difference between the agents should be readily apparent.

This design has a potential bias, of course. If a particular effect is not related to the drugs' pharmacology, but is rather an idiosyncratic response that occurs equally frequently with any of the drugs, propranolol would be at a disadvantage, because all patients in the study would be selected because they had that idiosyncratic response to it. The second drug could appear better even if the adverse effect in an unselected population would be equally frequent. Nonetheless, this kind of study could show, at a minimum, whether it is useful to try the second in an effort to eliminate a particular side effect; if there were no difference between the drugs in such a study there would seem little reason to do so.

If studies using this design have been carried out, I am unaware of them. Instead, patients with an adverse effect on one drug have usually simply been switched to another agent. When fewer patients complained of the adverse effect, a beneficial difference (e.g., on asthma) has been attributed to the second drug. Unfortunately, such a study is not really informative because it does not control for time effects, placebo effect or investigator effect. If you will forgive an undocumented anecdote, I have been told by a representative of one manufacturer, thinking of carrying out a study of his beta-blocker's effect on dreaming, that of 100 patients identified as having bad dreams on propranolol, only 10 still had them when they were considered in preparation for a randomized trial of the design suggested above. If an uncontrolled trial were carried out in such patients, i.e., if they were simply transferred to the second drug, that would look like a 90% success rate.

The data available on clinically important differences among beta-blockers is disappointing. Apart from the fundamental matters of effectiveness and safety, the most important information for a physician about drugs is the way in which they are similar to and different from closely related drugs. While information about such differences is not always easy to obtain, there seem good reasons to hope such questions will be explored more in the future than they have been to date.

There is an additional problem I should mention. It relates to the observation reported earlier today by Dr. Kaplan, one that we see confirmed in nearly all clinical trials, that elevated blood pressures tend to fall over time after entry into a study. A consequence of this is that if the treatments in a trial are titrated upward until some defined blood pressure end point is reached, patients seem to respond to the higher dose with a greater response. This may not be a correct impression, as the investigator may be seeing nothing more than the spontaneous downward drift of blood pressure. The true dose-response curve can be determined best from a parallel design study in which patients are randomized to several doses of the drug. When this has been done, it has often turned out that doses have been overestimated. In the case of atenolol, for example, it has become apparent that the very high doses used in Europe, 400-600 mg, give no greater antihypertensive effect than 100 mg, or perhaps even 50 mg.

With beta-blockers, failure to minimize dose seems so far not to be very costly, in that most side effects seem not to be dose related once a substantially beta-blocking dose is achieved, but it still appears important to know a dose beyond which titration is probably not useful and, in general, to limit exposure to an agent to an amount that provides benefit. Careful assessment of the relationship in properly designed trials should therefore be part of the evaluation of beta-blockers.

GENERAL GROUP DISCUSSION - Problems in Study Design

Moderator: Dr. Joel Morganroth

Dr. Sami: My question is for Dr. Temple. I am a Canadian and not really involved with the F.D.A.; but if you were presented with a drug, let's say a beta blocker, which had identical action to propranolol and identical side effects, identical efficacy in every respect, would that make a problem in approving this drug for clinical use or not?

Dr. Temple: You mean, does it have to be better or different?

Dr. Sami: Yes, better or different?

Dr. Temple: No.

Dr. Scriabine: I wonder if Dr. Temple would share with us some of the current problems that F.D.A. has in getting a drug approved after the Advisory Committee has recommended their approval.

Dr. Temple: As I had to explain in a long memorandum to the Commissioner who wondered what Dr. Cohn meant when he asked about that, there are a number of things which can delay final approval after an Advisory Committee meets on a drug. One is that it is not uncommon for additional data to have been presented to us recently that may need to be reviewed even though the Committee may have seen a summary of it. Another possibility is that we are working on something else and cannot get to it. A third possibility is that questions raised by the Committee may have required further submissions even afterward. And that sometimes recommendation for approval has certain either implicit or specific conditions in it; that is, assuming F.D.A. agrees that the data show this or things like that. I have no further answers than those--we would like to have them all out a month or so later, but that doesn't always work.

Dr. Harrison: We were talking about approval. The calcium antagonists are all chemically quite different, and I don't think analogous in any way to the beta blocking drugs. But it seems to me that some reduced expense, some reduction in number of studies required could be set up--you could set up some type of class response to the beta blocking drugs with some requirements for post-release surveillance for safety. It seems to me that there is some way there might be a tradeoff that would decrease the time to approval and yet still continue to provide some very necessary information that we might need and don't get for drugs. I am not a big one to be pushing post-release surveillance, but I think in this kind of situation you might have that happen with some drugs.

Dr. Temple: Let me be sure I know what you mean. You mean post-approval surveillance or more specific studies carried out?

Dr. Harrison: Well, either. Either you could set requirements about studies that would be continued--I mean once you knew that the drug was a beta blocking drug, had been demonstrated to be effective in a few studies and you could shorten the time to approval and you could also maybe tradeoff the continuing study and the post-surveillance study and get some ideas about safety down the line. It seems to me that that's another approach.

Dr. Temple: There are really two parts to that question. The amount of data that comes in an application are determined by first of all the amount that are needed to show that it really works in angina or hypertension or whatever, and there is a certain amount of exposure which people can argue about how much that should be that is deemed needed to see what its adverse effects are going to be. I would say that it is now much easier to show that an agent is an effective beta blocker in hypertension and that the number of studies would be fairly small for that. Most of the data that would be developed would be to show what its adverse effects are. Now could that be reduced--that's a hard question. There is no reason that I can think of that the next drug that comes along couldn't be as variant in its way as practolol was in its, and you want at least enough people tested to be sure that some very high level or relatively high level adverse effect like that isn't seen.

Dr. Harrison: But that came about very late and long after the drug had been approved and might not have been noticed had the clinical trial been started to look at the sudden death question and that is why I think post-surveilance kinds of data might be very helpful with some drugs.

Dr. Temple: I don't dispute that. I was just illustrating an example of how drugs that have seemed to be very closely related can have bizarre adverse effects. In fact, I would go a step further and say that almost every unusual adverse reaction that has occurred has occurred in a member of a class when other members did not have anything like that. So that the fact that they seem to be closely related is not, per se, reassuring since we don't know what side groups do the bad stuff.

Dr. Harrison: Well, what I am trying to do is to get your work down to a manageable level. I would like to see someone walk into your office with a new drug for approval with one single man carrying an armful of data forms and summaries rather than sending two trailer truckloads which you obviously can't get to with the limited staff that you have for months. I would like to see someone walk in and put it on your desk and say, here it is. That's why I think that the more I am in this business, the continued growth of the data forms and the data being collected, particularly beta blocking drugs in terms of safety, seems to me have gone far overboard. Maybe I am wrong, but I just have the idea that we have pushed a good thing too far.

Dr. Temple: The amount of studies done, for example, in the United States for atenolol was substantially smaller than that done for most other agents. We made use of data that already existed and, I would say, didn't insist that things be repeated over and over again. In fact, I don't know if you will recall it, but when the first proposals as to what was needed came in, several of us sat there and said, "Wait a minute, that's way too much to do; why don't you not do so much." If someone were asking, for example, what would not be a whole lot of studies needed, there would not be a whole lot of additional safety data to collect. So, I think you do learn whether you could take a brand new agent and approve it on the basis of 200 patients instead of the 750-1000 that now come in is really a different question, and I'm not sure it's reasonable to do that.

Dr. Cohn: I would like to return to science, actually, there are several of us in this room, including Dr. Temple, who are on a commission that is trying to simplify the drug approval process; and we spent yesterday embroiled in those discussions. So, I thought that we could get back to science today. The issue about the role of the sympathetic nervous system that Don Harrison brought up I think is a very interesting one and its role in support of cardiac function is one that I think remains somewhat unclear at the moment moreso than ever, perhaps, because of the increasing use of beta blockers even in people who have poor function and seem for some reason to tolerate them quite well; and I think we've all had that experience. I wonder whether it isn't true, of course, that you don't learn very much about the sympathetic nervous system. We didn't learn much about it until we developed methods for blocking it; and as we gain new drugs that do different things to receptors, we begin to get more insight into the role of the sympathetic nervous system. I think it is certainly clear that the sympathetic nervous system does some bad things even in heart failure and in the periphery and maybe in the heart as well. It may be playing some role in the sudden death issue that we discussed before. So, I think we are in a period when we cannot use preconceived ideas about what should be good and what should be bad. The observations have to be made. I guess that is support for continuing to study each of these drugs that comes along because each is different. I wonder if I could ask Bob Temple another question about how he would view the current trend now toward development of beta blockers that have other pharmacologic activities as well; and this gets back to the co-existence of alpha blocking actions, vasodilators actions and diuretic actions. It is clear that beta blockers are being used in this country very frequently at least in association with other drugs. They are being used with type I antiarrhythmics; they are being used with diuretics; they are being used with nitrates; they will probably be used with calcium channel blockers; and how do you view the goal to develop a single compound which has dual effects, that is beta blocking actions, plus one of these others. I'm not the least bit pessimistic that the chemist won't be able to come up with compounds that will do all these things. Should that be a high priority or do you think that there ought to be an effort to maintain relative pharmacologic purity in compounds?

Dr. Temple: That is a terrific question. You're probably substantially better equipped to answer it than I am. It doesn't seem to be a major advantage to have two properties in one molecule. It might agreeably be considered harder to titrate when a molecule than two separate entities. However, on the other hand it obviously also simplifies dosing; and for conditions like hypertension, common dogma is that the fewer drugs given the better off you are. What I am fairly convinced of is that the apparent great advantage of those combination molecules remains to be shown and in most cases will not turn out to be as exciting as people predicted. That's just a pessimistic gut reaction and it's also based on a couple of the early examples of those molecules that we've seen. I guess the other thing is that probably we've had such combinations all along and probably did not pay that much attention to them. I mean we keep learning new things about what agents do, and it often turns out that we have more receptors than we first thought about.

Dr. Harrison: I have a view about it. I think it's interesting chemistry; but I think in pharmacology you are going to see the side effects increase like problems with children--they double. Then you have actions in the drug and they go by factor of 9. In other words it's a square of the side effect question here so think as you put more and more of them together you are going to see the increasing incidence of intolerance to the drug. I think you showed that in a way with labetalol with one of the studies that you were doing where you made one prediction that went the other way in a patient that had pre-syncopal hypotension; and I think that you, as you start altering more of the body's mechanism with a drug, the side effect question will be the one that will kill you.

Dr. Woosley: In that same vein labelatol supposedly has a 20:1 ratio of beta to alpha and how many patients in the hypertensive population have a need for a 20:1 ratio. Well, hopefully, it is big enough for that company to treat some patients without, like you say, and excessive number of side effects; but when you start adding in two and three effects and it takes away the ability to dose to a determined dose response ratio for a drug, I think it would be a very shotgun approach with the likelihood that you are going to miss on most of these type molecules in a large percentage of the population.

Dr. Hjalmarson: I would like to comment on what was brought up by Don Harrison of problems with beta blockade in patients with congestive heart failure. I think it is very important to define what kind of failure we are talking about. One example he mentioned is that we had positive effects in patients with congestive cardiomyopathy and that could not be confirmed by workers in New Zealand. We have no patients where alcoholic cardiomyopathy is among our groups of at least 35 patients which we have controlled carefully well. Out of 16 patients he had studied he had 12 patients with alcoholic cardiomyopathy. Furthermore, we have reported that it takes about six months of continued treatment with beta blockade to get a marked or optimal improvement of heart function in these patients and some studies only lasted for one month. Another group of patients that I would like to comment about is patients with heart failure in acute myocardial infarction and our experience is that patients with a quite low heart rate at entry and heart failure respond poorly to beta blockade, and I had to be very careful to give beta blockade to these patients in contrast to patients having a higher heart rate and backward failure. We have a study under publication now in Acta Scandinavica performed by myself and Dr. Raites in Sweden where we randomized the patients with heart failure and tachycardia. They should have a PCW pressure of above 17, the material ranged between 17 and 33, and they should have a heart rate of about 85. They were randomized to either nitroprusside or metoprolol, and there was a marked and significant drop in filling pressure in the group of patients treated with metoprolol. Looking at the triple product as some kind of indication of oxygen consumption that was reduced similarly with the two drugs. Even in patients with acute myocardial infarction and ischemic congestive heart failure there could be a marked difference from patient to patient depending upon what kind of sympathetic drive he has to start with and whether that could be reduced by beta blockade.

Dr. Harrison: That assumes that the tachycardia is appropriate--I mean many people stay alive with heart failure because of the tachycardia. Once you get a more than about 30% of your heart infarcted, you have no change in stroke volume and so your cardiac output is totally dependent on heart rate. So if you knocked the heart rate down in those patients, you'd certainly be in difficulty.

Dr. Hjalmarson: May I comment on that. That was told us ten years back when we started to use beta blockade in acute myocardial infarction. The heart rate in acute myocardial infarction is an adaptation for the patient. He has to have that high heart rate due to his poorly functioning left ventricle. I am completely sure that it is not true in the majority of patients. We have much higher sympathetic drive than that is necessary in most of these patients with failure.

Dr. Harrison: I think we are off the subject a bit. I am not sure that I agree with you.

Dr. Morganroth: Let me ask Dr. Woosley to address another tolerance issue which is important in clinical use of these beta blocker agents and that is the risk of beta blockers crossing placenta. Do you have insight on what you might advise for further studies to define the use of these agents in pregnancy.

Dr. Woosley: There is an article on placental transfer of beta blockers, and I can't recall the data or anything except the title. So there is now some data on this, and I think there are standard ways to obtain that data with these drugs; and I think it is an important issue that may be a very important difference in drugs when you are treating young populations, as many of these drugs will be given to, so I think it is something we need more data on. I think there is some data already coming out.

Dr. Temple: My impression is that most of them do cross the placenta and most of them are at least slightly toxic to the fetus at the very high doses studied. I'm not sure we've seen any differences.

Dr. Fitzgerald: Just a supplementary comment really. There have been several studies of beta blockers on the relationship between the blood level in the mother and in the fetus particularly with propranolol. There was a recent carefully designed study on atenolol that showed there was equivalent blood levels in the fetus as in the mother with respect to time and also that there was no effect or the usual criteria for the well being of the fetus. About 12 years ago there were about 12-14 women with H.O.C.M. who got pregnant who were on beta blockers during the whole pregnancy and didn't seem to have any problems. So, I think there is a fair bit of information around to actually go and look through the European literature.

Dr. Woosley: I think there is also some data recently on the excretion of beta blockers in milk and its importance, potential importance, on nursing children. So I think that is another area that deserves further investigation.

Dr. Morganroth: Let me just finish this topic by asking Dr. Temple about the F.D.A.'s position on this subject. Should this issue be more clearly studied prior to approval of new agents?

Dr. Temple: Well, animal studies are always done both of excretion into the milk and toxicity to the fetus and that is usually reflected in labeling. There is usually no human data, and it is not easy to come by--I think the general idea is that unless necessary, the drug should be avoided and so you get a relatively small number of people exposed. But the right thing to do is that after a time recapitulate, see what is in order to see if you can modify the labeling. Whether it would be appropriate to avoid breastfeeding while you are on the drug and probably that's the best practice, it's not easy to do human studies of excretion into the milk. I guess you could do a short-term study on dose. I don't know if it requires more attention. I don't think so.

Dr. Sen: I just wanted to mention and draw your attention to the fact that there is a report of excretion of breast milk and fetal placental passage of metoprolol in the European literature by Andstrom.

Dr. Morganroth: I wonder if we could move to another topic--and that is to spend a few minutes on the issue that was raised earlier this afternoon. That is the question of sudden death versus pharmacological endpoints for the use of beta blockers in arrhythmias; and of course, this is also true for other antiarrhythmic agents. I wonder, Don, if you would comment on the importance of timeliness of such studies and how such studies, can be best performed. I wonder if you could also comment on the experience from other studies and what sorts of study designs or approaches one should take to this important problem.

Dr. Harrison: Well, I just owe a comment on the beta blocker studies. As you know, the study from Sweden in the three-month intervention has just been reported; and the timolol study has been just reported. Lord only knows, 20,000 other patients are still under study in a number of protocols for beta blocking drugs. I guess I believe the results of these studies will certainly answer the question about a secondary prevention trial post-myocardial infarction, I don't believe it will be an unanswered question when most of those studies are reported in the next year to 18 months. Where I came from and the places I was in Europe in eight countries, it seemed to be answered already in most of their minds; and I think many people feel that way.

I guess I believe that there is a group of very high-risk patients that have left ventricular dysfunction frequently have complex arrhythmias and frequently are left out of beta blocking trials, and in fact, that probably deems that a careful study with some of the newer antiarrhythmic drugs; and I guess that I believe it should be a selected high-risk group. I won't debate all of the ways that a high-risk group might be selected; but it might be selected on ventricular function plus some established levels of complex and frequent ventricular arrhythmias. To make the trial as functional as possible, I believe the question should be, "Can the marked suppression or total suppression of ventricular premature beats alter the life survival in this group of patients?", and I think whether it has to be a single class I agent or a cascade of class I agents so that you don't lose so many patients to dropout because of side effects. Perhaps the best way to go about this trial is to use the cascade type of effect so that you can keep most of the patients once they are allocated to an antiarrhythmic drug for a period of time. Now that raises a question as to whether placebo is ethical in such a study at this point in time, particularly if you know that they are having short runs of VT or even if you know they are having what I call sustained VT--greater than 10 or more consecutive premature beats--then that becomes very difficult to answer on ethical grounds. I don't believe that you can still on ethical grounds have a placebo group with such a high-risk group of patients to answer that question. Some of these patients may have been picked off in the beta blocking drug trials, and it may have been some of the patients that have survived. But I think that many of these are excluded from beta blocking trials. So I think it is time we have such a question answered, and I think we should use the drugs than can almost totally suppress VPCs if we can.

Dr. Levitt: In view of the fact that as you started out by saying that the beta blockers appear to be the only class of compounds that has data on the effect in preventing sudden death or in having an impact on mortality after acute myocardial infarction and from what we heard a little earlier about the relative lack of efficacy of beta blockers in terms of the doses that are used that in most studies you only get a 50% incidence of suppression of ventricular ectopic activity is going to be related to prevention of sudden death in this group.

Dr. Harrison: I don't know. That's the question as I see it; and I think there are people who have mortality of 20% in one year after myocardial infarction, so it is a very high mortality rate that we are talking about in these patients. I'm not talking about those patients who are routinely handled in a standard fixed dose trial with beta blocking drugs. I am talking about the very high-risk patients who had extensive myocardial infarction who are the ones who are resuscitated from VF or the ones that are showing up with recurrent VT at this point in time, and the question is not the one you have posed. The question is whether or not in this group of patients that suppression of arrhythmias as totally as possibly will, in fact, reduce death.

Dr. Levitt: That's the point that I was driving at. In selecting the antiarrhythmic drug for these patients you would use something like programmed electrical stimulation to determine which drug you would use?

Dr. Harrison: No, I don't think so. I would not. I think that programmed electric stimulation has yet to be proven as a technique which will lead to determination of efficacy. I think that there are several of these drugs around now that really will highly suppress VPCs and you can document that by oral trials. I mean they'll suppress more than 90%. So, I think that you've got an oportunity to try some of these drugs, and this would be the time to answer the question.

Dr. Morganroth: I think that the secondary prevention trials in acute myocardial infarction must be looked at totally separate from the primary prevention mode that Dr. Harrison was addressing. The mechanism for the decrease in "sudden death" in the secondary trial, may involve cardio-protective effects from recurrent ischemia, recurrent infarction, etc., and not necessarily the antiarrhythmic effect; in fact, most of those studies have had no arrhythmia monitoring at all to even judge group comparability. In terms of using electrical stimulation in chronic PVC patients I would totally agree with Dr. Harrison. I think that in such long-term outpatient trials that with the lack of clear correlation between invasive electrophysiologic studies and clinical long-term monitoring suppression and/or sudden death prevention one should not complicate the trial by having inhospital invasive expensive testing which will add enormously to costs and study complexity. I think Dr. Temple will comment on this.

Dr. Temple: It seems worthwhile to try to answer as many questions without overloading the study. Wouldn't it be reasonable to not test specific drugs--but test the treatment approach of suppression? Is that right?

Dr. Harrison: I said that but I could go the other way. I've been back and forth on this issue in the last few weeks as I have thought a lot about it. If you picked any of the available antiarrhythmic drugs at the present time, I am talking about available and approved by your office to be used, that you really would have to have a cascade because you would lose at least 30% of the patients which would make the size of the trial and the interpretation very difficult. I think using some of the other drugs, and I just mention amiodorone as a potential, although I'm a little queasy about amiodorone, it could be used without having to have a backup.

Dr. Temple: I guess everyone would agree that there is controversy about whether program stimulation or some reasonable endpoint on Holter is a better choice, but certainly there are some people who think that the program stimulation endpoint is meaningful. What about the possibility of comparing several treatment approaches using whatever drugs are necessary to implement it. Whether you could assign people to a placebo or not I think is a hard question, but you could assign them to legitimate approaches to therapy so one could be assigned to program stimulation selected drug. Another group could be sent back to the local physicians to do whatever they do.

Dr. Harrison: That's possible. It's not that I do believe in program stimulation. I don't believe in program stimulation induction at this point in time for recurrent ventricular fibrillation; but for recurrent ventricular tachycardia, yes I do in terms of selecting a drug. I think that at least in our hands we are now beginning to experience in spontaneous ventricular fibrillation that program stimulation has not been helpful in that group, but I think it has been helpful in the spontaneous VT. I believe that program stimulation is going to be helpful in some group, but I think that in dealing with this group you could do what you said that you could have several ways to enter the trial and drug be chosen on that basis.

Dr. Morganroth: Let me back up one step, Bob. You mentioned that it is difficult to assign placebo to a group. Why would that be the case unless you felt that there was actually evidence that treatment of ventricular arrhythmias in fact prevented sudden death. Obviously, I am not talking about the sick patient with VT in an ICU, but rather the patient with chronic complex arrhythmia that is not being hurt immediately by their arrhythmia. It seems to me that many physicians don't treat such patients and that using placebo would be the clearest way of really determining whether or not the treatment group is, in fact, having a different response.

Dr. Temple: I don't have any trouble with that. I think what my view would be based on what I've seen, but there are many different perceptions. I think there are institutions in which it would be very difficult to do that not because it is absolutely proved but because they would say it seems fairly likely that therapy is beneficial and you're talking about life and death here and, therefore, you're obliged to do something. A way out that has been taken in that setting is to send the patient back with good advice to his physician to do what we would ordinarily do. Whether that really solved the ethical problem or not is something you can debate. But it has been done.

Dr. Somani: I would like to bring to your attention the results of Michigan sudden death protocol. In this protocol the patients are admitted only if they have been brought into the hospital with ventricular fibrillation and resuscitated and in the last two years. Our data have been accumulated showing that if they are treated with an antiarrhythmic drug, they are sent back to their referring physicians and are being followed by multiple Holter report recordings every month. The data has now been analyzed to some extent and of the more than 50 possible factors, it appears that treatment with antiarrhythmic drugs, depending upon the choice of the physician, seems to be the only factor which decreases the recurrence of fibrillation. So the patients who are continuously receiving treatment by their physicians with any antiarrhythmic drug available at this time seem to be surviving longer than the patients who are not treated, and this appears to be the trend at this time from the analysis.

Dr. Harrison: Are these randomized?

Dr. Somani: They are not randomized; there is no placebo except that they are referred back to their original physicians, and it's the decision of the physician to prescribe antiarrhythmic therapy or not.

Dr. Morganroth: Are there any efficacy measures being obtained? Holter monitoring? Do you know the relationship between these measures and outcome?

Dr. Somani: The results seem to indicate that on Holter those who were totally suppressed with the antiarrhythmic agent seem to survive longer than those who did not have this response. That appeared to be the only factor so far in the multi-factorial analysis. So these types of studies are being done.

Dr. Woosley: I think Dr. Harrison and most people who are using investigational drugs now under the emergency protocols that many of you people have set up have at least 50 people that you could call into the hospital and who would die within two days of stoping their medicines or go onto sustained ventricular tachycardia or some horrible arrhythmia. So, I don't think there is any doubt that these medicines work in a subset of the population. But what everybody else is talking about is that asymptomatic population, the real problem out there, that often is not being treated and the real quandry that the cardiologist sees when he sees a patient one month post-MI, feels an irregular pulse, gets a Holter and sees a lot of complex ectopy. You look at your drug choices and you see drugs that could induce ventricular fibrillation in 5% to 13% of the population. You send them home on a drug, and they die, and you wonder "Well, is it because he didn't start taking the medicine quick enough or because he took the medicine?" and you send them home without treating them, and he dies, and you think "Well, maybe I should have put him on medication." So I think that's the population that needs the answer. I don't think there is any doubt that the drugs work; and I think what we really want to know is what level of arrhythmia suppression do we have to get. When we looked at our propranolol data, we found that and I've forgotten what else--we looked at the relationship between dose and suppression of PVCs and suppression of ventricular tachycardia and a lower dose will suppress ventricular tachycadia than is required to suppress all ectopy and I think there are few exceptions. But that, in general, is an observation that most people have made. So maybe we don't have to use a tremendously high dose of a drug to suppress all ectopy. The question that might fall out of that study is what dose is associated and what degree of suppression and what degree of survival.

Dr. Sami: I just want to add a comment to what Ray just said in addressing Dr. Harrison's proposal for placebo. There are not very many patients with marked ventricular dysfunction and complex ventricular arrhythmia who are asymptomatic. When you really look at ejection fractions, for example, patients with low ejection fraction are all very sick with their arrhythmias. We have tried in the study in Montreal--we've given placebo to those people on inhospital and continuous monitoring and none of these people can sustain more than 24 hours under placebo without really feeling the arrhythmia--feeling sick, feeling palpitations and dizziness. I also would like to just mention that we have completed a study in Montreal with encainide in patients with intractable and complex ventricular and LV dysfunction, and it seems really true that Holter monitoring recording and suppression of complex ventricular arrhythmia does have a bearing on mortality. Out of 14 patients who had initial response to the drug, two had a non-satisfactory response with continued couplets and short runs of VT and those two patients died within the first year. The other 12 who continued to have a good response and continued to have this on a long-term basis on repeated Holters every three months continued suppression of their run of ventricular tachycardia and couplets are all surviving for an average of ten months. So I think that there is hope there, and I don't think I would like to give those people placebo for a long-term period.

Dr. Morganroth: There are clearly two groups of patients. We have studied patients and reported on those with idiopathic congestive and ischemic cardiomyopathy, and in that group we detected a very large number who had complex arrhythmias that were entirely unaware of their arrhythmia. So the degree of symptoms obviously depends on the degree of their LV dysfunction. If you're dealing with an inhospital versus and outpatient population, I think you will find differences in terms of the nature of their response to their arrhythmia. I suspect that there are plenty of patients post-infarction with abnormal regional wall motion on echo and patients with mild-to-moderate congestive cardiomyopathy who on Holter will have triplets, maybe four or five beats in a row or more, lots of couplets, and fairly frequent PVCs that are entirely unaware of them; and I suspect that this group does, at least from our studies, have a high sudden death rate per year (20-25%) and that such a population of high-risk patients placed half on drug X or cascade and half on a placebo would answer this question within a year or two with a relatively low cost.

Dr. Woosley: Just to make a general comment. A recent mexilitine study was set up to try to study this question and used the intent-to-treat approach; and I think the study is often misquoted as I go to meetings, and the bottom line was that the survival was not influenced by mexilitine but the dropout was so high because of side effects that even though the patients had as a group deduction in PVCs the dropout rate was so high that it masked any potential benefit on mortality. So I think it just reinforces the need that whatever drug is chosen, like Don says, a cascade system or drugs with a very nice therapeutic index, will allow you to use an effective dose.

Dr. Temple: I would think once the principle that any approach works is established you could then start to compare various drugs and see if there are any important differences in tolerability or ultimate effect, like maybe having a long half-life keeps you from dying in the middle of the night.

Dr. Morganroth: Since Dr. Temple has had the last word, I guess we can adjourn this session.

REMARKS

BY

ARTHUR HULL HAYES, JR., M.D.
COMMISSIONER OF FOOD AND DRUGS

I want to thank you for inviting me to be here this evening. In a sense this is a homecoming because my professional life before becoming Commissioner dealt with cardiovascular drugs and beta blockers, as many as you know. So it's a double pleasure to be here this evening to represent THE FOOD AND DRUG ADMINISTRATION and to break bread with my colleagues.

One goal that I set for myself when I became Commissioner of FDA was that I would try to get out of Washington as much as possible to speak to the health professional community. I learned very quickly that Washington really is different from the rest of the country. It's not just that it is the national capital. But one's perception can grow narrow near the Potomac, and meetings like this help me broaden my perspective. And they also give me the opportunity to renew old friendships. I wasn't always Commissioner. I haven't changed.

I'm often asked what it's really like to be Commissioner of FDA. I had trouble finding quite the right description until I woke up at 4:30 on the morning of the wedding of Prince Charles and Lady Diana.

What impressed me most was watching Queen Elizabeth. Her day consisted of having people move her from one spot to the next, perhaps pushing some papers in front of her for signing, moving from meeting to ceremony without having much time to think, or even to know what's coming next.

Let me tell you, that's perfect training to be Commissioner.

On a more serious note, the Commissioner's job is a hectic one. FDA regulates products that account for 25 cents out of every dollar spent by a consumer in this country. That means not only all drugs and medical devices, but also foods, and cosmetics, and products that emit radiation, and other products as well.

I have marvelled, quite frankly, at how much the Food and Drug Administration does accomplish, considering the enormity of its mission.

Criticisms often occur because there is a lack of consensus on a particular matter, but the Agency nevertheless has to make a decision, and all those who agree with it often remain silent, while those who disagree make noise. FDA has a very strong scientific base, but it cannot treat problems the way we are accustomed in the academic setting. In the university, we can discuss an issue, and argue both sides, and try to develop more data, and change our minds a year later. At FDA, there is no such luxury. Decisions have to be made, not on the basis of tomorrow's new perspective, but on the basis of what we have before us today. We cannot defer regulatory decisions because all the scientific information isn't in yet. In short, action won't wait. FDA often is, and has to be, on the frontier of science. We have to make decisions that other people just as soon would not make.

And a lack of complete information is not the only obstacle. Decisions have be to made based on the requirements of the law and a long legal history of cases. FDA cannot do only that which is right and scientifically correct; it has to be legally correct as well. Add to that element of high public visibility, and 435 Congressmen and 100 Senators whose role is to oversee what we're doing on behalf of their constituents, and you can really see why FDA decisions often can be controversial.

In fact, when I sat down for my first meeting with the FDA staff, and started to go around the table to learn the latest developments, the very first thing I was told was that I was being sued. I knew I was in trouble when I looked at the personnel lists of FDA employees and found that the Office of General Counsel had 45 lawyers. I have learned since, that virtually every decision made by FDA is going to be controversial and disliked by some group or another, and that on many decisions I'll be sued. The only question is whether the suit is filed in 24 or 48 hours.

But it would be a mistake for anyone to think that, because of this constant controversy, because we have to make decisions when all the science is not yet in, because our decisions affect so many people that some are bound to oppose them, that the process is deficient. Quite to the contrary, the analyses I receive from the staff are usually first-rate, the ability of the Agency to carry out its mission is unparalleled, and the people at FDA are as capable as any staff anywhere.

Just to give you an indication of how the world misperceives, if you will, what FDA does, let me tell you a little story about a very distinguished scientist, who shall go unnamed, who visited me in my office this past summer.

We were talking about various parts of the organization and I was explaining what this group did and what that one did. My guest, with absolute sincerity, told me there was one office director he particularly wanted to meet: the Director of the Office of De-Regulation.

Well, I had to explain to him that we really didn't have any such office.

And I went on to tell him that I personally believe quite strongly in efficient and effective regulation. I can't see how the average American can figure out for himself or herself whether a drug is safe and effective, or whether a food additive is safe, or whether a particular X-ray machine is emitting too much radiation. There really does need to be some objective party that is concerned about the safety of the products that we use, and not only that but also about the labeling. The science today is too complex, the marketing systems too intertwined, to ask people to make these judgments by themselves.

By the same token, I also believe that regulation at any level should not be inhibitory to innovation and progress. I often ask myself whether some of the great innovations in medicine might have been abandoned early in their development if the researcher had to meet all of FDA's present regulations, and I fear that in some cases the answers might be yes.

So we have to strike a balance between regulations that make sense and that improve the public health and those that don't, between regulations that encourage innovation and those that inhibit it, between regulations designed to protect people and those designed to fulfill paperwork requirements, between those whose costs are justified and those that are not. To decide where to draw the line, let me assure you, is no easy task.

In my judgment, the system that now exists provides us with a good foundation--a good point of departure. The system works. We do have a safe and abundant and affordable food supply. Our drug supply and our medical devices are safe and effective. This is a tribute to the many men and women, not only in government but also in the private sector, who have dedicated their lives to making the system work.

Seventy-five years ago, when the first food and drug law was passed, it required essentially that foods and drugs be pure and honestly labeled. Today our society is more complex, more industrialized, and more sophisticated. Today we also are faced with rising costs, limited resources, and greater expectations than ever before. FDA is being asked to find more efficient and less costly ways to advance the health and safety of the American people.

I'd like to discuss with you this evening three initiatives that are intended to accomplish just that.

First, and this will be very brief, I want to report to you on an effort we are undertaking to review the regulations now on the books.

Secondly, I'd like to discuss what we are doing to try to bring more information to the public about the amount of sodium in the food supply, and how that relates to the treatment of hypertension.

And thirdly, I'd like to describe for you the steps I have taken to speed the review of new drugs and how that relates to the beta blockers and calcium antagonists.

On the regulations review, FDA now has about 3700 pages of regulations that impose requirements on products and the companies that make them and those that study them. These regulations range from telling how many eggs have to be in a product labeled as mayonnaise, to how many milliwatts of radiation a microwave oven can emit, to how to file a Freedom of Information request.

There has never been a comprehensive review of all these regulations to see whether they are effective and whether they are still serving their social purpose. And some of these regulations date back decades. FDA, along with other regulatory agencies, in response to the President's Executive Order on regulation, is now undertaking a massive review to evaluate these regulations.

My view is that a large number of these regulations will indeed be found to be useful. But some may not be, and we will modify or eliminate them. What I'd like to do is to create an atmosphere, a regulatory atmosphere, that provides protection to consumers and meets their expectations for safe and effective products, while at the same time provides maximum flexibility for companies not only to market their products as they see fit, but also to develop new products. Our society cannot permit the government to inhibit innovation.

My second topic is sodium, a subject that has interested me professionally for long time. Those of you who treat patients with hypertension know, as I do, the frustration of trying to keep people on a sodium-reduced diet. The variety of foods is limited, and it is difficult for people to know how much sodium is in many of the processed foods they eat.

We have launched a program whose goal is to expand the variety of low sodium foods available to hypertensive patients, and to label foods better as to sodium content.

I have met with the major manufacturers of processed foods to seek their voluntary cooperation. I believe that the best approach is to spell out for the companies what we are seeking, and to provide them the support and assistance they need. I have told them, though, that if we do not achieve voluntarily some measurable progress toward lower sodium foods and better labeling, then I will consider the need for a mandatory program.

To accomplish my goal, I need the support not only of the food processors but also of the health care community. We need to redouble our efforts to educate patients about the relationship between hypertension and sodium. We need to encourage further research into this disease, which affects as many as 60 million Americans. We as health professionals need to communicate to the food industry the urgency of our concerns.

I look forward to the day when Americans will be as conscious about their sodium intake as they are about their calorie intake, when restaurants will offer low sodium meals as well as low calorie meals, when hypertensive patients can shop intelligently for low sodium diets, and still have a wide variety of foods.

I believe that a voluntary approach to public health concerns like this-- rather than a heavy-handed regulatory approach--can work. I have learned in my brief time as Commissioner that many people in the private sector are willing to cooperate with the government on voluntary programs to improve the public health.

One very recent example that comes to mind is the agreement by Merrell Dow Pharmaceuticals to issue a voluntary patient package insert for Bendectin, the drug prescribed for pregnant women. The need for patient information was identified by one of our expert advisory committees and Merrell Dow just last month volunteered to produce a brochure for users of this drug. I was delighted by the spirit of cooperation that the company demonstrated, and am looking forward to similar responses from the food industry in the sodium area.

Let me move on now to the third area I'd like to discuss with you, the drug approval process. This has been the single most controversial subject I've had to deal with since becoming Commissioner.

The questions discussed at this symposium are a paradigm of the drug questions to be resolved by the FDA.

The 1962 Kefauver-Harris Drug Amendents and its attendant regulations began a new era in the FDA. Adequate and well-controlled clinical trials have revolutionized the approach of investigators to untried therapies. Today's physician can call on more rational drugs whose mechanisms of action are better understood, and whose labeling is more accurate than were the drugs of 20 years ago.

In that 20-year span, the technological revolution in science and medicine has changed the entire approach to new drug development. New ideas, new opportunities, new scientific understanding and expectations and new problems-- require new solutions. Doctors, patients, the pharmaceutical industry, and indeed the Congress all expect the drug approval standards, the regulatory procedures, and our drug policies to be in step with scientific advances. It makes sense that the entire drug approval procedures also need to be addressed in the light of criticism and the current movement for general regulatory reform.

I am committed now to the most thorough review of the intricate and complex details of the entire evaluation and approval process since the 1962 Amendments.

I start with a fundamental premise, that the general standard for drugs in this country is essentially sound and well-reasoned. As physicians, we must insist that all drugs be shown, through scientific evidence, to be safe and effective. Our modern scientific capabilities necessarily make the drug development process longer. But we cannot sacrifice good science in our efforts to save time. We cannot tolerate the sale of second-rate drugs. The consequences to our medical system and to the public would be devastating.

I believe also that FDA's role goes beyond simply preventing the sale of unsafe or ineffective drugs. We are part of the Public Health Service. The mission of this organization is disease prevention and health promotion. Obviously, making new drugs readily available is also an important constituent of that worthy goal.

Drugs can alleviate and cure diseases that once disabled or killed millions. The potential for new treatments is unlimited. I believe that FDA has an important role to play as an Agency to promote the public health. That includes doing whatever is needed to encourage the marketing of better medicines.

I must say that this idea is not new to FDA since my arrival. In fact, I found when I arrived at FDA this past spring that several improvements had already been made in this drug approval process.

For example several years ago the Agency established a priority review system for important new drugs. Any drug that represents a significant therapeutic advance is reviewed with priority attention.

And the Agency has established a comprehensive advisory system through which outside medical experts provide advice on the study and approval of new drugs.

FDA also has developed, with the help of the scientific community and industry, guidelines on how to design studies to test 28 classes of drugs in humans.

The most significant effort was the establishment in 1979 of an internal working group to redraft the drug approval regulations. I am now reviewing the recommendations of this group and in the coming months we will propose changes to streamline the system significantly. One specific goal is to reduce the enormous paperwork burden on industry.

Since I've become Commissioner, there have been several important initiatives in this direction.

Two Congressmen, James Scheuer of New York and Albert Gore of Tennessee, have formed a commission to study the drug development and approval process. The chairman of this commission is Dr. Gilbert McMahon of the Tulane Medical School. FDA is working closely with this commission to provide information and assistance.

And I have established my own task force, which I chair, whose mission is to look beyond the process itself and to study the legislation policies and management systems that have formulated the present drug development system. We will take a fresh look at the entire system from beginning to end. Among the many issues we will look at are FDA's criteria to approve new drugs, the use of foreign data and how best to use advisory committees.

Let me make clear that this effort is designed to speed the review and approval of new drugs. That doesn't automatically mean that it will hasten the approval of a specific drug. A new drug can be approved only when there is clear and, in the language of the law, "substantial evidence of safety and effectiveness." By law we cannot approve drugs before that evidence is available.

The process of gathering and reviewing that evidence can be extremely complex. As an example, consider the regulatory history of the two classes of drugs that are the subject of this symposium. FDA's review of the beta blockers and calcium antagonists has been a cause celebre for Agency critics. The Agency's role in the development of these drugs does, in fact, raise important questions of regulatory policy.

When I came to FDA last spring, I set about to satisfy my curiosity on the history of these drugs. I'd like to share with you the story from FDA's standpoint.

The first beta blocker, propranolol, was approved in this country in 1967.

But it was not until 1978 that the major indications for beta blockers--angina and hypertension--were not approved until 1973 and 1976, respectively.

The long interval between beta blockers was, to a large degree, the result of FDA's "beta blocker policy," formulated in 1972. That policy required that any beta blocker would have to undergo complete carcinogenicity testing in two species to determine that the drug was not carcinogenic before human studies of more than 30 days duration could begin. Planning and conduction two 20-year carcinogenicity studies is usually a three-year undertaking. So there is no denying that the Agency's policy had considerable effect on the development of new beta blockers.

FDA believed there were serious grounds for concern at the time: One beta blocker--pronethalol--was clearly carcinogenic. And two others--alprenolol and practolol--looked like they might have a similar problem, although the data were less definitive. So it appeared there might be a general tendency of beta blockers to be tumerogenic.

FDA's concern was shared by two special outside advisory committees. In fact, their recommendatioins formed the basis of FDA's beta blocker policy, which resulted from what appear to be legitimate and reasonable health concerns.

After the policy was announced in 1972, no new applications for these drugs were received until late 1976, when Ciba-Geigy filed for approval of metoprolol. Safety and efficacy were documented by the results of many excellent controlled trials, all but two of which, incidentally, were conducted outside the United States. Approval was granted in 1978.

Since then, nadolol and atenolol have also been approved. The atenolol approval relied heavily on data from European studies. Timolol and pindolol are currently in the late stages of review. Timolol, of course, has laid claim to its own indication--prevention of post-infarction death. This is obviously an exciting development, if the claim is substantiated by the data.

FDA's beta blocker policy has succeeded in identifying two beta blockers that were carcinogenic before there was significant exposure to them in this country.

There is no question that this discovery was a benefit. But it now appears that, while certain individual beta blockers have a tendency toward carcinogenicity, these drugs as a class do not. We therefore need to consider whether the drugs should continue to be treated differently from other drugs in this regard.

What has been the cost of FDA's beta blocker policy, in terms of new drug development? I think it would be difficult to contend that any of the beta blockers represent a major therapeutic advance over the original, but there are some minor advantages. For example, cardioselective beta blockers may permit treatment of patients with accompanying bronchospastic disease, and they also seem to offer advantages in diabetics. And the longer half-life agents may prove more effective in single daily doses for angina. But most of the pharmacologic differences remain unexplored; teasers to the clinician with--as yet--thin back-up data.

Even fewer answers are available on the other group of cardiovascular drugs of major interest--the calcium antagonists. The literature is finally beginning to include reports of controlled trials of these agents and some applications are in the review process. But their ultimate role in therapy, their advantages over alternatives, and the differences among individual calcium antagonists are yet to be determined.

I know FDA has received a lot of "bad press" because of a perceived delay in approving these drugs. And you may share those views. But the fact is that calcium antagonists have come to FDA for approval only recently, and even then, the accompanying data have been incomplete.

For example, the original owner of nifedipine--Delbay--never conducted clinical trials on the drug, so far as we know. Pfizer--the present owner and the moving force behind the studies we do now have--took over the IND in mid-1978. Notable activity on verapamil and diltiazem began at about that time.

The nifedipine application was submitted in April 1980, but it included almost no long-term data for any use, and no controlled trials on vasospastic angina. About half of the 500 patients treated had received the drug for just one day. Since then, there have been many major additions to the nifedipine application, including extensive safety data submitted this past July.

Applications for verapamil and diltiazem came to FDA in February of this year, but a great deal of essential data were not available until this past several months that our reviewers have been getting the kind of data they need to review these drugs adequately.

It remains to be sen how important the calcium antagonists really are, though I remain optimistic about them. Whether they will prove more effective than beta blockers for exertional angina is unknown, but the side effects are clearly different, perhaps representing a gain over the beta blockers in some circumstances.

In vasospastic angina, there have been few comparisons with adequate doses of organic nitrates, and at least one study has showed no difference between nifedipine and isosorbide. Whether this is actually the case can only be determined through additional study.

Those of you in this audience whose work has contributed to a better understanding of the beta blockers and the calcium antagonists merit recognition.

But, as you can see, the review process is indeed complex, especially when it must try to keep pace with emerging technologies such as the beta blockers and calcium antagonists. And this is precisely why we must devote continued attention to the task of improving the drug review system.

In developing the needed changes, we will solicit ideas from industry, from academia, from the professions and from anyone who has constructive

suggestions. We already have formally requested the opinion of members of

Institutional Review Boards and others on what role IRBs should play in regulating

the early phases of drug research. I want to learn directly from those who work

every day with these issues whether IRBs are capable of taking on more

responsibility for early clinical research, and whether they're interested. I

welcome, indeed need, your comments on this.

Another area of focus will be the so-called orphan drugs. These are drugs

that are of little commercial interest, either because they are for relatively rare

diseases or because they cannot be patented. The Pharmaceutical Manufacturers

Association has formed a commission to study ways to bring these drugs to market

and I have pledged FDA's assistance to that commission in anyway possible.

Drug evaluation carries with it the dual responsibility of protecting the

public from drugs that are unsafe or ineffective, while at the same time assuring

that drugs that offer significant therapeutic gains are identified and brought to

market as quickly as possible.

In this country, as in much of the world, the pharmaceutical industry and

the academic scientific community share the responsibility for rational drug

development. The responsibility for performing good studies and from submitting

the data promptly rests with the private sector. And I must tell you that the

quality of the applications we receive remains the single most important factor

influencing the speed of review and approval of new drugs.

As the regulator, FDA has a responsiblity to make its requirements clear,

to review the data carefully, and to conduct this review efficiently and in the

public interest. This is our goal. The task is not an easy one. We have made

progress. And we will make more.

In undertaking this assignment I have been fortunate to have available to

me a large number of people from the health professions who have willingly given me their time and their thoughts and their ideas and their commitment. I have come to appreciate the need for open and continuous communications between FDA and its constituencies, one of the most important of which is the health professions.

I want you to knw that I meet regularly in Washington and other cities with representatives of organizations representing health professionals. This includes not only organizations like the AMA but also speciality organizations. I value highly my opportunities to meet with them. These meetings give me a chance to bounce some ideas off them and also to get a sense of what my colleagues in the health professions think about certain issues, not after they've been decided, but while they're very much under discussion.

All of us as health professionals--no matter where we work--share common goals. We want the best care for patients. We want to keep costs down. We want patients exposed only to safe and effective drugs and medical devices.

For us at FDA to do the work that we are assigned we need the support of people like you. FDA is, I believe, an integral part of the health care chain in this country. It is up to all of us to make sure that every link in that chain is strong.

Thank you.

BETA BLOCKER IN SUDDEN DEATH PREVENTION

JAMES A. SCHOENBERGER, M.D., MODERATOR

The support of biomedical research is a societal responsibility of the highest order. Unfortunately, in today's world, this view is not shared by all, and there is a serious challenge to the continuing financial committment to permit the level of research to expand as new opportunities present themselves. In the United States, taking into account the erosion of support by inflation, the amount available to research and training of young investigators has been reduced to alarming levels. New ways must be sought to increase the level of research support, particularly that research which tests the applied value of therapeutic procedures such as the pharmacologic treatment of disease.

Since pharmacologic manufacturers stand to gain from such research when it proves the value of any drug treatment, they should be permitted to become active financial partners with other concerned groups such as the government and voluntary health agencies in support of research. Certain safeguards should be established, if such a cooperative partnership is to maintain rigorous scientific integrity. Among these safeguards are:

1.   The research data must be obtained by a precise protocol adhered to by all investigators involved in the study.

2.   In multicenter studies, the data should be collected by an independent, free standing, coordinating center, and analyses should be carried out by standard biostatistical techniques.

3.   Endpoints of the study should be adjudicated by an independent, blinded group of qualified investigators.

4.   A review committee consisting of qualified investigators with no interest or active participation in the trial should review the data periodically for safety and effectiveness, and should have binding power to alter the study or terminate it if necessary.

DO BETA-BLOCKERS PROLONG LIFE?

LARS WERKÖ

The question posed in the title of my talk has not really been
answered. It has, however, been approached in a number of studies in
patients who have had an acute myocardial infarction. From some of
these studies a tentative answer might be that in some patients with
an acute infarction decreased mortality and morbidity has followed
treatment with some β-adrenergic blocking agents, namely alprenolol,
practolol, timolol, and metoprolol. Whether this is true also for
other β-blockers and for all patients with myocardial infarction is
still open to doubt. An important question requiring further studies
is whether this decreased mortality following the acute heart attack
will mean a decreased cardiac death rate also in patients with angina
or high blood pressure treated with the same β-blockers already befcre
they developed an acute myocardial event.

Already soon after the emergence of the β-adrenergic blocking drugs it
was suggested that they might protect the heart and cardiovascular
system from excessive adrenergic influences. Some open studies on the
effect of propranolol in patients with acute myocardial damage gave,
however, conflicting results. The small but well controlled study of
alprenolol in patients up to two years after an acute myocardial
infarction showed a significant reduction of mortality (Fig 1). This
was followed by similar positive results in the larger multicenter
practolol study. Encouraged by these results a large number of studies
have been started. The results have, so far, been variable and many
studies have been terminated prematurely because of negative results.
Table 1.

234

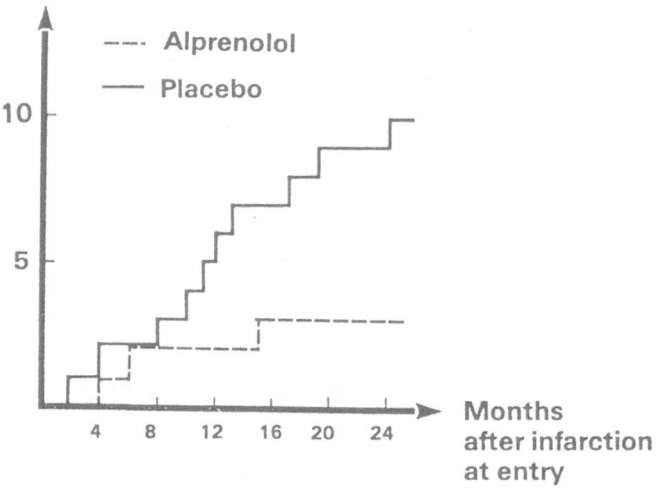

Fig 1 Cumulative number of deaths in the alprenolol study.
(Wilhelmsson et al, 1974)

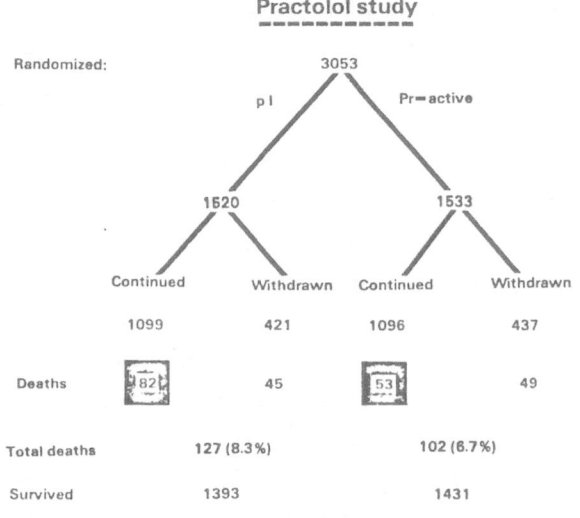

Fig 2 Number of patients, randomization and outcome of the
large multicenter practolol study (Barber et al 1975).

PROSPECTIVE STUDIES

Drug	No of patients	Start after AMI	Duration	Total death pl / active		Authors
PROPRANOLOL 20 mg x 4	454	Day 1	3 wks	24	31	Norris et al (1968)
ALPRENOLOL 100 mg x 4	87	Day 1	1 yr	3	3	Reynolds & Whitlock (1972)
ALPRENOLOL 200 mg x 2	230	4 wks	2 yrs	14	7	Wilhelmsson et al (1974)
ALPRENOLOL 100 mg x 4	162	3 wks	2 yrs	11	5'	Ahlmark et al (1974)
PRACTOLOL 200 mg x 2	3053 (2282)	2 wks	14 mts	124 (83	96 54)·	Multicenter Int Study (1975, 1977)
PRACTOLOL 300 mg x 2	298	Day 1	2 yrs	46	41	Barber et al (1975)
ALPRENOLOL 200 mg x 2	282	Day 1	1 yr	29	13	Andersen et al (1979)
	198	Day 1	1 yr	35	48	
ATENOLOL 50 mg x 2	388	Day 1	1 yr		19	Wilcox et al (1980 a)
				19		
PROPRANOLOL 40 mg x 3					17	
OXPRENOLOL 40 mg x 3	315	Day 1	6 wks	10	14	Wilcox et al (1980 b)
PROPRANOLOL 40 mg x 3	720	1 week	6 mts (3-9)	27	28	Baber et al (1980)
TIMOLOL 10 mg x 2	1884	1-4 wks	17 mts (12-33)	152	98	The Norwegian Multicenter Study (1981)
METOPROLOL 1395	Day 1	3 mts	62	40		Hjalmarson et al (1981)

Table 1: Prospective studies of the influence of beta-blockers on
the mortality after an acute myocardial infarction (AMI).
Many are negative but have been too small or been terminated
prematurely.

During 1981 two important large well controlled, double-blind studies
have been reported, one of them studying the effect of timolol in
patients 1-24 months after the acute attack (Fig 3), the other using
metoprolol from the first day until 3 months after the acute event
(Fig 4). Both these studies have clearly demonstrated decreased
mortality and morbidity in the patients treated with active drug
compared to placebo.

Nevertheless the reports of these trials will certainly be scrutinized
in depth before the results are generally accepted. The Norwegian trial
reported in April 1981 has already been the object of many comments,
most of them rather positive but some clearly critical. The Swedish
study published this month has not yet been looked at in the same
searching fashion but will certainly also be discussed in a similar
critical vein. The importance of such a critical analysis immediately
after the results of clinical trials of treatment of patients with
acute myocardial infarction have been published is obvious to all
cardiologists who have seen the rise and fall of many new ways of
treatment of coronary heart disease.

Clinical intervention trials in patients with acute myocardial
infarction have always been particularly difficult. This has been the
case whether the intervention has aimed at anti-thrombotic therapy,
treatment of arrhythmias, blood lipid lowering measures of interference
with patelet aggregation. It has also been the case whether the trial
has encompassed patients with a heart attack during the acute phase or
the treatment or secondary prevention has been aimed at patients after
such an acute episode. This has led to marked differences of opinion
between different clinicians regarding the value of any or all of these
ways of treating a patient who has just experienced an acute myocardial
infarction.

Anti-thrombotic therapy, anti-arrhythmic treatment, blood lipid lowering
measures or interference with platelet aggregation have thus all been
advocated based on insufficient data, been favoured by some, criticized

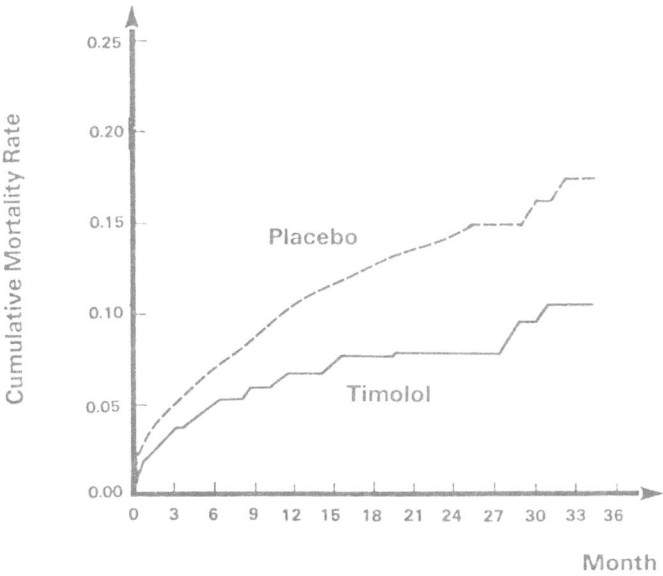

Fig 3a   Cumulative mortality in the timolol study.
Number of patients and randomization.

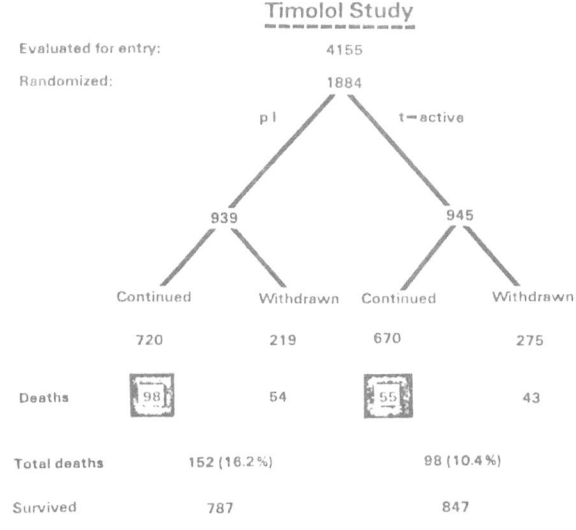

Fig 3b   Outcome of the timolol study.
(Norwegian multicenter study group 1981)

238

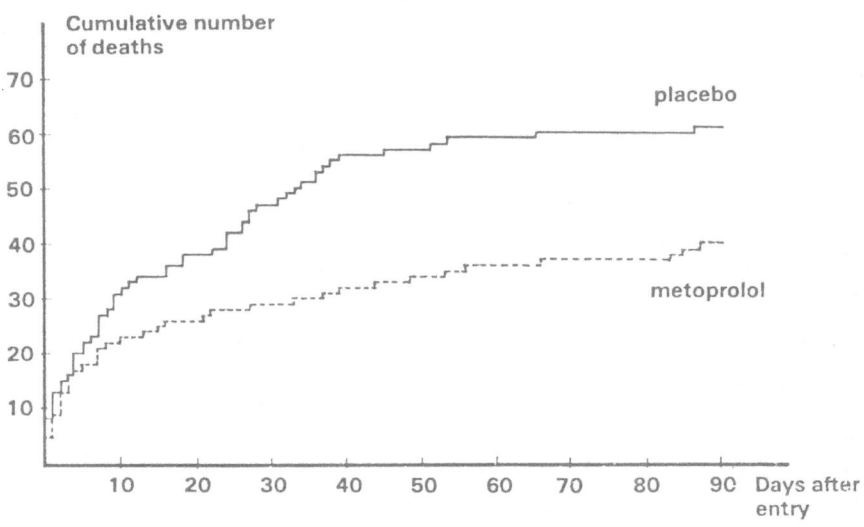

Fig 4a Cumulative number of deaths in the metoprolol study.
        Number of patients and randomization.

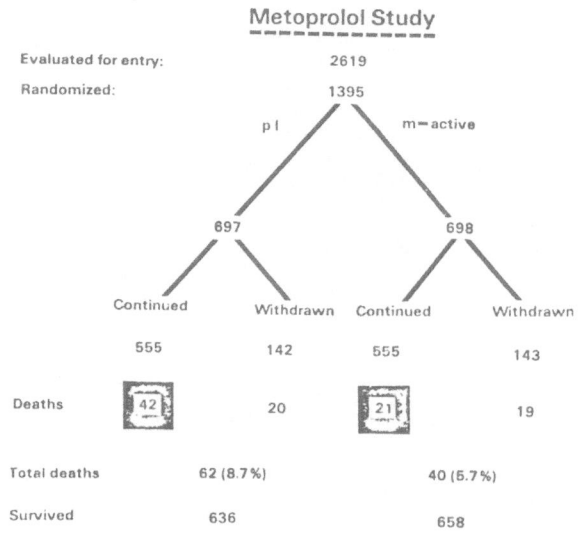

Fig 4b Outcome of the metoprolol study.
        (Hjalmarson et al 1981)

by some and finally discarded by most as not scientifically supported by the data at hand.

There are, however, special problems doing clinical trials with β-adrenergic blocking agents in patients with myocardial infarction. Some of them are due to the properties of this class of medicines, some of them are due to the complexity of the clinical disorder.

The rather wide-spread pharmacological action of β-blockers leading to unwanted adverse reactions and all the contraindications to β-adrenergic blockers require that many patients must be excluded from the trial from its start. Several patients will also drop out during the trial. Another confounding effect is that it is virtually impossible to conduct a perfectly double-blinded study as the pulse lowering effect of the active drug usually will show up and may be noted by the trialists. As there by now are rather firm indications of a beneficial effect of β-blockers in many cardiovascular disorders, this may lead some clinicians to misuse the protocol with a devastating effect to the results of the trial.

Earlier studies with β-adrenergic blockers have consequently suffered the same or similar inadequacies as other intervention trials. The two most recent ones seem to have been able to overcome these inherent difficulties. They may give more adequate guidance both regarding the treatment of the post-infarction patient and the proper design of a trial after an acute myocardial infarction.

As to the complexity of the disease to be treated - acute myocardial infarction and several of its sequels - it may suffice to point out the varying patho-anatomic picture, the varying background factors, and the lack of strict correlation of any of these to the clinical picture of the disorder.

Some of the special problems inherent in studies of post-infarction patients are thus due to the circumstance that acute myocardial infarction is not a simple disease entity lending itself to easy standardization. The pathological process in the coronary arteries

may be different and may be extremely varying in extent. The same may
be said for the extent, localization and evolution of the myocardial
damage. The background factors of importance for the disorder may be
different and may also play a different role in the two sexes and at
different ages.

As it is impossible to stratify the clinical series for all such
differences it will be necessary to have a large clinical series,
uniformly studied and analysed in a way to minimize the inequalities in
treated and control series. This was pointed out by Mitchell regarding
the Norwegian timolol trial where treatment was started 7 to 28 days
after the acute attack in 1884 patients, 945 taking timolol and 939
placebo. This large series of patients with confirmed myocardial
infarction from a catchment area of 1.3 million inhabitants was
randomized and "the differences between the treatment groups at entry
tended to be small". Notwithstanding the trialists efforts and comments
Mitchell points out that the placebo group was significantly older, had
more previous hypertension, more previous diuretic treatment, more heart
failure and cardiomegaly, and more arrhythmias during the index event,
all factors of importance for the long-term prognosis. The authors have
tried to address this problem by adjusting for the largest differences
and other factors considered to be prognostically important and claim
that it does not influence the results. This has not stopped Mitchell
from putting question marks on the study. On the other hand, in the
Swedish metoprolol trial, the patients on active drug were slightly
worse off regarding prognostic indices than the placebo patients. Even
so the ideal trial ought to contain so many patients that randomizing
should create two groups of exactly the same prognostic profile.

The two Scandinavian studies do not cover exactly the same time period
after the acute myocardial event. They were independently planned and
conducted and fill thus almost completely the requirements put forward
by Sheila Gore, statistician to the British MRC when she discussed
supportive evidence. The very close results of these trials in a
Norwegian and a Swedish population sample re-inforces the positive outcome to a considerable degree. In a way the Swedish study thus answers

new set of questions that Mitchell wanted to ask after reviewing the data of the Norwegian.

Studies started by and sponsored by a pharmaceutical company are also the target for special criticisms. There is thus a widespread belief that any data "controlled and analysed" by a pharmaceutical manufacturer must by itself be doubtful. It is quite clear that a pharmaceutical manufacturer has a commercial interest to promote his products. This does not have to mean, however, that he is more biased than any of the academic clinicians who may have their reputation at stake when the results of large studies do not confirm with their stated beliefs. The USDGP was not sponsored by any industry, but by official and academic institutions (and scientists working there). It is still the most obvious large scale trial of the efficacy of certain treatments where lack of clinical judgement and biased interpretations of results have led to more confusion than clarity. This does not mean that some companies and especially if working together with clinicians willing and eager to promote a certain theory of their own have not overextended their data and tried to prove results that the data at closer scrutiny do not support. When analysing results from large scale clinical trials it should be done only on the merits of the data, not against the background biased of who produced the data.

All these problems regarding past and present studies of β-blockers necessitate an unusual stringent protocol for the trial. They require an absolute adherence to the details of the agreed protocol, which is notoriously difficult in multicenter studies. It is thus necessary that participating centers are selected with utmost care, that the study is closely monitored at each center with frequent and irregular visits and that the analysis of the results take into consideration the problems mentioned.

The analysis of the results of a clinical trial should comprise all patients selected with the intention to treat, and not only those completing the trial,

- the patient series should be large enough to get two really comparable series of patients;

242

ON-GOING PROSPECTIVE TRIALS WITH BETA-BLOCKERS AFTER AMI

Center	Drug	No of pts	Duration
Multicenter France	ACEBUTOLOL	550	1 year
Belfast North Ireland	METOPROLOL	400	2 years
Stockholm Sweden	METOPROLOL	250	2 years
Amsterdam Netherlands	METOPROLOL	600	1 year
Multicenter USA	METOPROLOL	3000	1 year
Multicenter Europe	OXPRENOLOL	4000	1 year
Multicenter USA	PROPRANOLOL	4200	1 year
Multicenter Norway	PROPRANOLOL	800	1 year
Multicenter	PINDOLOL	700	1 year
Multicenter England	SOTALOL	1600	1 year
		16100	

Table_2: Ongoing trials with beta-blockers after an acute myocardial infarction.

- the end points should be defined in an unambiguous manner
  before the study starts;

- both total death rate as well as cardiac death rates should
  be analysed;

- all clinical conditions of importance for selection and
  analysis, such as angina and myocardial infarction, should
  be well defined beforehand, and

- the length of study and number of patients should be
  determined at the start and adhered to.

Such rigid criteria may be considered to be close to impossible to use.
What may be important is also that they may be a far cry from the
ordinary clinical appearance of patients with various cardiovascular
disorders and pain in the chest. It is, however, dangerous to
compromise on them beforehand. The Norwegian timolol trial and the
Swedish metoprolol trial have demonstrated that it is possible to use
such rigid rules. They should thus be reinforced in the analysis of
the many contemporary studies aiming at changing the mortality or
morbidity after an acute myocardial infarction, or at preventing such
an event.   (Table 2)

It may very well be necessary that a close cooperation should be
created between governmental agencies and/or institutes, university
departments and the pharmaceutical industry to be able to recruite
the large resources needed for studies like these. It may also be
outside the possibilities of any one of these interested parties to
conduct such a study by themselves. How a cooperation should be
organized ought to be seriously discussed, and why not here?

REFERENCES

Ahlmark G, Saetre H & Korsgren M: Letter: Reduction of sudden deaths
    after myocardial infarction. Lancet 2: 1563, 1974.

Andersen MP, Bechsgaard P, Frederiksen J, Hansen DA, Jürgensen HJ,
    Nielsen B, Pedersen F, Pedersen-Bjergaard O & Rasmussen SL:
    Effect of alprenolol on mortality among patients with definite
    or suspected acute myocardial infarction. Lancet 2: 865, 1979.

Baber NS, Wainwright Evans D, Howitt G, Thomas M, Wilson C, Lewis JA, Dawes PM, Handler K & Tuson R: Multicentre postinfarction trial of propranolol in 49 hospitals in the United Kingdom, Italy and Yugoslavia. Br Heart J 44: 96, 1980.

Balcon R, Jewitt DE, Davies JPH & Oram S: A controlled trial of propranolol in acute myocardial infarction. Lancet 2: 917, 1966.

Barber JM, Murphy FM & Merrett JD: Clinical trial of propranolol in acute myocardial infarction. Ulster Med J 36: 127, 1967.

Barber JM, Boyle D McC, Chaturvedi NC, Singh N & Walsh MJ: Practolol in acute myocardial infarction. Acta Med Scand, Suppl 587: 213, 1975.

Briant RB & Norris RM: Alprenolol in acute myocardial infarction, a double-blind trial. NZ Med J 71: 135, 1970.

Clausen J, Felsby M, Schönau Jörgensen F, Lyager Nielsen B, Roin J & Strange B: Absence of prophylactic effect of propranolol in myocardial infarction. Lancet 2: 920, 1966.

Gore SM: Assessing methods - art of significance testing. Brit Med J 1981, 283, 600.

Hjalmarson Å: Myocardial metabolic changes related to ventricular fibrillation. Cardiology 65: 266, 1980.

Hjalmarson Å, Ariniego R, Herlitz J, Holmberg S, Málek I, Svedberg K, Waagstein F, Waldenström A, Waldenström J, Vedin A, Wilhelmsen L & Wilhelmsson C: Limitation of infarct size in man by the beta$_1$-blocker metoprolol. Circulation 60, Suppl II: 164, 1979 (Abstract).

Hjalmarson Å: Betablocker. Current status in prevention of sudden coronary death. N Y Acad of Science, May 1981 (to be published).

Hjalmarson Å, Elmfeldt D, Herlitz J et al: A double-blind trial of metoprolol in acute myocardial infarction. Effect on mortality. Lancet 1981.

Lambert DMD: Hypertension and myocardial infarction. Br Med J 3: 685, 1974 (Abstract).

Mitchell JRA: Timolol after myocardial infarction: An Answer or a new set of questions? Br Med J 1981, 282, 1565.

Multicentre International Study: Improvement in prognosis of myocardial infarction by long-term beta-adrenoceptor blockade using practolol. Br Med J 3: 735, 1975.

Multicentre International Study: supplementary report: Reduction in mortality after myocardial infarction with long-term beta-adrenoceptor blockade. Br Med J 2: 419, 1977.

Multicentre Trial: Propranolol in acute myocardial infarction. Lancet 2: 1435, 1966.

Norris RM, Caughey DE & Scott PJ: Trial of propranolol in acute
    myocardial infarction. Br Med J 2: 398, 1968.

Norwegian Multicenter Study Group: Timolol-induced reduction in
    mortality and reinfarction in patients surviving acute myocardial
    infarction. N Engl J Med 304: 801, 1981.

Reynolds JL & Whitlock RML: Effects of a beta-adrenergic receptor
    blocker in myocardial infarction treated for one year from onset.
    Br Heart J 34: 252, 1972.

Romo M: Factors related to sudden death in acute ischaemic disease.
    Acta Med Scand, Suppl 547: 1, 1973.

Sleight P: Beta-adrenergic blockade after myocardial infarction
    (editorial). N Engl J of Med 1981, 304, 837.

Snow PJD: Effect of propranolol in myocardial infarction.
    Lancet 2: 551, 1965.

Thaulow E: The effect of timolol on platelet aggregation in coronary
    heart disease. In: Symposium on Acute and Long-term Management of
    Myocardial Ischemia, Oslo April 3-5, 1981 (to be published).

Vedin JA, Wilhelmsson C, Bolander AM & Werkö L: Mortality trends in
    Sweden 1951-1968 with special reference to cardiovascular cause of
    death. Acta Med Scand, Suppl 515: 1, 1971.

Waagstein F & Hjalmarson ÅC: Effect of cardioselective beta-blockade on
    heart function and chest pain in acute myocardial infarction.
    Acta Med Scand, Suppl 587: 193, 1975a.

Waagstein F & Hjalmarson ÅC: Double-blind study of the effect of
    cardioselective beta-blockade on chest pain in acute myocardial
    infarction. Acta Med Scand, Suppl 587: 201, 1975b.

Wilcox RG, Roland JM, Banks DC, Hampton JR & Mitchell JRA: Randomized
    trial comparing propranolol with atenolol in immediate treatment of
    suspected myocardial infarction. Br Med J 280: 885, 1980a.

Wilcox RG, Rowley JM, Hampton JR & Mitchell JRA: Randomized placebo
    controlled trial comparing oxprenolol with disopyram phosphate in
    immediate treatment of suspected myocardial infarction.
    Lancet 2: 765, 1980b.

Wilhelmsson C, Vedin JA, Wilhelmsen L, Tibblin G & Werkö L: Reduction
    of sudden deaths after myocardial infarction by treatment with
    alprenolol. Preliminary results. Lancet 2: 1157, 1974.

Editorial: Beta-blocker after myocardial infarction. Lancet 1981, 1,
    873.

Clinical Trials to Prevent Sudden Death: What are the Problems in Study Design?

Stewart J. Ehrreich, Ph.D., Philip L. Dern, M.D., Mary Johnson, Ph.D.

INTRODUCTION

The clinical trial is the most definitive tool for evaluating the efficacy and safety of beta-blockers in preventing sudden death among post-infarction patients. Since these intervention trials necessarily involve large-scale data collection and long-term patient follow-up, the need for proper planning is especially critical. It is necessary to insure that the time, effort and expense will yield valid results that will ultimately withstand the close scrutiny of the scientific community. Factors influencing the conduct of a trial and the interpretation of results may be subtle and difficult to anticipate in the design stage. Nevertheless, general principles of trial design combined with the experience from previous beta-blocker trials should serve as a useful guide. Our discussion today will focus on some of the problems which have arisen in the design of beta-blocker trials and what their implications are for future studies.

Sample size estimation and recruitment potential:

First, the size of the study and the recruitment potential of participating clinics are major factors to be considered in the planning phase. Many trials which do not carefully consider sample size requirements turn out to lack the power or ability to detect

drug effects of fairly substantial magnitude and clinical importance.
Methods for estimating sample size in follow-up studies are available
(with corrections for drop-outs and drop-ins) and these are based on
preliminary estimates of the event rates from previous experience.
If faulty estimates are used it is clear that errors in the sample
requirement will occur with a consequent difficulty in establishing
statistically significant study treatment effects. Likewise,
unrealistic expectations regarding the ability of the clinical
centers to actually recruit subjects, given all the eligibility
requirements which must be met, may lead to difficulty in achieving
sufficient numbers to establish significant effects.

Examples of problems related to sample size may be found in
previous clinical trials with beta blockers (See table I). In the
multicenter post-infarction trial of propranolol reported by Barber
etal (1) 1,000 subjects were apparently thought to be required for
each of 2 treatment groups, in order to give adequate power to detect
a 50% reduction in 3 month mortality (from 4% in the placebo group to
2% in the propranolol group). This assumed reduction was based on
the earlier practolol trial results (2). In fact, only 720 patients
were entered into the trial; 95% confidence limits on the observed
treatment difference showed that a reduction in mortality as large as
50% could not be determined by results of this small trial. Another
example may be found in the Practolol Multicenter Trial reported by
Green etal, (2). The estimated number of patients needed was based
on the assumption that the mortality rate over the first year in the
placebo group would be about 8%, that half of these deaths would be
sudden and that practolol would reduce these by half giving a total

mortality reduction of 25%. A target of 2,000 patients was planned
for each group, allowing for drop-outs. In actuality, the trial had
to be terminated prematurely because of literature reports citing
serious adverse reactions with long-term practolol use. About 1,000
fewer patients were recruited and less than 2,000 patients total had
been followed 12 months.

Despite this failure to achieve the required sample size, the
group difference in mortality turned out to be 33% instead of 25% as
originally postulated, and significant results emerged from the trial.

For beta blocker trials, actual availability of suitable patients
with MIs who are willing to participate will often preclude any
efforts to establish short-term or long-term recruitment goals.
Preliminary ("pilot") studies might be used to estimate actual
accrual rates in the study centers. However, under the pressure to
get on with the trial itself, enthusiasm for such pre-trial estimates
may be limited. Unfortunately, some studies deal with lagging
recruitment by accepting a smaller number of subjects than originally
planned or by relaxing the inclusion criteria. A preferred solution
to recruitment problems would be to extend the time for recruitment
or, in multicenter studies, to add recruiting centers. These require
neither modification of admission criteria or diminution of power.
Addition of more clinics (if recruitment lags) often means less
involvement of principal investigators in formulation of trial policy
and presents a risk that protocol procedures may not be uniformly

followed and that problems in pooling results may occur.

The most reasonable approach to insure adequate patient numbers is to maintain strict scientific criteria in obtaining pre-trial estimates of sample requirements and ability to recruit, and to view this preliminary work as an integral part of the trial design itself.

Endpoint (response variable) specifications

In a sudden death protocol, the end-point would seem rather simple to define, but recent analysis of the Anturane study indicates the pitfalls in the "obvious" sudden death endpoint (3). Some trials have equated "death in less than 24 hours after onset of symptoms" with sudden death and then have simply presented findings for intervals of 1 hour, 2 hours, 2-12 hours, 12-24 hours (2). A trial with a goal of testing an hypothesis regarding the mechanism of the primary response variable, sudden death, would ideally use a more restrictive endpoint that incorporates the mechanism. A particular problem with the endpoint "sudden death" is in the documentation of associated phenomena such as "myocardial infarction, which have criteria that are considerably more complex than those for "death" alone. The clinical diagnoses may be incomplete in subjects withdrawn or in those dying unobserved, and autopsy rates even for subjects not withdrawn may be low.

Patient eligibility and treatment selection

The selection of a target population and details of the treatment regimen are other potential problems in designing a beta-blocker trial. The study population should be carefully defined in the protocol and correspond to unambiguous eligibility criteria that can be uniformly applied. The impact that inclusion and exclusion criteria will have on study design, ability to generalize, and subject recruitment must be taken into account. It must be kept in mind that the study population is the subset of the general population defined by the eligibility criteria. As previously noted, when such subjects are actually sought, few may be found. In addition, the entry criteria themselves may be incompatible with each other in subtle ways that may only be noted as the trial progresses. A good case can be made for a pre-trial application of the criteria to judge their usefulness in a smaller sample of patients.

In the case of published reports (Table I) on possible prevention of sudden death by beta blockers, the general class of patients included those who:

(A) Were positively diagnosed as having had a myocardial infarction through the existence of "very probable" ECG changes defined by W.H.O.

(B) Exhibited serum enzyme levels (SGOT,LDH) at least twice the accepted upper normal limit for the hospital laboratory concerned for LDH and at least three times for CPK.

Variations on these eligibility criteria were seen in each of the clinical studies. The generalizability of findings is thus specific for each trial and depends on how well the entrance criteria were defined and applied.

Patients were treated at different times after onset of myocardial infarction in the various beta blocker studies (1-4 weeks). This therefore provides a potentially serious problem in generalizing results of each study. Obviously, the immediate post

M.I. period is critical in terms of the potential for early arrhythmia (or fatal arrhythmia) development. A <u>beta</u> blocking agent may be particularly important in the prevention of such attacks and early intervention with drug at the proper dose level and treatment schedule could be paramount. Alternatively, early treatment could be ineffective or deleterious. If, however, prevention of a second M.I. or sudden death is a metabolic, vascular or other delayed phenomenon, not amenable to the electrophysiological effects of the drug, it is conceivable that even delayed treatment would be of benefit.

While usually not discussed in depth, the <u>dose</u> of <u>beta</u> blockers together with the proper <u>interval</u> between doses may be a very critical choice in study design. While earlier studies may show the average dosage required to produce a given level of <u>beta</u> blockade, what sort of dose would be best suited to prevent sudden death? Similarly, would 120 mg/day of propranolol (1) be enough?

It would be unfair to attribute the inconclusive nature of some of these trials to inappropriate selection of drug treatment given the state of knowledge at the time they were initiated. Nevertheless the outcome of a study taking thousands of patients and several years work, not to mention the enormous cost, could potentially depend upon such variables.

Blinding

Assurance of the "double blindness" of long term trials with drugs such as <u>beta</u> blockers, is also a worrisome problem. This difficulty has already been discussed by Mitchell (4) and others (5).

Patients taking adequate doses of <u>beta</u> blockers usually exhibit a bradycardia within several days of dosing. Indeed, the physician

might question the adequacy of therapy should no cardiac slowing
occur.

While this is not generally recognized by all patients it
certainly would be discovered by the health professional making the
periodic clinical examinations. Thus the blindness of the study
would be difficult to protect. Although this may not directly
influence the frequency of arrhythmia, second infarction or death,
the possibilities for bias introduced by differences in patient
management are considerable. The use of observers blind to pulse
rate would be a conventional suggestion perhaps worth considering if
back up "safety valve" could be assured to maintain a standard of
medical care.

Post Randomization Phenomena

A. Withdrawals

The approach to patients who withdraw from a study also presents
a problem in the design of beta-blocker trials. Since many patients
drop-out of these trials for drug-related reasons (e.g. bradycardia),
there is the potential for bias in assessing the drug's effect on
mortality in only those patients who tolerate the drug well enough to
remain on study. The protocol should address this issue both in
terms of the planned analysis and planned efforts for data
collection. For example, the design of the Blocadren trial (6)
called for complete ascertainment of deaths among all randomized
patients, regardless of withdrawal status. With this information, it
was possible to look at the drug's effect on mortality in 2 ways: (1)
the "intention-to-treat" approach, counting all deaths, whether they

occurred while on treatment or after premature withdrawal, and (2) the "per protocol" approach, counting only fatalities observed while the patient was on treatment or within 28 days of withdrawal. If the ascertainment of deaths among withdrawn patients is accurate and complete, the "intention-to-treat" analysis can be fairly convincing since it represents a conservative estimate of a beta-blocker's effect on mortality, counting deaths during treatment as well as those occurring after withdrawal. Unlike total mortality, the most clear-cut end-point, the interpretation of results for specific causes of death and nonfatal events is more problematic. For example, even though sudden death may be precisely defined, it is not easily verifiable among withdrawn patients whose deaths are often unwitnessed. One may also question the accuracy of the diagnosis for nonfatal events which occur even a short time after dropping out of a trial. Steps need to be taken in designing methods for follow-up to assure that all events to be used in the evaluation of a drug are reported reliably not only in patients who adhere to the drug regimen, but also in those who fail to complete it. In addition, a method for providing independent verification of key endpoints should be established in advance.

B. Extra-trial medications as procedures

Part of the ethical basis of a clinical trial is that subjects' medical management will not be unduly compromised by adherence to the protocol. Thus mechanisms are built into trials to allow withdrawal, change in treatments, and use of non-study medications.

Where the clinical trial involves a number or a sequence of

treatments, as in the "stepped care" trials of antihypertensive drugs (7), an orderly sequence of drug layering is built into the protocol. It remains to be seen how the detailed analysis of such trials will be carried out although it is clear that those designing such trials believe, probably correctly, that such analysis will be easier, or indeed possible, if therapy is so structured. However, in trials of a single dose of one agent, the concomitant therapy is usually left unstructured, presumably partly for supposed ethical reasons. The analysis and inferences from such trials is a challenging problem justifying considerable attention in the planning stage.

C. Subgroup analyses and Multiple endpoints

One well-known, but commonly overlooked problem with the design of beta-blocker trials is the failure to anticipate multiplicities in the analysis. If the entry criteria for the trial are very broad, it is tempting to divide the large, heterogeneous sample into smaller subgroups of patients for which the drug is hoped to be of benefit. The search for significant subgroups is usually pursued most vigorously when the overall drug effect is non-significant. The drug effect may be examined in subsets of the data cross-classified by a variety of patient characteristics, e.g. age, race, sex, previous medical history, and other baseline factors which may or may not have been considered, a priori, to have prognostic value. If we approach the data from the viewpoint of hypothesis-testing and neglect problems of multiplicity, the results can be misleading. Obviously, the more significance tests that are conducted on the data, the greater the possibility of drawing erroneous conclusions. Even if we look at the drug effect in only 10 classes of patients defined by age, sex, and some baseline factor, there is a 40% chance that at least 1 of the 10 subgroups would turn up significant at the 5% level, purely by chance, even if the drug had no therapeutic value.

Evidence of a drug effect in an isolated subgroup of patients from a large trial can be very misleading. Statisticians warn that, unless the main overall comparison is significant, investigators should be conservative in their interpretation of significant subgroup results. However, such results draw attention to subsets of patients who appear to benefit from the drug and so, generate new hypotheses to be tested in more well-focused trials. In the practolol trial by Barber et al (8) patients with acute MI overall showed no reduction in total mortality that could be attributed to the drug. But, in a subgroup of 53 patients with an initial heart rate over 100 beats/min., mortality was "significantly" lower in the practolol group than the placebo group up to 1 year after entry. The finding is suggestive but would have to be confirmed in a trial designed to consider this patient population were this considered to have high priority. Likewise, in the multicenter trial of practolol, a reduction in overall mortality was noted only in patients whose pre-entry infarcts were sited anteriorly and whose blood pressures at entry were below the mean for the trial as a whole. It is difficult to rule out the possibility that these findings represent false-positive results due to multiple comparisons or that they reflect possible baseline imbalances within subgroups that could account for the observed drug effect. On the other hand it is equally difficult to exclude them as being real effects.

It is often possible, in the design of the study, to cut down on multiplicity problems arising from multiple subgroups and multiple end-points. Both the class of patients and the end-points to be considered should be clearly specified in the initial protocol. Stratified randomization can be used in the design to achieve baseline balance between treatment groups and to reduce the variability in group comparisons if the stratification is used in the analysis. The Blocadren trial used this method by randomizing patients in each clinic within 3 strata defined in the protocol on the basis of patient history and specific characteristics of the entry infarction. The consistency of Blocadren's effect on mortality across the 3 prognostic groups lends additional credibility to the overall positive findings from that trial. To avoid "ransacking the data" for significance in the final analysis, hypotheses concerning subgroups should be specified before data collection begins, they should be based on reasonable expectations and the experience of previous trials, and they should be limited in number. Morbidity and mortality end-points for analysis should be clearly defined beforehand and uniformly applied during the course of the trial.

CONCLUSIONS

Given the difficulties with classical clinical trials of phenomena with relatively small endpoint rates the question of reducing the number of subjects or the length of the study while still allowing an adequate design is under investigation (9).

While the cost of large randomized double blind trials is

enormous, the potential benefit to great numbers of patients, may
well be worth the expense. Considering the problems encountered in
previous beta-blocker trials, and the protocol modifications commonly
made, it is clear that the preparation of a protocol for a long term
clinical study is a difficult and important task worthy of detailed
attention by the investigator and his best consultants.

TABLE I

CHRONOLOGY OF BETA-BLOCKER CLINICAL TRIALS

COMPOUND	TRIAL (REFERENCE)	# PATIENTS	RESULTS*	MAJOR PROBLEMS
Propranolol	Snow 1965 (10)	91-93	(+)	Too few patients
Propranolol	Balcon 1966 (11)	114	(−) (14 vs 13 deaths)	Too few patients
Propranolol	Clausen 1966 (12)	110	(−) (19 vs 16 deaths)	Too few patients
Alprenolol	Wilhelmsson 1974 (13)	274	(+) (7 vs 14 deaths)	Too few patients Late entry
Practolol	Green 1975 (2)	3,038	(+) (94 vs 117 deaths)	To few patients Author estimates 2,000 needed
Alprenolol	Anderson 1979 (14)	282	(+) (13 vs 29 deaths)	Too few patients (+) under age 65 (−) over age 65
Propranolol	Barber 1980 (1)	720	(−) (27 vs 28 deaths)	Premature Cessation of Trial
Timolol	Von Der Lippe 1981 (6)	1,884	(+) (98 vs 152 Deaths)	-------

* (+) Overall positive
  (−) Overall negative
  Deaths reported as treated vs placebo group.

REFERENCES

1. Barber, N.S. et al Multicenter post-infarction trial of propranolol in 49 hospitals in the United Kingdom, Italy, and Yugoslovia. Br. Heart J. 44, 96, 1980.
2. Multicenter International Study. Improvement in programs of myocardial infarction by long term beta adrenergic blockage using proctolol. Br. Med. J. 3, 735, 1975.
3. Temple, R. and Pledger, G. Sulfinpyrazone in the prevention of sudden Death after myocardial infarction. New Engl. J. Med. 302, 250, 1980.
4. Mitchell, JRA Timolol after myocardial infarction: an answer or a new set of questions? But. Med. J. 282, 1565, 1981.
5. Anonymous. Beta Blockers after myocardiol infarction. The Lancet April 18, 1981 p. 873.
6. Van Der Lippe et al. Timolol-induced reduction in mortality and reinfarction in patients serviving acute myocardial infarction. New England J. Med. 204, 801, 1981.
7. Five-years findings of the hypertension detection and follow up program J.A.M.A. 242,262, 1979.
8. Barber, J.M. et al Proctolol in acute myocardial infarction. Acta Med. Scand. Suppl. 587, 1975, 298.
9. Fundamentals of Clinical Trials. Friedman, L., Fineberg, C.D and DeMets, D.C. John Wright, Boston, 1981.
10. Snow, P.J.D., Effect of propranolol in myocardial infarction. Lancet 2, 920, 1965.
11. Balcon, R. et al A controlled trial of propranolol in acute myocardial infarction. Lancet 2, 917, 1966.
12. Clausen, J. et al Absence of prophylactic effect of propranolol in myocardial infarction. Lancet 2, 920, 1966.
13. Wilhelmsson, C. et al. Reduction of sudden deaths after myocardial infarction by treatment with alprenolol. Lancet 2, 1158, 1974.
14. Andersen, M.P. et al. Effect of alprenolol on mortality among patients with definite or suspected acute myocardial infarction. Lancet 2, 865, 1979

WHO SHOULD FUND CLINICAL TRIALS?

C.D. FURBERG

The former Director of the NIH, Dr. Fredrickson, made the following
statement last year at the meeting of the Clinical Trials Society (1): "I do
not believe that the ordinary research budget of the National Institutes of
Health can support many of the clinical trials that should be done in the
future. The NIH can best concern itself with clinical trials that will either
bring novel medical techniques to practical application for the first time, or
will provide new insights into the mechanism or natural history of disease.

I do believe, however, that NIH should be prepared to play a
catalytic role in assuring the scientific quality of trials that have a
primarily economic motivation."

Clearly the question of who should fund clinical trials has no simple
solution. This is even more an issue in times when resources are strained.
The thoughts presented here for discussion are those of the author alone. As
funding relates closely to the responsibility for organizing and managing a
trial, both aspects will be addressed.

In discussing funding, it is important to bear in mind what kind of
clinical trial we are considering. Clinical trials can be divided into two
broad categories, namely treatment and prevention trials. This is a simple
view and the distinction between the two is not always clear. The response
variable in short-term treatment trials is often a symptom, e.g. the
alleviation of exercise angina. In prevention trials the objective is to
change the likely course of a disease by reducing the incidence of a non-fatal
complication or postponing death. A typical example is a long-term study of
an antiarrhythmic agent to prevent sudden cardiac death in survivors of a
myocardial infarction. Depending on the outcome, prevention trials may have
wide-ranging health implications and are, therefore, important to the general
public. Studies of some drugs can have treatment as well as preventive
aspects, e.g. a long-term beta-blocker trial of symptomatic patients with

coronary heart disease. The two objectives may be, firstly, to assess any symptom relief and, secondly to evaluate the effect of the drug on coronary mortality.

Treatment Trials

The main objective of a treatment trial is to evaluate the symptomatic effect of a drug when compared with placebo or with another agent that is already proven. If the study results are favorable, the main beneficiary, other than the patient, is the pharmaceutical sponsor. For a single trial cost is a relatively minor issue as these studies are usually small in size and of short duration. It seems appropriate, therefore, that industry should continue to fund this type of trial. The question of who manages these is not critical.

A special case are studies of the so-called orphan drugs. This category includes medication that offer poor prospect for adequate economic return of an investment. Among these are drugs not covered by patent, e.g. aspirin. Society may have an interest in the evaluation of such agents for the treatment of either rare or certain common conditions. When it is obvious beforehand that the cost of a trial cannot be recovered by the sponsor and yet the trial is deemed medically essential, society will almost certainly have to share the financial burden.

Industry is also likely to be the major beneficiary of treatment trials comparing two or more drugs. Cost is again a relatively minor factor. The selection of drugs for comparison and their dosage is critical because if all have a beneficial effect, almost any study outcome can be obtained by manipulating these two factors alone. There are also methodological considerations. Two drugs can never be shown to be equally effective in the strict sense. Lack of a statistically significant effect does not necessarily mean equivalence. Large sample sizes are usually required for adequate statistical power. By setting up small underpowered trials, unable to assess clinically important differences in efficacy, one has a good chance of being able to claim "equality." It seems appropriate that industry should fund comparative treatment trials, but as credibility is a factor and even the appearance of a conflict of interest should be avoided, these trials would be best managed by a research group that does not have a vested interest in the result.

Prevention Trials

Prevention trials also fall into the same two basic categories as treatment trials. They often address questions of public health importance. Selection of a particular preventive measure for testing is best based on scientific rather than commercial considerations. As most prevention trials are collaborative, long-term endeavors, cost is a key factor. It may be argued that because industry and society both stand to gain, funding in these instances should be shared. As credibility is of particular concern, management of the trial ought to be controlled by a disinterested group.

Comparing the preventive effect of two or more drugs can be major undertaking. If the objective is to determine whether a new drug is of similar benefit to an established proven drug, the main beneficiary will be the manufacturer of that drug. On the other hand, if the new drug proves superior to the standard medication, the public will also benefit. In this instance, an element of cost sharing seems to be reasonable. Adequate safeguards to ensure credibility of the results are important.

Cooperation

No drugs could be developed and tested without a close cooperation between pharmaceutical companies and independent investigators. Funding and trial management have usually gone together resulting in a possible conflict of interest. This has been more of an issue in prevention rather than treatment trials. However, the climate is perhaps changing. We are seeing large-scale multicenter trials supported by pharmaceutical companies but managed entirely by non-industry groups.

So far collaboration between industry and government has been limited. The National Heart, Lung, and Blood Institute has only gone as far as accepting donation of medication for some of its large prevention trials. Even at this level, cooperation can be sensitive. The special interest of all involved parties must be understood so as to protect the integrity of the trial.

Pharmaceutical companies should refrain from using their contribution for promotional purposes until the study has been completed. In accepting financial assistance or drug supply it must be clear that the government is not endorsing any product. In return the government should give appropriate recognition of any contribution and, in addition, make study data available if requested for the filing of a New Drug Application.

Summary

   Cooperation between industry and government should be fostered. Third-
party payers should also be involved as they are potential beneficiaries of
well-designed and conducted clinical trials.

   This goal should be pursued and I am optimistic that an effective
mechanism for co-sponsoring clinical trials can be developed. A more open
exchange of information between industry and the government sector would be a
good place to start.

REFERENCES

1. Fredrickson DS. 1981. Sorting out the doctor's bag. Controlled Clin
    Trials, 1: 263.

GENERAL GROUP DISCUSSION - Beta Blockers in Sudden Death Prevention

Moderator: Dr. James Schoenberger

Dr. Schoenberger: I am going to take the chairman's prerogative to start the questioning by asking a question that is bothering me. Dr. Werkoe, from what we heard yesterday, the F.D.A. is not permitted to give class approval of beta blockers if one or two have been shown to be effective in certain clinical conditions. We now have evidence that timolol and metoprolol are effective in reducing mortality following myocardial infarction. You gave us an excellent review of the problems which those trials introduced, but certainly there are enough trials already ongoing that it is possible that we may get two or three more which will give us positive results. The question then comes if we are obligated to test each drug separately to see whether it also has this benefit, the problem which I see arising is the difficulty of recruiting patients for clinical trials when physicians are aware that drugs are available which do significantly reduce mortality; and given that problem, how are we going to fight our way out of that? How can we revise the protocols to take into account the awareness that we now have that some drugs are effective in trying to devise a method of testing new drugs.

Dr. Werkoe: I really don't know how to answer that question. I think you should ask the F.D.A. again about how they look at the problem. It certainly is going to be very difficult to do more studies whilst you have some of the results out in the open but on the other hand as was said repeatedly yesterday, we don't know everything about how the beta blockers act and especially not in the very complex situation of acute myocardial infarction or the post-MI patient. So I really don't think that we can say that it is just beta blockade or just the beta I blockade that is working in these patients. It may be that these drugs have some other effect, too. I think we have to look at the data very carefully before making up our minds. Another thing which is very important is, 'are the effects as good in all kinds of patients with myocardial infarction'; and again we have to look very carefully at the data and probably do more studies in subsets of patients in order to see if they should be treated or not.

Dr. Schoenberger: That is not an entirely satisfactory answer from my standpoint because unfortunately practicing physicians are not as critical about the evidence as you are, and some of them make up their minds from the therapeutic standpoint on very flimsy evidence. Since they control the patients for the most part in this country and if they refuse to withdraw beta blocker therapy from the patient, we have to live with this fact; and we have to redesign the protocols to take that into account. It is going to make for a real problem. Those of us who are actively engaged in recruitment of patients for these trials I think would affirm what I am saying, that we may be in a very difficult era.

Dr. Kaplan: Having seen your review of statistical requirements, which I think are probably very obvious to people who have been doing the variety of clinical studies, I also recall the slide of Dr. Werkoe's that showed the number of small studies particularly with metoprolol which are now in process. Now maybe none of the members of the panel should answer this; maybe someone from Ciba-Geigy should answer this. How can we justify the spending the money that is eventually going to cost us all for these trials which inherently are going to be inadequate? We are all talking about the need for adequate trials for this sort of problem, and yet we see the evidence that there must be another 10 inadequate trials in process all begun after all of the appropriate information has long been available.

Dr. Hjalmarson: I would like to comment about these small studies. They were in fact not designed mainly to show an effect on mortality, they just happened to have listed that they would like to look into that, and I think that is really wrong information in that project protocol. You can say beforehand that they will never show any effect.

Dr. Werkoe: I would also like to correct the fact that you said you should ask Ciba-Geigy. Ciba-Geigy has the metoprolol on license in this country, and the only big study they are making here is going to be hopefully large enough. The drug is produced by Astra and sold by Astra all over the world outside the U.S.; so Ciba-Geigy has some studies going on in places, but the main responsibility is the United States.

Dr. Schoenberger: I would like to try an answer to that question, too, as a non-statistician. I think if you have a dramatic enough effect on the endpoint, you may not need a large sample size, so you can't just look at the sample size and say that no results cannot be significant. I think if you got a 75% reduction in mortality you wouldn't need a lot of patients to show that it was significant. I do think, however, that the point that Dr. Werkoe made about the problems that we get with small sample size in terms of trying to get two identical groups randomized is more pressing with small sample sizes; but certainly as we found out in the AMIS trial, a large sample size does not obviate this difficulty either.

Dr. Sami: I really have two questions concerning long-term trials and I would like the help of the panel in answering some of these. We know already from a fair body of information about post-myocardial infarction prognosis about some of the risk factors that help identifying patients who are really at high risk of sudden death post-myocardial infarction. We also know that there are some criteria that when present in patients post-myocardial infarction can give those patients an excellent prognosis for the following two years. I am referring to many studies that have been done on this subject. Some of those factors are angina post-myocardial infarction, significant ST depression on exercise testing, and presence of complex ventricular arrhythmia in association with poor left ventricular function. Why not select a population that is really known to be at high risk and eliminating those people who are healthy anyway and who will only serve to dilute the results between any significant intervention for long-term prevention and that would diminish the need for having much larger numbers of people? This is the first question. The second really is what do we do with coronary bypass graft surgery? One of the important things about the Swedish and the Norwegian studies is the question that there was very little intervention in those people in terms of coronary angiogram and exercise testing in patients and sending patients with angina post-myocardial infarction to coronary angiography and surgery--when we find that they have significant vessel disease, for example, how do we handle this in terms of North American long-term trials?

Dr. Schoenberger: Those are two very difficult questions and Dr. Dern has expressed a willingness to take the first one and we'll see if we can get a volunteer for the second one.

Dr. Dern: I'd just like to say that the idea of selecting patients at high risk is certainly a reasonable way to increase the rate of the event that you are interested in, because one of the problems in these mortality studies, particularly as you fractionate upon the endpoint into subsets, let's say death in less than so many hours, with associated findings A, B, C and in the absence of X, Y, Z, you can see you get these very small strata, and the incidence rates with such an endpoint are going to be very small. You are getting down to an epidemiologic type of frequency of endpoint and you wonder about such things as retrospective trials which we are not faced with at this point. These are very small rates and one of the ways to get the rates up is to select patients beginning at higher risk. and I think that in general is a good idea. The only problem I would say is what about patients at somewhat lesser risk who might be adversely affected. You don't get the whole picture if you are going to select only those patients at the very highest risk. You lose out on the information that there may be some patients who at a little lesser risk really would be adversely affected by the treatment; but on the other hand, that might be the price one has to pay to get sufficiently high incident rates of the endpoint to be able to do a trial with a practical sample size. So I would agree with you.

Dr. Goldstein: I think one of the problems that you get into when you do cut your sample size to a very high risk group is that when you end up with your study, how do you interpret that information for the public in general. I think it is very hard for the general commission to identify all those very sophisticated characteristics of the patient population at risk. I think one of the problems we have even in the clinical trials themselves, and for instance in BHAT, is that we end up with a group of people who some people might say are not typical of all the people who go through the coronary care unit. Yet we have made the characteristics as broad as possible so that they can be truly applicable to a large population. If you cut it down even smaller, I think one the criticisms of the trial would be, 'so what, who are you?' Who are you talking about? It may not be applicable to the significant population. I think in terms of the question of coronary surgery, it obviously is a major problem in North American trials. In BHAT we have just dealt with it as some of the noise in the study. We have tried to exclude those people who might be candidates for coronary bypass surgery from entry into the study itself. Nevertheless, there have been a significant number of people who have angiography and coronary bypass surgery. Whether that will have an effect on the overall mobidity-mortality trial, of course we don't know at this point; but we will analyze it, as Dr. Werkoe points out, once they are in the trial, they are in the trial regardless of what interventions have taken place.

Dr. Furberg: There is also another issue. I am for studies of subgroups. You get smaller samples. It also makes more sense; I think we have been almost naive in our approach of treatment of post-MI patients. We had studied unselected groups pretty much of six large-scale trials of antiarrhythmics. Five of them pretty much took any post-MI patients regardless of the prevalence of arrhythmias. Only one looked at the subgroup with complex arrhythmias and, in fact, that is the only one that showed some promise. So that is another reason for going with subgroups.

Dr. Watanabe: Dr. Ehrreich reviewed for us many programs involved in this type of study, but my personal bias is that probably the single most important issue in this type of topic is the definition of sudden cardiac death. Some people take death 24 hours from the onset of the event and others take only one hour. I would like to know if there is a consensus of opinion between our distinguished panelists; and if not, could they try to reach a consensus.

Dr. Goldstein: It is an issue that I had some strong feelings about. I think it depends upon the population that you are studying and the availability of information. I think it also depends upon the question you are trying to ask. My own particular feeling is that clinical trials, such as we are talking about, do provide an opportunity in which one can examine the temporal characteristics of mortality and come up with fairly good insight into it. I think that if one is looking for an antiarrhythmic agent, I think one would want to know about instantaneous death certainly within one hour, probably instantaneous; whereas, if one is looking at a drug with a mechanism like a beta blocker or a calcium blocker which has an effect perhaps on ischemia, one might look at a longer time span. My own feeling about the definition of sudden death would be fairly simple because I think once you make it more complex, one gets into the trouble like the Anturne trial where there were some people who had EKG evaluations. Some had autopsy information and a whole host of things which were not applicable or available to the whole population. Witnessing of the death is very important and, for my own personal definition, witnessed within one hour comes to grips with the issue as clearly as possible. I think one could look at other subgroups, but my own particular definition would be witnessed death within one hour.

Dr. Hjalmarson: I think it is very important that the main object should be total mortality. When we start to cut it down into hours, it really will make it very tricky; and I can, for example, mention that sudden death in a multicentered study with practolol was two hours. One can ask why was it two hours? Perhaps it was so that within one hour there was no effect. If you take 24 hours or four hours, there was no effect either. So I think it is very important that its total mortality and even instantaneous death might not be arrhythmic death. We have a very high proportion of autopsy performed in our studies in the metoprolol study, and we have a very high number of patients with rupture--even in patients not during the just first few days of the infarction but even later on. Onset of severe pain at home and then suddenly dropping dead unwitnessed, autopsy showed rupture. So I think it is very important to have a lot of information about these patients.

Dr. Temple: Just a follow up to Dr. Sami's question about enriching the study population for people who are at the highest risk. Dr. Dern and Dr. Werkoe can correct me, but I believe the timolol trial did, in fact, do that in that it calculated its sample size based on the highest of the risk groups and what it did though, instead of confining the study to the high-risk group, it carried the other people along and randomized them anyway. I think that the expectation was that most of the action would be in the high-risk group; and, indeed, it was. It turns out that if you carry along people who are lower risk and don't contribute that many deaths, the statistical cost is not very great. You don't dilute things out too badly. You don't pay a terrible price if you have most of the action going on in the subgroup, and it does give you a chance to answer the question--Does it go the other way? You don't answer it definitively, of course, but you get a look at the question in the people with milder disease. In the case of timolol if you start doing post-hoc analyses, you could reach the conclusion that it is probably not as valuable in terms of total number of bodies saved to treat the people without the higher risk factors at the beginning; and yet, you are pretty reassured that it doesn't go the other way, that they are not in some way harmed and that, if anything, they seem to have some slight advantage. I think that choosing sample size on the basis of a subgroup like that makes a lot of sense. There is something attractive about carrying the others along, too, to get, if not a statistically valid assessment of how the other subgroups do, at least a gander at it.

Dr. Dern: I think this relates also to the question of how you get patients to submit to a trial when there are many treatments around that are thought to be effective. It is by including people in the trial who are not certain would not be harmed that you can approach this fact. For example, it should be possible to deal with the private physician in the following terms and say "Look, we're not absolutely sure that this treatment is going to be the best for your particular patient; and if we are not absolutely sure, your best medical procedure would be to give that patient a 50% chance of getting the right treatment for that particular patient." If you start limiting your patients in the trials to the more severely ill, you might conceivably have more difficulty getting patients, particularly if you should offer some treatment that is less attractive on the basis of the present experience.

Dr. Copen: Most of the trials done so far are double blind and, consequently, an arbitrary dose of beta blockers have been chosen. I would like to ask some of the panelists whether any of them are getting a clinically effective beta blocking dose. It seems unlikely that patients are getting toxic doses, but I really don't have a good feeling for how many are getting a clinically effective dose, and the second question that comes up is 'what happens when this drug gets approved?' Do we recommend treating with the arbitrary dose used in the clinical trials, or are we titrating each patient with exercise testing or isuprel to a clinically effective beta blocking dose?

Dr. Goldstein: Its obviously a very difficult question and I guess of 200 people in the audience here, none of us would probably agree on what an effective dose is. Perhaps, you know what it is; and we would be delighted to hear about it. What we did in BHAT, because of the obvious bias in terms of rate response, we have used the blood level determination. In the initial design of the trial, we felt that dose ranging was a very important characteristic of giving a beta blocker in the clinical situation. We had to take that out of the hands of the physicians for fear it would bias them, and we used a pre-determined blood level during a particular period of the dose therapy. After 3 days of propranolol at 40 mg/3 times a day, we drew blood levels and divided those people into groups of less than 20 nannograms and over 20 nannograms; and those people who were on the low blood level side were increased to a dose of 240 mg daily and those on the high side were treated at 180 mg. That was an attempt to deal with dose ranging, taking it out of the physician's hands. What we will recommend at the end if the drug is effective is another question, and I think it will have to be anybody's decision at that point.

Dr. Schoenberger: I think the question is extremely complicated and incapable of an easy answer, as Dr. Goldstein has said, because it is also possible that the dose which we are using may be above that which is ideal. For example, there are those who have criticized the aspirin trial on the basis that the doses used were excessive and depressed prostacycline generation; and this may have caused the negative effects. I don't know the answer to the question, but I think we could go on infinitely doing clinical trials. Perhaps, we ought to go on and see.

Dr. Copen: Its likely that the majority of the patients in these studies are having post-myocardial infarction exercise tests, so it is not part of the protocol. Indeed, I am participating in one of these studies; and it is hard to get away without having the post-myocardial infarction exercise test. It would seem that it might be useful for some of the people in these protocols to see if they could be back and pull out a few hundred or a thousand exercise tests which obviously weren't part of the protocol and then see if we could identify the group that seems to have a clinically effective dose.

Dr. Kostis: My question is regarding the duration of treatment. Since beta blockers have side effects, including effects on metabolism, that may affect coronary disease and since the beneficial effect appears to be mainly in the beginning of these trials, do we continue the treatment for life? Do we stop it after a certain interval; and if it is stopped then, have we merely postponed the high risk of death early after infarction or have we abolished it by giving it early?

Dr. Furberg: You bring up a very important question. The trials that have been conducted have been going on for a year up to two years, and the information on which we have now to base a decision is limited. What we do beyond one or two years if all the trials come out positive and we agree with the conclusion that the drugs do prolong long life is a judgement call and to be sure we need to follow people longer in our trials. Today, there is a tendency rather than have larger samples and go over shorter duration, if you want an answer sooner. I think it would be desireable to have our trials run a little bit longer so we can answer the question for how long should we treat the patients. Another question is: When should we start treatment?--all the trials we have discussed today initiated treatment within a month of the infarct. We have no information whether starting 6 months or 2 years after the infarct is beneficial, and that is a question no one has looked at; and I guess we should put our efforts to that.

Dr. Kostis: Would it be possible or ethical to randomize the treatment group to a treatment and placebo group and the placebo group to a treatment and placebo group at the end of the study and see if the patients who were initially in the treatment group and randomized two years later into a placebo group have lower rates of mortality or very high, as if they were only a month after infarction?

Dr. Furberg: I think in theory that sounds appealing, but on the other hand it is going to depend on the outcome of your trial. You are going to have to report the results when your trial is over; and if you report positive results, I don't think you are going to get cooperation from physicians to randomize them into a second phase of the trial.

Dr. Schoenberger: I would like to comment, too. I think that, unfortunately, most of what clinicians do has never been subjected to to proper clinical trial; and so, your question has very broad implications.

Dr. Cohn: Having completed a soon-to-be-published trial on acute myocardial infarction, I have some comments about the selection of high-risk patients for specific forms of therapy. We went into this trial feeling that one would like to identify the highest risk group in order to demonstrate the most effective way for efficacy of the therapeutic intervention. We certainly discovered to a far greater extent than previously recognized that acute myocardial infarction is a terribly heterogeneous disease in which one can predict at the moment of entry into the hospital, especially if you use invasive hemodynamic monitoring, a mortality rate which will vary tenfold from one group to another. So, we really can identify a high-risk group. It is clear that in that group the number of events is going to be higher, and there really is an advantage in looking at a form of therapy. We would all agree that we are dealing with a disease in which mortality is probably multifactorial and we are dealing with drugs, whose mechanism of action are really not understand in the disease process. So, we really do not, or I think cannot, have a preconceived idea that the therapy we selected to try is necessarily going to work in the highest risk group; and, in fact, in our nitroprusside trial we got some surprises. It may very well be that in a certain high-risk subset group, nothing is going to do anything. We have to really carry out these studies with an understanding that there are multiple possible mechanisms of death taking place and that the therapy we are testing may only be acting on one of them. I would like to ask the panel where we are now since we have developed to the point that the beta blockers look so effective in several of these studies; yet I think that most of us would agree that if they are effective, they must only be working by 1 or 2 or 3 or multiple possible mechanisms of mortality. Are we in a position where we are going to have to start carrying out studies of several drugs together to see whether there is an additive effect? That is, there are aspirin studies, platelet aggregation studies, beta blocker studies and nitrate studies--all these things possibly playing a role. Is that the next step, carrying out several studies together to see whether one can get an additive effect by attacking more than one mechanism?

Dr. Schoenberger: I think that is essentially what I was driving at with the question with which I opened this discussion. Mainly, that we may have to, in order to obtain cooperation with practicing physicians, put all patients on a beta blocker if there is a strong preponderance of evidence that it is favorable and add additional drugs to that.

Dr. Werkoe: I think it is very important to stress that myocardial infarction is a very complex disease, and it has been too simple to say that it is a sequel of coronary artery disease because it isn't only the question of the disease in the coronary arteries. It is also the question of the myocardial damage and the state of the myocardium and how large the damage in the myocardium is, etc. The beta blocker is probably working on the myocardial level and not on the vessel level. For example, somebody asked what about all these patients who are submitted to surgery--I think you have an excellent chance to look, as far as I know, there hasn't been any too convincing evidence that you prolong life with surgery, but

278

why not randomize all the surgery patients after surgery into two groups: one group to be treated with the placebo and one with beta blockers in order to see whether you can add to the surgical intervention with a beta blocker and then randomize them into surgery or no surgery. That is one way, and it certainly is possible to use several different approaches to treatment in such a multifactorial disease as myocardial infarction.

Dr. Furberg: Dr. Cohn was arguing against studies of subgroups, and I would like to expand a little bit on that. I think he is right. We don't know the mechanism of action for sure. I think we should study more on selected groups of post-MI patients that would apply to nitroprusside, to beta blockers. If we try that approach and we don't find any overall significant effects, we see a trend; and I think it makes some sense in the next generation to start looking at subgroups. I think you could also make a case that antiarrhythmic drugs should only be studied, or primarily be studied, in people with complex arrhythmias. I think we need both. I think I would be fully in favor of the broader approach initially to get information on as many patients as possible with the condition; and then, maybe in a later phase, go for subgroups.

Dr. Dern: I would also like to support that notion, and I think it is in the analysis of the trials that are available now in terms of subgroups. For example, which subgroups having, perhaps, very little or no effect of a treatment will provide the information necessary to start trials with the subgroups of clinical interest and a perspective basis because at the moment, one can certainly find areas in all of the trials that have been published in certain subgroups in which their drug effects are quite minimal or even reversed; and these findings are no more than interesting observations, but they do provide the hypotheses to be tested in future studies.

Dr. Hjalmarson: I think it is important to remember that there are two events that could happen for a patient to have had an infarction. That is, either to die or to get a new infarction. We can quite well predict the patients who are more likely to die than other subgroups who have a small risk of death; but it is impossible to predict a new infarction, and I think that most of these interventions we have to have as objectives even though the main objective is mortality. We have to keep account also how many patients got a new infarction, for that will be of importance for prognosis even later on.

Dr. Schoenberger: Even recognizing, as I am sure you do, how difficult it is to precisely define new infarction in the face of the previous infarction , it is a soft endpoint at best.

Dr. Michelson: Once the first drug is approved in this country for an indication which is post-myocardial infarction, to facilitate further recruitment, would it be acceptable to the F.D.A. to design a study without a placebo group? To actually design a study that would compare drug A to drug B and then alternatively, when the drug B is not another beta blocker, would it be acceptable, as Dr. Schoenberger suggested initially, to have both groups on whatever drug that turns out to be--whether it is timolol, metoprolol, or another drug. Then bring in another drug which has purportedly a different mechanism of action, whether it is an anti-platelet effect or whether it is superimposed on half of the people receiving the beta blocker and the other half only receiving the beta blocker.

Dr. Ehrreich: Dr. Mitchell in his critique of the timolol study did mention that at least as far as ethical considerations are concerned that he would suggest, for now, using a timolol group and then timolol plus drug X, etc. At this stage obviously we don't know if the drug itself is responsible for the effects or whether it is beta blockade or whatever. I think this question was even brought up at the Advisory Committee meeting where timolol was discussed, and the individuals who ran the study in Norway were asked the question, "Is this an effect of timolol or is it an effect of beta blockade?", and the answer was "We don't know". I think until we know more certainly the answer to the question, as far as I would be concerned, you still don't know whether you can get away without a placebo group.

Dr. Michelson: Many of us are happy that a drug has been shown to decrease mortality or re-infarction by a certain fixed percentage, but I don't think any of us are satisfied with that as our goal. I think we would rather have it be 100%; and even if you told me the drug reduced it by 37%, I would still be looking for a drug that makes it 38 or 39 or 40%. It is nice, however, to go back to referring doctors and let them know that, in fact, their patient is getting a drug that they have read about in the newspaper. At least that or something like that could potentially be better.

Dr. Schoenberger: I don't think anyone wished to add to that.

Dr. Scriabine: I would like to ask a question concerning the organization that is supposed to run future studies. What is the definition of dependent organizations? An academic group which has their large grant from one pharmaceutical company is not really independent. If the government organizations are not going to run that, then the only alternative I think is pharmaceutical manufacturer associations where one competitor is watching over the other. It probably is better than an acacdemic group or contact house.

Dr. Furberg: In this context it is a relative term. I think ideally you would have a group independent of a pharmaceutical sponsor run the trial, but there has to be some flexibility depending upon the level of involvement of all the sponsors. I am not saying that the industry doesn't have independent credible persons--I am sure they do. However, I think we have to work on this issue. I am favoring more openess and more collaboration, and maybe we can get away from this whole question of independence. If you had more insight and more knowledge of what we each do and could share information and could meet early on to discuss design analyses and interpretation, I think we would be much better off and, maybe, get away from the independence issue.

Dr. Schoenberger: I would like to add to what is being discussed. There are other potential partners for carrying out these trials, particularly in the voluntary sector. The American Heart Association is extremely interested in studies which demonstrate the efficacy of treatment for the population at large and is another group that I think could be effective partners in the conduct of these trials.

Dr. Temple: I guess the key is to make sure everybody is underpaid and then there is no problem. I think obviously there is no problem in seeing whether a second kind of intervention adds to the first by their adding that or placebo to the group, but the size of the studies gets very large once you have eliminated a substantial number of deaths. An even more difficult problem is how, if you really wanted to and if you once believed that some beta blockers have been shown to reduce mortality, do you test other beta blockers to see if they do, also. The problems of a positive controlled study in that setting are really enormous, apart from the power question which is bad enough. These studies are not always 100% reproducible every time you do them; and you know that if you tried to reproduce a study carried out in Sweden or Norway, you would wonder whether you had precisely the same population, whether it would have been large enough to show and whether the risks in the population you picked would have been large enough

to have shown a difference. If there were one there in the first place and if a
placebo was present, it's an enormous task to know how to do that; and I guess I
would ask the question, apart from some commercial considerations which I
realize are formidable, "Is it in anybody's interest to do that?". Suppose it turned
out that the community decided that beta blockers probably have this
characteristic, but you can never really be sure, so that in deciding to treat
somebody, you dance with the girl who brought you; and in people who can't
tolerate the drug, it has been shown that the clinician makes the decision to use
the other drug, with no real certainty that he is going to be helping, though the
probabilities are that he will be. Suppose the situation just stayed that way
forever? How bad would that be? What amount of resources should be devoted to
trying to do positive controlled studies with additional beta blockers with a fair
risk that you won't know what you have shown?

Dr. Dern: With respect to the question again on testing different drugs and
combinations, I would like to point out that in all of the beta blocker trials that in
effect one has done that because of the associated host randomization therapy.
Therefore, a good question is to what extent could one systematize the treatment
that is given in addition to the beta blockade. There are many drugs that are
given in addition to the primary agents that are studied. The beta blockers are
given in unsystematic ways, hoping that everything will balance out through some
kind of miraculous effects if we don't pay any attention to them--that they will go
away; but almost in any trial that you can think of, a particular drug has an
association with other agents; and we are already into that problem. The
difficulty is that these other agents have been given in an unsystematic way, due
to the ethical considerations and so forth. I think we are already into that issue;
we do not have pure beta blocker trials to my knowledge.

Dr. Schoenberger: It seems to me that we have to interject an element of common sense here, because there never will be a perfect clinical trial. There will always be people who will point out flaws in the design or conduct of the trial or lack of generalization of the trial to the general population; and if we become such scientific purists, we'll never treat anybody for anything. I think somewhere between that extreme of purism and that rampant pragmatism which is now existent at least in the U.S., lies a happy mean which seems plausible and prudent.

Dr. Fitzgerald: I would like to echo the chairman's comments about common sense. The result of the Norwegian trial using timolol is due to its chemical entity or to defined chemical classes of beta blockers, and I think a certain amount of pragmatism and common sense is called for here. It is my impression that the beta blockers have been around for about 21 years; so we are talking about some very mature material. There was a very considerable amount of animal experimental data which I think should be put into the equation with due common sense. I would like to hear what the panel says, because I would like to suggest that trials at the present time would lead me to the conclusion that if you have adequate beta blockade in the post-infarction situation, you are likely to have a better effect than giving a placebo alone. I think in the end the experts have to come off the fence and really declare themselves; and if we are just saying it is a chemical entity unrelated to a pharmacological class, I think we have some difficulties. I believe that there are more important questions raised here to which we now need to address ourselves. Particularly, how do we get at the hard core of patients who don't respond to beta blockers? I believe that is the next most important question. I do believe there could be a case for saying "Look, let's accept it,". But what's going to happen when all the results are out that Professor Werkoe showed? We could be in a state of complete chaos in 18 months' time, with six more negative trials. But assuming that isn't the outcome, I would like to hear a statement from the panel. Do they believe it is due to beta blockade or due to the fact that it is a chemical entity?

Dr. Werkoe: If you look at the positive trials, what is common to all of them is that they are beta I blockers; and it is quite certain that there is at least a 95% chance, if not more, that it is blocking of the beta I receptors that is the effective mechanism that has shown up in these trials.

Dr. Goldstein: Timolol has beta II also.

Dr. Werkoe: What is common to all of them is the beta I blockers. They all have different spectra besides that, but beta I is common to them all.

Dr. Goldstein: I think that the case is getting stronger. There is no question that beta blockers are a potent agent in the post MI patient. I think most of us would like to see a little more positive information. The drug comes from a strong physiologic background. There is a lot of bench information to indicate its potency in preventing and limiting myocardial infarct size. The information from the metoprolol trial tends to further strengthen the case and hopefully sodalol trials and others coming down the road will continue to support that. I would share the same anxiety that you have--I certainly hope they all go the same direction.

Dr. Furberg: I agree with Dr. Fitzgerald, but I don't think we should stop here. I think we need to move on and approach the hard core group that does not respond to beta blockers; and I think that if we in six months to one year's time to had the answer as to whether these drugs generally work, I don't see any problem from a methodologist point of view to adding a second drug. I think we have to do that for ethical reasons--offer beta blockers as a standard treatment and compare the added second drug to the intervention group.

Dr. Epstein: I think it would be a pity to get off the fence. I think we are at a very exciting point. We have a lot more to learn; and I think you in your initial remarks, Dr. Schoenberger, raised an important issue and I would also go along with Dr. Furberg. Facts are: #1, it looks like beta blocking drugs are going to increase survival unless catastrophes occur which was just pointed out. #2, your original point. There are a lot of pharmaceutical companies that would like to be able to say that their drug, although it has not been so tested, should have class approval. I would be against this. Nevertheless, capitalism is a good thing because you can learn alot with the economic motivation to do repetitive studies; but what I am concerned about is, if you do a radionuclide study in a patient before they are discharged, the mortality in a patient with an ejection fraction less than 40% is about 20T during that first year; and if the ejection fraction is above 40%, the mortality is 1 and 2%:--high risk and low risk as Dr. Cohn pointed out. Now to me intuitively, it seems not rational to think that the patient with a low ejection fraction is going to be benefited by beta blocking agents. He may, but he may not. But what Dr. Furberg was saying is let's get at the patients who are not responding to beta blockers, but we don't know which patients these are. We know that the broad category of patients who have acute myocardial infarction are responding but at this point at least to my knowledge it doesn't. Another comment made is that there are so many subgroups in these thousands of patients that maybe it would be a good idea to convene a conference of all the participants of all the studies and let them search out the subgroups for hypotheses. Then we could say it looks like these are the patients who did and these did not, and then let's bring in the pharmaceutical houses who have not yet had a positive study and say these are the hypotheses which we should examine

286

over the next few years. Then we will have the critical answers of maybe doing a
radionuclide study post-discharge or a 24-hour Holter and say these are the
patients in whom beta blockers work. These are the patients who should be
getting other forms of therapy. I would not like to throw in the towel and say
everyone should be on beta blockers. It seems to me that it is too heterogeneous a
group, and we don't know who might benefit and who might experience a
deleterious effect from beta blockers.

Dr. Schoenberger: I think those are excellent suggestions, and my hope would be
that the practicing physician doesn't take it out of our hands as he well can do.

Dr. Furberg: Just a brief reply to Dr. Epstein. The meeting you are talking about
is already planned. The Institute is going to go ahead with a workshop on beta
blockers after the propranolol trial has been completed. They will try to get
everyone together to sit down and address the questions that you raised and all the
others that have been brought up today.

Dr. Biddison: I would like the panel to briefly consider the treatment of high-risk
coronary patients with beta blockers. If we accept that they have, perhaps, one or
a combination of three major factors (#1--complex ventricular arrhythmia; #2--
previous myocardial infarction, as in the timolol study; and #3--those who have
low ejection fractions as commented on by Dr. Epstein including congestive heart
failure. Many of these patients would not be applicable of treatment with beta
blockers. Are we really going to be able to get at our high-risk patient and treat
them with beta blockers?

Dr. Hjalmarson: I think that in the real high risk group of patients we can't give
beta blockade, but I think that group will be quite small. If we talk about acute

myocardial infarction, I think we have to leave out about 20% of infarctions being too severe to be given beta blockade. If we talk about post-infarction, and some of these have died, then you have, perhaps, 10% of all patients who can't be given beta blockade; but still that is the highest risk group.

Dr. Schoenberger: We are living in exciting times. The availability of potent drugs has changed medicine from what it was not too many years ago when a person had less than a 50% chance of benefiting from an encounter with a physician to the point where we are truly able to alter the natural history of disease. We are plagued from the problems of all clinical trials; namely, that they raise more questions than they answer, the fact that perhaps the results are not truly generalizeable, and that we are still plagued by a lack of the understanding of the precise mechanisms by which the actions which we have observed occurred. Finally, I think there seems to be a good consensus that in the next 5-to-10 years we are going to have to look at new methods of financing these expensive trials because they do seem to be expensive; and in the process of looking for alternate sources of financing, we have to maintain the scientific integrity of these studies.

CALCIUM CHANNEL BLOCKERS/HISTORICAL PERSPECTIVES

JEROME WEINSTEIN, M.D.

The basis for our interest today in the calcium channel
blockers originated almost 100 years ago in 1883 with
Ringer's[1] classical experiments demonstrating that extracellular calcium is necessary for muscle to contract. During
the next seventy years investigations into the physiology of
muscle contraction defined more precisely the role of calcium.
The reports of Locke and Rosenheim[2] in 1907 and Mines[3] in 1913
identified extracellular calcium as the "coupler" of intermediary in the excitation-contraction process. In the late
50's and early 60's the experiments of Luttgau and
Neidergerke[4,5] indicated that an intracellular calcium pool
participated in myocardial contraction and that a functional
relationship existed between the intracellular pool and
extracellular calcium. Additional studies in the 60's by
Winegrad and Shanes[6] and the Fabiatos[7,8] confirmed the
existence of intracellular Ca^{++} compartments and the effect
of the influx of extracellular calcium ions on the release of
intracellular Ca^{++} from stored pools. In the 1970's Katz,[9,10]
Langer[11] and the Fabiatos[7] described the role of intracellular
Ca^{++} in the interaction between actin and myosin that results
in contraction. Again in the 70's research from a number of
laboratories[12-19] described the slow inward calcium current
that follows depolarization and rapid Na^+ influx, and identified specific transmembrane channels for this current.

Interest in compounds that could interfere with calcium
activity (the calcium antagonists) began in the 1960's.

Investigations into the mechanism of excitation-contraction coupling demonstrated that a number of substances could interfere with excitation-contraction coupling by antagonizing the effect of calcium. In 1965 Kaufman and Fleckenstein[20] demonatrated that Ni^{++} and Co^{++} selectively impair contractility. It is interesting to note that a year later cobalt-containing beer was identified as the etiology of chronic heart failure among heavy beer drinkers in Canada. Fleckenstein and co-workers were able to inhibit excitation-contraction coupling with as many as 30 substances that acted as calcium antagonists. These included Ba^{++}, Sr^{++}, Mn^{++}, adrenergic beta receptor blocking agents, barbituric acid and local anesthetics. These antagonize Ca^{++} interaction at one or several sites to modify coupling. There are many sites for calcium interaction (Figure 1.) that are critical to the E-C coupling mechanism.

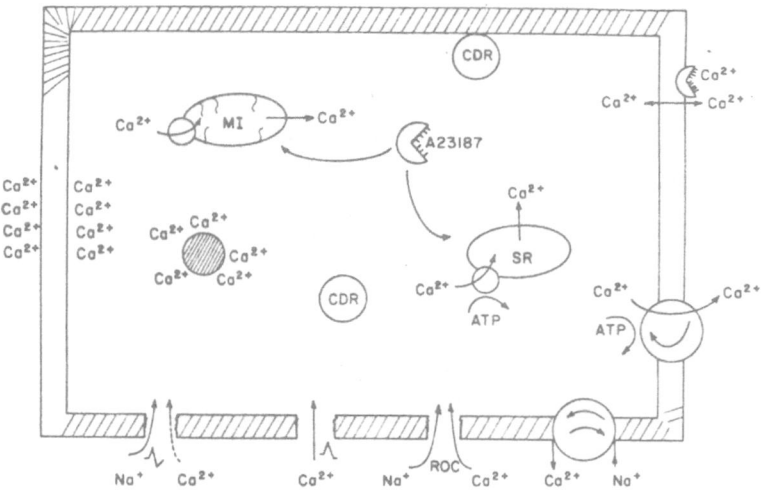

Schematic representation of Ca^{2+} entry, exit, mobilization and storage mechanisms. Shown are Ca^{2+} entry through discrete channels, Ca^{2+} entry through the Na channel, the Na^+-Ca^{2+} exchange pump, the Ca^{2+}-ATPase and direct entry by an ionophoremediated process. Within the cell Ca^{2+} binding to membranes and intracellular proteins including calmodulin (CDR) is shown, in addition to Ca^{2+} uptake processes within mitochondria (MI) and sarcoplasmic reticulum (SR). Each of the sites of Ca^{2+} interaction represents a potential site for Ca^{2+}-antagonist action.

FIGURE 1.

Thus, calcium antagonists may be active at a variety of target sites and therefore constitute a large and pharmacologically heterogeneous group. Our interest today however is to address a class of compounds that specifically inhibit the slow inward Ca^{++} current by antagonism of Ca^{++} fluxes at cellular membrane sites. Katz and Reuter[21] pointed out that this class of drugs is appropriately termed "calcium channel blockers" rather than calcium antagonists.

The family of calcium channel blocking compounds are listed in Figures 2. and 3. The Group A compounds inhibit Ca^{++} dependent myocardial excitation-contraction coupling by at least 90% before affecting the fast Na^+ channel.

Group A			
Verapamil (mol.wt. 454.59)	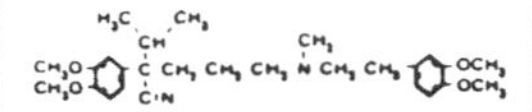	Hydrochloride = Isoptin Knoll A.G. Ludwigshafen, F.R.G.	Fleckenstein (1968 & 1971); Fleckenstein et al (1967 & 1969)
Compound D-600 (gallopamil, mol.wt. 485.59)	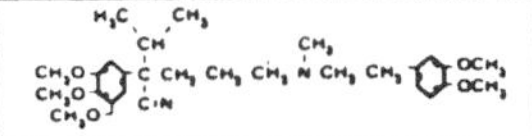	Hydrochloride Knoll A.G. Ludwigshafen, F.R.G.	Fleckenstein (1971); Fleckenstein et al (1969)
Nifedipine (mol.wt., 346.34)	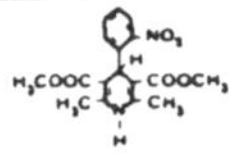	Adalat, Bay a 1040 Bayer A.G. Leverkusen, F.R.G.	Fleckenstein (1971); Fleckenstein et al (1972 & 1975); Grün and Fleckenstein (1972)
Niludipine (mol.wt. 490.55)	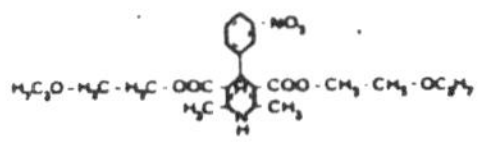	Bay a 7168 Bayer A.G. Leverkusen, F.R.G.	Fleckenstein (1979)
Nimodipine (mol.wt. 418.45)	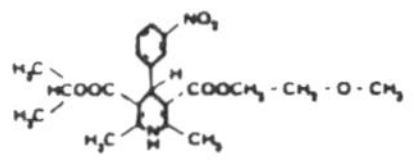	Bay e 9736 Bayer A.G. Leverkusen, F.R.G.	
Diltiazem (mol.wt. 414.52)	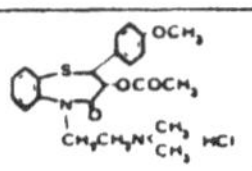	Hydrochloride = Herbesser Tanabe Seiyaku Ltd. Osaka, Japan	Nakajima et al (1975)

FIGURE 2.

The Group B compounds are less Ca^{++} specific. These influence the rapid Na^+ influx at levels of inhibition of Ca^{++} dependent E-C grouping as low as 50%. The B compounds also inhibit Mg^{++} influx which is not affected by the A compounds. In the columns on the right are the pharmaceutical firms that developed these compounds and the early reports identifying their specific Ca^{++} blocking action.

Group B			
Prenylamine (mol.wt. 329.46)	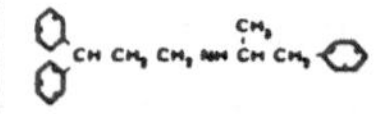	Segontin Farbwerke Hoechst A.G. Frankfurt/Main, F.R.G.	Fleckenstein (1968 & 1971) Fleckenstein et al (1967 & 1969)
Fendiline (mol.wt. 315.46)	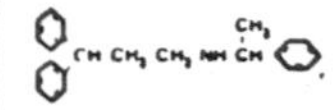	Hydrochloride = Sensit Dr. Thiemann A.G. Lunen, F.R.G.	Fleckenstein et al (1977)
Terodiline (mol.wt. 281.0)	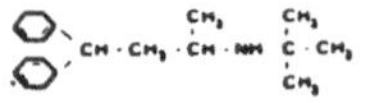	Hydrochloride = Bicor Kabi A.B. Stockholm, Sweden	Fleckenstein-Grün (1978)
Perhexiline (mol.wt. 277.50)	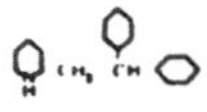	Maleate = Pexid Richardson-Merrell, Inc. Cincinnati, OH, U.S.A.	Fleckenstein-Grün et al (1976)

Figure 3.

The first reports of the effects of calcium channel blockers dealt with their negative inotropic effects. In 1960 Lindner[22] published his work with prenylamine. In 1962 and 1967, Haas[23,24] demonstrated the negative inotropic effects of verapamil and its methoxy derivative, D-600. However, it was Fleckenstein[25] at the Physiological Institute of the University of Freiburg in 1964 who first described the basis for the mechanism of action of these compounds--namely a selective loss of contractility as occurs with calcium deficiency. Subsequently, experiments with tracer labelled material and the use of the voltage clamp technique have shown that these substances block the influx of calcium across the cell membrane of the excited heart muscle fiber without affecting the Na^+ influx of the action potential.

The unpublished observations of Kolhardt, Physiological Institute, Freiburg, 1970 (Figure 4.), were presented by Fleckenstein at the meeting of the European Section of the International Study Group for Research into Cardiac Metabolism in London (9/6/70).

The earliest interest for therapeutic application of the calcium channel blockers was as coronary vasodilators. In 1972 Grün and Fleckenstein[26] reported on the excitation-contraction uncoupling of vascular smooth muscle by nifedipine, verapamil, D-600 and prenylamine. Reports of clinical trials in the late 60's and early 70's in Japan and Europe with

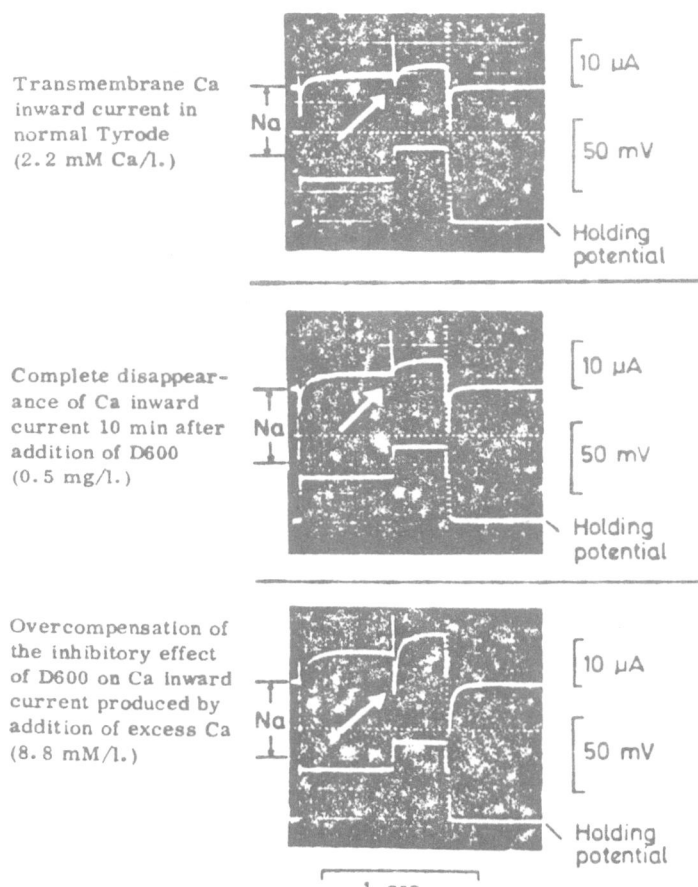

Transmembrane Ca
inward current in
normal Tyrode
(2.2 mM Ca/l.)

Na

10 µA

50 mV

Holding
potential

Complete disappear-
ance of Ca inward
current 10 min after
addition of D600
(0.5 mg/l.)

Na

10 µA

50 mV

Holding
potential

Overcompensation of
the inhibitory effect
of D600 on Ca inward
current produced by
addition of excess Ca
(8.8 mM/l.)

Na

10 µA

50 mV

Holding
potential

1 sec

FIGURE 4.

nifedipine,[27-31] verapamil[32-34] and prenylamine[35-37] demonstrated efficacy of these compounds in angina pectoris. With
increased appreciation in recent years of the role of coronary
spasm in atherosclerotic coronary disease[38] as well as in
Prinzmetal's angina, the therapeutic benefit of the calcium
channel blockers in angina pectoris could be identified as a
spasmolytic effect. Additionally, studies in Japan[39] reported
in 1975 and in the U.S.[40-50] between 1978 and 1980 established
that calcium channel blockers such as nifedipine, verapamil
and perhexilene are specific treatments in Prinzmetal's
variant angina.

Interest in the use of calcium channel blockers in the management of cardiac arrhythmia followed reports on the effects of these agents on the sinus and A-V nodes and A-V conduction by Zipes and Fischer,[51] Cranefield[52,53] and Watanabe[55] in the U.S. in 1974 and by Japanese investigators such as Ono[54,56,57] and Narimatsu[58] between 1976 and 1979. Most of the general clinical experience with this class of drugs has been obtained with nifedipine, verapamil, perhexilene, and diltiazam, but verapamil has emerged as the most important in this group in the treatment of arrhythmia.

Although the antiarrhythmia properties of verapamil were reported as early as 1962,[59] it required the development in the 70's of the voltage clamp methods[60,61] in the in vitro studies and the techniques of intracavitary recording[62-64] and programmed stimulation to elucidate the mechanisms. With these techniques the re-entrant nature of a variety of arrhythmias was revealed, the significance of the slow calcium depolarizing current in re-entrant arrhythmia was elucidated and the therapeutic significance of verapamil as a slow channel blocker in these arrhythmias was identified.

As early as 1970 with I.V. verapamil[65] and 1972 with peroral nifedipine,[66] clinical studies demonstrated that calcium blockers could be effective antihypertensive drugs. Later in the 70's, investigations into the role of vascular muscle sodium and calcium ion exchanges[67-69] in hypertension (reported in 1976 and 1977) offered a basis for the pharmacologic mechanisms of these compounds in reducing peripheral vascular resistance. Subsequently, a substantial literature[70-79] was generated from studies in Japan and Europe supporting the clinical efficacy of nifedipine (mainly) and verapamil[80] (to a lesser extent) in hypertension.

In 1976, Kaltenbach[81] in Germany reported on the initial success with verapamil in the treatment of hypertrophic cardiomyopathy. Subsequent reports from Kaltenbach[82,83] and studies in the U.S.[84,85] confirmed the benefits of calcium channel blockade with verapamil in hypertrophic cardiomyopathy.

The latest chapter, as the history of the calcium channel blockers develops, relates to the possibility that intervention with these agents can protect ischemic myocardium. Fleckenstein[86] in 1971, Shen and Jennings[87] in 1972, Katz and Reuter[21] and Henry[88] in 1979 reported their observations indicating that calcium influx into ischemic cells results in injury to intracellular organelles. These studies demonstrated that accumulation of intracellular calcium during ischemia contributed to cell death.[89,90] Clark and Henry[91] were able to demonstrate that the calcium blocking effect of nifedipine protected against cell injury due to Ca^{++} accumulation associated with ischemia, and Naylor et al[92] demonstrated a similar protective effect with verapamil as well as with nifedipine and propranolol. These studies suggest potential application of Ca^{++} blockers as cardioplegics during open heart surgery as well as a potential to limit infarct size during evolving myocardial infarction. Additionally, a number of reports from animal investigation suggest that nifedipine, verapamil, and diltiazem may limit infarct size by improving myocardial perfusion and, as a result of reduced contractility and reduced afterload (and PVR), reduce oxygen demand.[93-106]

It does appear that in the 80's the calcium channel blockers will add impetus to the research into the pathophysiology and the treatment of cardiovascular disorders as resulted from the emergence of the β-blockers during the previous decade.

In the United States at this time verapamil has been approved by the FDA for the treatment of arrhythmias, and verapamil, nifedipine and diltiazam are under review for approval in the treatment of angina pectoris.

REFERENCES

1. Ringer S: A further contribution regarding the influence of the different constitutents of the blood on the contraction of the heart. J Physiol (London) 4: 29-42, 1883.
2. Locke FS, Rosenheim O: Contributions to the physiology of the heart. The consumption of dextrose by mammalian cardiac muscle. J Physiol (London) 36: 205-20, 1907.
3. Mines GR: On functional analysis by the action of electrolytes. J Physiol (London) 46: 188-204, 1913.
4. Lüttgau HC, Niedergerke R: The antagonism between Ca and Na ions in the frog's heart. J Physiol (London) 143: 486-97, 1958.
5. Niedergerke R: Movement of Ca in frog heart ventricles at rest and during contractions. J Physiol (London) 167: 515-29, 1963.
6. Winegrad S, Shanes AM: Calcium flux and contractility in guinea pig atria. J Gen Physiol 45: 371-93, 1962.
7. Fabiato A, Fabiato F: Calcium and cardiac excitation-contraction coupling. Ann Rev Physiol 41: 473-84, 1979.
8. Fabiato A, Fabiato F: Calcium release from the sarcoplasmic reticulum: a brief review. Circ Res 40: 119-30, 1977.
9. Katz AM: Contractile proteins of the heart. Physiol Rev 50: 63-158, 1970.
10. Katz AM, Bailin G, Krichberger MA, Today M: Regulation of myocardial cell function by agents that increase cyclic AMP production in the heart. In: Fishman AP, ed. Heart Failure. Washington, D.C. Hemisphere Publishing Corp.; 11-28, 1978.
11. Langer GA: Heart: excitation-contraction coupling. Annu Rev Physiol 35: 55-86, 1973.
12. Noble D: The initiation of the heartbeat. Oxford: Clarendon Press, 1975.
13. Reuter H: Properties of two inward membrane currents in the heart. Annu Rev Physiol 41: 413-24, 1979.
14. Reuter H: Divalent cations as charge carriers in excitable membraines. Prog Biophys Mol Biol 26: 1-43, 1973.
15. Vitek M, Trautwein W: Slow inward current and action potential in cardiac Purkinje fibers: the effect of Mn^{2+}ions. Pfluegers Arch 323: 204-18, 1971.
16. Mascher D, Peper K: Two components of inward current in myocardial muscle fibers. Pfluegers Arch 307: 190-203, 1969.
17. Diamond JM, Wright EM: Biological membranes: the physical basis of ion and nonelectrolyte selectivity. Annu Rev Physiol 31: 581-646, 1969.
18. Williams RJP: The biochemistry of sodium potassium, magnesium and calcium. Q Rev Chem Soc 24: 331, 1970.
19. Rosenberger L, Triggle DJ: Calcium, calcium translocation and specific calcium antagonists. In: Weiss GB, ed. Calcium in Drug Action. New York: Plenum Press, 3-31, 1978.

20. Kaufmann R, Fleckenstein A: Ca^{++}-competitive elektro-mechanische Entkoppelung durch Ni^{++}-und Co^{++}-Ionen am Warmblutermyokard. Pflüg.Arch.ges.Physiol. 282: 290, 1965.

21. Katz AM, Reuter H: Cellular calcium and cardiac cell death. Am J Cardiol 44: 188-90, 1979. (Editorial)

22. Lindner E: Phenyl-propyl-diphenyl-propyl-amin, eine neue Substanz mit coronargefässerweiternder Wirkung. Arzneim Forsch 10: 569, 1960.

23. Haas 'H, Härtfelder G: α-Isopropyl-α-((N-methyl-N-homo-veratryl)-γ-aminopropyl)-3,4-dimethoxyphenylacetonitril, eine Substanz mit coronargefässerweiternden Eigenschaften. Arzneim Forsch 12: 549, 1962.

24. Haas H, Busch E: Vergleichende Untersuchungen der Wirkung von α-Isopropyl-α-((N-methyl-N-homoveratryl)-γ-amino-propyl)-3,4-dimethoxyphenylacetonitril, seiner Derivate sowie einiger anderer Coronardilatatoren und β-Receptor-affiner Substanzen. Arzneim Forsch 17: 257, 1967.

25. Fleckenstein A: Die Bedeutung der energiereichen Phosphate für Kontraktilität und Tonus des Myokards. Verh. dtsch.Ges.inn.Med. 70: 81, 1964.

26. Grün G. Fleckenstein A: Die elektromechanische Entkoppe-lung der glatten Gefässmuskulatur als Grundprinzip der Coronardilatation durch 4-(2-Nitrophenyl)-2,6-dimethyl-1, 4-dihydropyridin-3,5-dicarbonsäure-dimethylester (Bay a 1040, Nifedipin). Arzneim Forsch 22: 334, 1972.

27. Hayase S, Hirakawa S, Hosokawa S, Mori N, Kanyama S, Iwasa M: Hemodynamic and therapeutic effect of BAY a 1040 in patients with ischemic heart disease. Arzneim Forsch 22(2): 370-3, 1972.

28. Kimura E, Mabuchi G, Kikuchi H: The clinical effect of 4-(2-nitrophenyl)-2,6-dimethyl-3,5-dicarbomethoxy-1, 4-dihydropyridine (BAY a 1040) on angina pectoris evaluated by sequential analysis. Arzneim Forsch 22(2): 365-7, 1972.

29. Kobayashi T, Ito Y, Tawara I: Clinical experience with a new coronary-active substance (BAY a 1040). Arzneim Forsch 22(2): 380-9, 1972.

30. Loos A, Kaltenbach M: Effect of nifedipine (BAY a 1040) on work electrocardiogram of angina pectoris patients (Ger). Arzneim Forsch 22(2): 358-62, 1972.

31. Raff WK, Kosche F, Lochner W: Nifedipine, a coronary-vasodilating substance with prompt sublingual effect. Arzneim Forsch 22(1): 33-9, 1972.

32. Neumann M, Luisada AA: Am J Sci 251: 552, 1966.

33. Sandler G, Clayton GA, Thornicroft S: Br Med J 1: 660, 1968.

34. Livesley B, Catley PF, Campbell RC, et al: Br Med J 1: 375, 1973.

35. Cardoe N: Prenylamine lactate ("Synadrin") in patients with angina pectoris. Brit J Clin Pract 22: 299, 1968.

36. Stoker JB: Effect of prenylamine in angina pectoris. Brit J Clin Pract 22: 384, 1968.

37. Winsor T, Bleifer K, Cole S, et al: A double-blind, double-crossover trial of prenylamine in angina pectoris. Amer Heart J 82(1): 43-54, 1971.

33. Mudge GH Jr, Grossman W, Mills RM Jr, Lesch M, Braunwald E: Reflex increase in coronary vascular resistance in patients with ischemic heart disease. N Engl J Med 295: 1333-7, 1976.
39. Endo M, Kanda I, Hosada S, Hayashi H, Hirosawa K, Konno S: Prinzmetal's variant form of angina pectoris: re-evaluation of mechanisms. Circulation 52: 33-37, 1975.
40. Muller JE, Gunther SJ: Nifedipine therapy for Prinzmetal's angina. Circulation 57: 137-9, 1978.
41. Antman E, Muller JE, Goldberg S, et al: Nifedipine therapy for coronary-artery spasm: experience in 127 patients. N Engl J Med 302: 1269-73, 1980.
42. Heupler FA Jr, Proudfit WL: Nifedipine therapy for refractory coronary arterial spasm. Am J Cardiol 44: 798-803, 1979.
43. Mizuno K, Tanaka K, Honda Y, Kimura E: Suppression of repeatedly occurring ventricular fibrillation with nifedipine in variant form of angina pectoris.
44. Goldberg S, Reichek N, Wilson J, et al: Nifedipine in the treatment of Prinzmetal's (variant) angina. Am J Cardiol 44: 804-10, 1979.
45. Waters DD, Theroux P, Dauwe F, et al: Ergonovine testing to assess the effects of calcium antagonist drugs in variant angina. Circulation 60(Suppl II): 248, 1979. (Abstract)
46. Theroux P, Waters DD, Affaki GS, et al: Provocative testing with ergonovine to evaluate the efficacy of treatment with calcium antagonists in variant angina. Circulation 60: 504-10, 1979.
47. Freedman B, Dunn RF, Richmond DR, Kelley DT: Coronary artery spasm--treatment with verapamil. Circulation 60 (Suppl II): 249, 1979. (Abstract)
48. Severi S, Davies G, L'Abbate A, Maseri A: Long term prognosis of variant angina with medical management. Circulation 60(Suppl II): 250, 1979. (Abstract)
49. Mizgala HF, Crittin J, Waters DD, Theroux P: Results of immediate and long-term treatment of variant angina with perhexiline maleate. Circulation 60(Suppl II): 181, 1979. (Abstract)
50. Raabe DS Jr: Treatment of variant angina pectoris with perhexiline maleate. Chest 75: 152-6, 1979.
51. Zipes DP, Fischer JC: Effects of agents which inhibit the slow channel on sinus node automaticity and atrio-ventricular conduction in the dog. Circ Res 34: 184-92, 1974.
52. Cranefield PF, Aronson RS, Wit AL: Effect of verapamil on the normal action potential and on a calcium-dependent slow response of canine cardiac Purkinje fibers. Circ Res 34: 204-13, 1974.
53. Wit AL, Cranefield PF: Effect of verapamil on the sino-atrial and atrioventricular nodes of the rabbit and the mechanism by which it arrests reentrant atrioventricular nodal tachycardia. Circ Res 35: 413-25, 1974.

54. Ono H, Hasimoto K: Ca^2 antagonism in various parameters of cardiac function including coronary dilatation with the use of nifedipine, perhexiline, and verapamil. In: Winbury MM, Abiko Y, eds. Ischemic Myocardium and Antianginal Drugs. New York: Raven Press; 77-88, 1979.

55. Watanabe AM, Besch HR: Subcellular myocardial effects of verapamil and D-600: comparison with propranolol. J Pharmacol Exp Ther 191: 241-51, 1974.

56. Himori N, Ono H, Taira N: Simultaneous assessment of effects of coronary vasodilators on the coronary blood flow and the myocardial contractility by using the blood perfused canine papillary muscle. Jpn J Pharmacol 26: 427-35, 1976.

57. Ono H, Himori N, Taira N: Chronotropic effects of coronary vasodilators as assessed in the isolated, blood-perfused sino-atrial preparation of the dog. Tohoku J Exp Med 121: 383-90, 1977.

58. Narimatsu A, Taira N: Effects on atrio-ventricular conduction of calcium-antagonistic coronary vasodilators, local anesthetics and quinidine injected into the posterior and anterior septal artery of the atrio-ventricular node preparation of the dog. Naunyn Schmiedebergs Arch Pharmacol 294: 169-77, 1976.

59. Melville II, Shister HE, Huq S: Can Med Assoc J 90: 761, 1964.

60. Fozzard HA, Beeler GW: Circulation Res 37: 403, 1976.

61. Hauswirth O, Singh BN: Pharmacolog Rev 30: 5, 1979.

62. Scherlag BJ, Lau SH, Helfant RH, et al: Circulation 39: 13, 1969.

63. Durrer D, Schoo L, Schulenberg RM, et al: Circulation 36: 644, 1977.

64. Wellens HJJ: In: Electrical Stimulation of the Heart in the Study and Treatment of Tachycardias, Stenfert Kroese BV, HE Leiden, 1971.

65. Brittinger WD, Schwarzbeck A, Wittenmeier KW, et al: Klinishexperimentelle Untersuchungen uber die blut-drucksenkende Wirkung von Verapamil. Dtsch Med Wochenschr 95: 1871-7, 1970.

66. Murakawi M, Murakawi E, Takekoshi N, et al: Antihypertensive effect of nifedipine, a new coronary dilator. Jpn Heart J 13: 128-35, 1972.

67. Blaustein MP: Sodium ions, calcium ions, blood pressure regulation, and hypertension: a reassessment and a hypothesis. Am J Physiol 232: C165-73, 1977.

68. Zsoter TT, Wolchinsky C, Henein NF, Ho LC: Calcium kinetics in the aorta of spontaneously hypertensive rats. Cardiovasc Res 11: 353-7, 1977.

69. Wei J-W, Janis RA, Daniel EE: Calcium accumulation and enzymatic activities of subcellular fractions from aortas and ventricles of genetically hypertensive rats. Circ Res 39: 133-40, 1976.

70. Aoki K, Kondo S, Mochizuk A, et al: Antihypertensive effect of cardiovascular Ca^{2+}-antagonists in hypertensive patients in the absence and presence of beta adrenergic blockade. Am Heart J 96: 218-26, 1978.

71. Bartorelli C, Guazzi M: Cardiovascular effects in man of nifedipine: therapeutic implications.

72. Guazzi M, Olivari MT, Polese A, et al: Nifedipine, a new antihypertensive with rapid action. Clin Pharmacol Ther 22: 528-32, 1977.

73. Kuwajiami I, Ueda K, Kamata C, et al: A study of the effects of nifedipine in hypertensive crises and severe hypertension. Jpn Heart J 19: 455-67, 1978.

74. Ueda K, Kuwajima I, Ito H, et al: Nifedipine in the management of hypertension.

75. Laaser U, Meurer KA, Kaufmann W: On the clinical evaluation of therapy with nifedipine in association with various antihypertensive drugs. Arzneim Forsch 27: 676-81, 1977.

76. Lederballe Pederson O, Mikkelsen E: Acute and chronic effects of nifedipine in arterial hypertension. Eur J Clin Pharmacol 14: 375-81, 1978.

77. Olivari MT, Bartorelli C, Polese A, et al: Treatment of hypertension with nifedipine, a calcium antagonistic agent. Circulation 59: 1056-62, 1979.

78. Guazzi MD, Fiorentini C, Olivari MT, et al: Short- and long-term efficacy of a calcium-antagonistic agent (nifedipine) combined with methyldopa in the treatment of severe hypertension. Circulation 61: 913-9, 1980.

79. Aoko K, Yoshida T, Kato S, et al: Hypotensive action and increased plasma renin activity by Ca^{++} antagonist (Nifedipine) in hypertensive patients. Jpn Heart J 17: 479-84, 1976.

80. Dieckmann L, Hosemann R: Zur blutdrucksenkenden Wirkung von Verapamil--Untersuchungen und Erfahrungen bei Kindern. Munsch Med Wochenschr 116: 515-20, 1974.

81. Kaltenbach M, Hopf R, Keller M: Treatment of hypertrophic obstructive cardiomyopathy with verapamil, a calcium antagonist. Dtsch Med Wochenschr 101: 1284-7, 1976.

82. Kaltenbach M, Hopf R, Kober G, et al: Treatment of hypertrophic obstructive cardiomyopathy with verapamil. Circulation 60(Suppl II) 76, 1979. (Abstract)

83. Kaltenbach M, Hopf R, Kober G, et al: Treatment of hypertrophic obstructive cardiomyopathy with verapamil. Br Heart J 42: 35-42, 1979.

84. Rosing DR, Kent KM, Borer JS, et al: Verapamil therapy: a new approach to the pharmacologic treatment of hypertrophic cardiomyopathy: I. Hemodynamic effects. Circulation 60: 1201-7, 1979.

85. Hanrath P, Mathey D, Kremer P, et al: Effect of verapamil on left ventricular relaxation and filling in hypertrophic cardiomyopathy. Am J Cardiol 45: 393, 1980. (Abstract)

86. Fleckenstein A: Specific inhibitors and promoters of calcium action in the excitation-contraction coupling of heart muscle and their role in the prevention of production of myocardial lesions. In: Harris P, Opie L, eds. Calcium and the Heart. New York: Academic Press; 1971.

87. Shen AC, Jennings RB: Myocardial calcium and magnesium in acute ischemic injury. Am J Pathol 67: 417-40, 1972.

88. Henry PD: Protection of ischemic myocardium by treatment with nifedipine.

89. Henry PD, Shuchleib R, Clark RE, Perez JE: Effect of nifedipine on myocardial ischemia: analysis of collateral flow, pulsatile heat and regional muscle shortening. Am J Cardiol 44: 817-24, 1979.

90. Christlieb IY, Clark RE, Nora JD, et al: Marked limitation of ischemia--reperfusion injury by nifedipine. Circulation 58(Suppl II): 100, 1978. (Abstract)

91. Clark RE, Christlieb IY, Henry PD, et al: Reduction of consequences of ischemia and preservation of myocardium with nifedipine. Am J Cardiol 43: 361, 1979. (Abstract)

92. Nayler WG, Ferrari R, Williams A: Protective effect of pretreatment with verapamil, nifedipine and propranolol on mitochondrial function in the ischemic and reperfused myocardium. Am J Cardiol 46: 242-8, 1980.

93. Schmier J, Bruckner UB, Mittmann U, Wirth RH: Intra-coronary collaterals and intramyocardial blood distribution in dogs following nifedipine administration compared with controls.

94. Clark RE, Christlieb IY, Henry PD et al: Nifedipine: a myocardial protective agent. Am J Cardiol 44: 825-31, 1979.

95. Hattori S, Weintraub WW, Agarwal JB, et al: The effects of nifedipine on ischemic myocardium: preservation of contraction during partial coronary occlusion. Am J Cardiol 45: 485, 1980. (Abstract)

96. Selwyn AP, Welman E, Fox K, et al: The effects of nifedipine on acute experimental myocardial ischemia and infarction in dogs. Circ Res 44: 16-23, 1979.

97. Wende W, Bleifeld W, Meyer J, Stuhlen HW: Reduction of the size of acute, experimental myocardial infarction by verapamil. Basic Res Cardiol 70: 198-208, 1975.

98. Smith HJ, Singh BN, Nisbet HD, Norris RM: Effects of verapamil on infarct size following experimental coronary occlusion. Cardiovasc Res 9: 569-78, 1975.

99. Singh BN, Smith HJ, Norris RM: Reduction in infarct size following experimental coronary occlusion by administration of verapamil. In: Roy PE, Rona G, eds. Recent Advances in Studies on Cardiac Structure and Metabolism. Volume 10. The Metabolism of Contraction. Baltimore: University Park Press; 435-52, 1975.

100. Reimer KA, Lowe JE, Jennings RB: Effect of the calcium antagonist verapamil on necrosis following temporary coronary artery occlusion in dogs. Circulation 55: 581-7, 1977.

101. DeBoer LWV, Strauss HW, Kloner RA, et al: Autoradiography with ^{99}Tc labeled albumin microspheres, a new method for delineation of ischemic tissue at risk of infarction: demonstration of the protective effect of verapamil. Am J Cardiol 45: 485, 1980. (Abstract)

102. Sherman LG, Liang C, Boden WE, Hood WB Jr: Effects of verapamil on performance of ischemic myocardium in conscious dogs. Circulation 60(Suppl II): 29, 1979. (Abstract)
103. Smith HJ, Goldstein RA, Griffith JM, et al: Regional contractility: selective depression of ischemic myocardium by verapamil. Circulation 54: 629-35, 1976.
104. Weishaar R, Ashikawa K, Bing RJ: Effect of diltiazem, a calcium antagonist, on myocardial ischemia. Am J Cardiol 43: 1137-43, 1979.
105. Nagao T, Matlib MA, Franklin D, et al: Effects of diltiazem, a calcium antagonist, on regional myocardial function and mitochondria after brief coronary occlusion. J Mol Cell Cardiol 12: 29-43, 1980.
106. Nayler WG, Grau A, Slade A: A protective effect of verapamil on hypoxic heart muscle. Cardiovasc Res 10: 650-662, 1976.

COMPARATIVE CLINICAL PHARMACOLOGY OF SLOW CHANNEL BLOCKING AGENTS

ROBERT E. KATES, Ph.D.
Division of Cardiology
Stanford University Medical Center
Stanford, California

The development of new slow channel blocking agents represents a major step forward in the field of cardiovascular pharmacology as well as clinical cardiology. These agents, also referred to as calcium antagonists, have been the subject of several recent reviews (1-3). While these drugs are chemically and pharmacologically dissimilar, they all have one property in common; they inhibit slow channel activity in isolated cardiac tissues and vascular smooth muscle. Clinically, they are all potent vasodilators, but their cardiac effects are a net result of direct actions on the heart and reflex responses subsequent to peripheral vasodilatation.

This review will be concerned with three slow channel blocking agents, diltiazem, nifedipine and verapamil. Since following chapters will deal specifically with the electro-physiologic and clinical differences of these drugs, these two features will not be emphasized here.

Diltiazem is a benzothiazepine derivative which has been evaluated extensively for the treatment of angina. As shown in Table 1, diltiazem is similar to verapamil in that it inhibits conduction through the A-V node, is a local anesthetic and at high concentrations appears to inhibit the fast sodium channel. The net effect on heart rate is minimal, and while no change has been reported by some investigators (4), a mild decrease in rate has been observed by others (5).

The pharmacokinetics of diltiazem have not been extensively studied. The major deficiency in the literature is an absence of data following intravenous administration, and the lack of adequate data relating to the absolute bioavailability of the oral formulation. Diltiazem is extensively metabolized following oral administration, and less than 4% of a dose is excreted in the urine as unchanged durg (6). A major metabolic pathway involved in the metabolism of diltiazem is deacetylation. Limited data suggest that this metabolite accumulates in the plasma of patients during chronic oral therapy, but that the levels of desacetyl diltiazem (Table 3) remain considerably below those of the parent drug. It appears, however, that this metabolite disappears very slowly from the plasma (7). Its activity, though not specifically defined, has been reported to be 40 to 50% of that of the parent compound (7)

Table 1. Pharmacologic differences of slow channel blocking agents.

Drug	Heart Rate[a]	AV Node Conduction	Local Anesthetic	Fast Channel
Diltiazem	0 or ↓	↓	yes	↓
Nifedipine	↑	0	no	0
Verapamil	↑ or ↓	↓	yes	↓[b]

    a.   effects are for intact animal or human subjects where net response is a result of direct cardiac effects and reflex response due to peripheral vasodilatation.

    b.   primarily due to the + isomer.

Studies with radiolabeled diltiazem have shown that, like verapamil and nifedipine, it is well absorbed following oral administration. However, no reports have appeared in the literature which permit one to draw conclusions as to the absolute bioavailability of diltiazem. Systemic availability is subject to extensive intersubject variability, and it has been reported that no relationship exists between daily dose and steady state plasma levels of diltiazem during chronic therapy (7). This is an area which requires further study.

The elimination half-life of diltiazem, following oral administration, has been reported to range between 4.4 and 6.9 hours (see Table 2).

We recently administered single intravenous bolus doses (.25 mg/kg) of diltiazem to three patients who were undergoing cardiac catheterization. Sufficient blood samples were drawn to facilitate pharmacokinetic interpretation of their diltiazem

plasma concentration decay curves. The half-lives we observed
ranged from 2.2 to 5.4 hours. The values for clearance and
steady state distribution volume were also calculated and are
tabulated in Table 2. It should be emphasized that these data
are from three patients only, and should be considered preliminary. Further studies involving intravenous diltiazem are
needed.

Table 2. Comparison of pharmacokinetic characteristics of
slow channel blocking agents.

	Drug		
	Diltiazem	Nifedipine	Verapamil
Bioavailability (%)	---	---	22 ± 7.7
Clearance (ml/min/kg)	15.7 ± 7.0	---	13.3 ± 7.7
$t_{\frac{1}{2}}$ (hr)	2-8	---	8.2 ± 6.1
Vd_{ss} (ℓ/kg)	3.92 ± 1.05	---	4.3 ± 1.9
Urinary Excretion (%)	<4	<1	<4
Protein Binding (%)	80-86	92-98	87-93

The plasma protein binding of diltiazem has been reported
to be 85-87%. No drug interactions involving displacement of
diltiazem have been reported. However, it has been shown that
coadministration of diazepam with diltiazem leads to a 20% to
30% reduction in diltiazem plasma levels (7). Whether this is
due to plasma protein displacement or some other mechanism is
not presently known.

Nifedipine differs from diltiazem and verapamil in that
it does not delay conduction through the atrioventricular node,
is not a local anesthetic and does not affect the fast sodium
channel (Table 1). It inhibits the slow inward current without
altering the kinetics of slow channel depolarization (8).
Nifedipine does not have any direct antiarrhythmic effects.
In the intact animal, or human subject, nifedipine exerts a

minimal negative inotropic effect which is clinically
insignificant.

Table 3. Metabolites of slow channel blocking agents.

Drug	Metabolite	Relative Activity	Relative Plasma Concentration
Diltiazem	desacetyldiltiazem	.4 - .5	.1 - .3
Nifedipine	hydroxymethyl-pyridine carboxylic acid	---	---
Verapamil	norverapamil	.25	∿1

The pharmacokinetics of nifedipine have not been well
studied. One reason for this appears to be instability of the
drug leading to chemical analysis difficulties. Nifedipine is
either extensively metabolized in the body or undergoes
spontaneous chemical rearrangement or decomposition in the
blood. The primary metabolite of nifedipine is a hydroxymethyl-
pyridine carboxylic acid (9). This compound is reported to
have no significant pharmacologic effects. Less than 1% of an
orally administered dose of nifedipine is excreted unchanged
in the urine (Table 1).

The extent of binding of nifedipine to plasma proteins has
been reported to range from 92 to 98% (10).

The limited pharmacokinetic data which has been reported
for nifedipine was obtained following administration of
^{14}C-labeled drug. The reported elimination half-lives for
nifedipine are obtained from determinations of total plasma
radioactivity and do not reflect the actual disappearance of
unchanged drug (11). These same studies showed that nifedipine
is well absorbed following oral administration, but no conclusions regarding the systemic bioavailability could be made.
Extensive studies are still needed to elucidate the absorption
and disposition kinetics of this drug.

Verapamil is a synthetic papaverine derivative which has
been the object of numerous investigations over the past several
years. Verapamil is a compound with an asymmetric center, and
studies have shown that the optical isomers exert different
electrophysiologic effects (12). As shown in Table 4, the

- isomer is considerably more potent than the + isomer with respect to most responses measured. The effect on coronary sinus blood flow is the only effect where the potency of the + isomer approaches that of the - isomer. It has been suggested that the + isomer of verapamil may be responsible for the local anesthetic and fast channel blocking properties of this drug.

Table 4. Comparison of pharmacologic properties of the optical isomers of verapamil[a].

Effect	Relative - isomer	Potency + isomer
increase coronary sinus blood flow	1.5 - 2.0	1
decrease AV node conduction	6 - 10	1
decrease heart rate	5.4	1
decrease $\dot{M}VO_2$	14.9	1
decrease developed tension of papillary muscle	15.3	1

[a]from reference number 12.

Verapamil can decrease the heart rate by directly suppressing the SA node, however, this may be compensated for by the reflex increase in heart rate due to peripheral vasodilatation which verapamil produces. As shown in Table 1, the net response can be either an increase or decrease in heart rate. The overall affect of verapamil is the sum total of the effects of both isomers. In the case of intravenous administration, the two isomers appear in the blood in equal amounts. Following oral administration this may not be the case.

The absorption and disposition kinetics of verapamil have been well studied (15,16). Following oral administration, verapamil is extensively metabolized and less than 4% of an administered dose appears in the urine as unchanged drug. A major metabolite of verapamil is the n-demethylated product, norverapamil, which accumulates in the plasma during chronic oral administration. This metabolite has been shown to possess about 25% of the potency of verapamil as a peripheral vasodilator (17). The electrophysiologic properties of this

compound have not been reported. Following long-term infusions
of verapamil, only low levels of this metabolite appear in the
plasma.

The disposition kinetics of both oral and intravenous
verapamil have been reported in normal healthy subjects (13),
patients with chronic atrial fibrillation (14) and patients
with liver disease (15,16). These reports are based on plasma
level measurements of racemic verapamil, and do not address
the question of differential kinetics of the two optical
isomers.

The total body clearance of verapamil is variable and a
range of 7.7 to 34.4 ml/min/kg has been reported (14) for
patients with atrial fibrillation. In patients with hepatic
cirrhosis, the clearance may be decreased by as much as a
half to a third. In this group of patients, verapamil
half-lives have been reported to range from 9.7 to 26.6 hours.

Verapamil accumulation during long-term dosing is
greater than one would predict from single oral dose studies.
It has been reported (14) that the mean concentration of
verapamil during long-term dosage was twice the mean level
that would be predicted from single dose data. This suggests
that either bioavailability increases or clearance decreases
during chronic oral administration of verapamil. If the
latter is true, then less frequent dosing may be clinically
acceptable for long-term oral therapy.

While the absorption of verapamil is complete following
oral administration, the systemic bioavailability is only
about 22% (17). In addition to the extensive first pass
extraction of orally administered verapamil, the hepatic
extraction may be stereoselective, with preferential clearance
of the more active - isomer. This was first suggested by
Eichelbaum and co-workers (18), and findings of several other
investigators tend to support this hypothesis. Rinkenberger
and co-workers (19) observed a disparity in the comparative
efficacy of oral and intravenous verapamil. They reported
that oral effectiveness could not be predicted from response
to i.v. administration. This agrees with the observations

of Eichelbaum that plasma levels of verapamil must be 2 to 3 times higher after oral than after intravenous administration to produce the same degree of prolongation of the PR interval. Further studies are needed to elucidate the role of these isomers and the significance of stereoselective first pass extraction of verapamil.

The plasma protein binding of verapamil has been extensively studied (20,21). In normal subjects, the extent of binding is 89.6% $\pm$ 0.17%. The binding of verapamil is reduced in patients undergoing cardiac catheterization to 83.3% $\pm$ 3.0%, following heparinization. Several drugs, when present in high concentration, have been reported to displace verapamil in vitro (21). The most dramatic displacement occurred with disopyramide. When present in a concentration of 12 $\mu g/ml$, the binding of verapamil was reduced to 74%. It is unlikely that this interaction is of any clinical significance.

In summary, an understanding of the clinical pharmacology of diltiazem, nifedipine and verapamil is still incomplete. In order for these agents to be employed in an optimal manner to maximize their clinical efficacy further studies will need to be conducted. In the case of diltiazem and nifedipine, very basic information is still needed regarding their pharmacokinetics and bioavailability. The unraveling of the role of the optical isomers of verapamil and the stereoselective aspects of the first pass clearance of this drug promises to be an exciting challenge with the reward being new knowledge which will facilitate the clinical use of this drug with a high level of sophistication.

REFERENCES

1. Henry PD. 1980. Comparative pharmacology of calcium antagonists: Nifedipine, verapamil and diltiazem. American Journal of Cardiology 46:1047-1058, 1980.
2. Ellrodt G, Chew CYC, Singh BN. 1980. Therapeutic implications of slow-channel blockade in cardiocirculatory disorders. Circulation 62:669-679.
3. Singh BN, Ellrodt G, Peter CT. 1978. Verapamil: A review of its pharmacological properties and therapeutic use. Drugs 15:169-197.

310

4. Kusukawa R, Kinoshita M, Shimono Y, Tomonaga G, Hoshino T. 1977. Haemodynamic effects of a new anti-anginal drug, diltiazem hydrochloride. Arzneim-forsch (Drug Res) 27: 878-884.
5. Kinoshita M, Motomura M, Kusukawa R, Kawakita S. 1979. Comparison of haemodynamic effects between β-blocking agents and a new antianginal agent, diltiazem hydrochloride. Japanese Circulation Journal 43:587-598.
6. Rovei V, Gomeni R, Mitchard M, Larribaud J, Blatrix Ch, Thebault JJ, Morselli PL. 1980. Pharmacokinetics and metabolism of diltiazem in man. Acta Cardiologica 35: 35-45.
7. Morselli PL, Rovei V, Mitchard M, Durand A, Gomeni R, Larribaud J. 1978. Pharmacokinetics and metabolism of diltiazem in man (observations on healthy volunteers and angina pectoris patients)in Bing RJ, ed., New Drug Therapy with a Calcium Antagonist: Diltiazem. Hakone Symposium 1978, Excerpta Medica 487:152-167.
8. Kohlhardt M, Fleckenstein A. 1977. Inhibition of the slow inward current by nifedipine in mammalian ventricular myocardium. Naunyn Schmiedebergs Arch Pharmacol 298:267-272.
9. Bossert F. 1975. The chemistry of nifedipine, in Lochner W, ed., 2nd International Adalat Symposium, Berlin, Excerpta Medica, p. 20-26.
10. Schlossmann K, Medenwald H, Rosenkranz H. 1975. Investigations on the metabolism and protein binding of nifedipine, in Lochner W, ed., 2nd International Adalat Symposium, Berlin, Excerpta Medica, p. 33-39.
11. Horster FA, Duhm B, Maul W, Medenwald H, Patzschke K, Wegner LA. 1972. Klinische untersuchunges zur pharmakokinetik von radioaktiv markiertem 4-(2'-nitrophenyl)-2,6-dimethyl-1, 4-dihydropyridin-3, 5-dicarbonsaüredemethylester. Arzneim-forsch (Drug Res) 22:350-334.
12. Satoh K, Yanagisawa T, Taira N. 1980. Coronary vasodilator and cardiac effects of optical isomers of verapamil in the dog. Journal of Cardiovascular Pharmacology 2:309-318.
13. Dominic JA, Bourne DWA, Tan TG, Kirsten E, McAllister RG. 1981. The pharmacology of verapamil. III. Pharmacokinetics in normal subjects after intravenous drug administration. Journal of Cardiovascular Pharmacology 3:25-38.
14. Kates RE, Keefe DLD, Schwartz J, Harapat S, Kirsten EB, Harrison DC. 1981. Verapamil disposition kinetics in chronic atrial fibrillation. Journal of Clinical Pharmacology and Therapeutics 30:44-51.
15. Somogyi A, Albrecht M, Kleims G, Schafer K, Eichelbaum M. 1981. Pharmacokinetics, bioavailability and ECG response of verapamil in patients with liver cirrhosis. British Journal of Clinical Pharmacology 12:51-60.
16. Woodcock BG, Rietbrock I, Vohringer HF, Reitbrock N. 1981. Verapamil disposition in liver disease and intensive care patients: Kinetics, clearance, and apparent blood flow relationships. Journal of Clinical Pharmacology and Therapeutics 29:27-34.

17. Eichelbaum M, Somogyi A, Unruh GE, Dengler HJ. 1981.
    Simultaneous determination of the intravenous and oral
    pharmacokinetic parameters of d, l-verapamil using stable
    isotope-labeled verapamil. European Journal of Clinical
    Pharmacology 19:133-137.
18. Eichelbaum M, Birkel P, Grube U, Gütgemann U, Somogyi A.
    1980. Effects of verapamil on P-R intervals in relation
    to verapamil plasma levels following single IV and oral
    administration and during chronic treatment. Klin
    Wochenschn 58:919-925.
19. Rinkenberger RL, Prystowsky EN, Heger JJ, Troup PJ,
    Jackman WM, Zipes DP. 1980. Effects of intravenous and
    chronic oral verapamil administration in patients with
    supraventricular tachyarrhythmias. Circulation 62:996-
    1009.
20. Keefe DL, Yee YG, Kates RE. 1981. Verapamil protein binding
    in patients and in normal subjects. Journal of Clinical
    Pharmacology and Therapeutics 29:21-26.
21. Yong CL, Kunka RL, Bates TR. 1980. Factors affecting the
    plasma protein binding of verapamil and norverapamil in
    man. Res Com Chem Path Pharmacol 30:329-339.

THE ELECTROPHYSIOLOGIC DIFFERENCES OF CALCIUM ANTAGONIST DRUGS

L. SEIPEL and G. BREITHARDT

INTRODUCTION

In 1967, FLECKENSTEIN et al (27) assumed that the new compounds prenylamine and verapamil were inhibitors of the action of calcium. The concept that these so-called Ca-antagonists are inhibitors of the slow channel, is now widely accepted (16, 46, 61, 88, 100). These drugs are affecting structures in which impulse propagation is mediated by the slow channel, i.e. the sinus and A-V node. In addition, they may depress action potentials and slow conduction in diseased myocardial or Purkinje fibers. As a consequence, SINGH and VAUGHAN WILLIAMS (90) postulated a new class of antiarrhythmic action (class 4). However, some recent investigations have questioned this uniform concept for all Ca-antagonists (3, 15, 21, 28, 42, 48, 61, 62, 88). In the following paper the electrophysiologic differences will be discussed with regard to experimental and clinical studies.

EFFECT OF CA-ANTAGONISTS ON THE SINUS NODE

In the isolated preparation, slow channel blocker depress sinus node (SN) automaticity and sinoatrial conduction (3, 15, 40, 44, 47, 57, 65-67, 73, 97, 99). The same effect has been demonstrated if verapamil is delivered via the sinus node artery (30, 52). In contrast to these results in isolated preparations, most studies in the intact animal could not demonstrate this depressive effect on sinus node activity (1, 14, 51, 55, 65). Only in high doses a marked sinus depression ensued in the dog (57, 65). In one study (79) a depressant effect of verapamil in therapeutic doses was observed.

Most studies in man could not show any significant effect on SN automaticity or calculated sinoatrial conduction time. Sometimes an increase in heart rate was observed (4, 5, 7, 8-10, 33, 35, 37, 39, 44, 45, 68, 69, 77, 86, 87, 89). There are only few opposite results (6, 13). Even under treatment with high oral doses, no significant change in heart rate was observed (41, 49). Only after intoxication with extremely high doses, bradycardia or atrial standstill occurred (20, 25, 70).

Table 1: Effect of different Ca-antagonists on sinus node (SN) function in patients without SN-dysfunction.
[1] n = 14   [2] n = 7   - = $<$ 5 %   ( ) not significant

	n	A-A	SNRT	CSNRT	SACT
Verapamil 0.1 mg/kg iv	20	-10.0 %	-	(+10.4 %)	(+20.2 %[1])
D 600 0.03 mg/kg iv	10	-	(+5.6 %)	(+20.1 %)	-
Tiapamil 1.0 mg/kg iv	10	-	-	(+16.1 %)	(+9.1 %[2])
Diltiazem 0.15 mg/kg iv	8	(-5.8 %)	-	(+6.8 %)	

Table 1 shows that there are no significant changes in cycle length (A-A), sinus node recovery time (SNRT) and calculated sinoatrial conduction time (SACT) after iv application of different Ca-antagonists in therapeutic doses. However, when given in patients with sick sinus syndrome, the same drugs sometimes cause a marked depression of sinus node activity (8-10, 13, 58, 85, 87, 92). Figure 1 demonstrates this dual effect of verapamil on the sinus node in patients with and without SN-dysfunction. Whereas in normals no significant change of SNRT is observed, the drug leads to a sometimes dangerous prolongation of SNRT or to a complete atrial standstill in patients with a sick sinus syndrome.

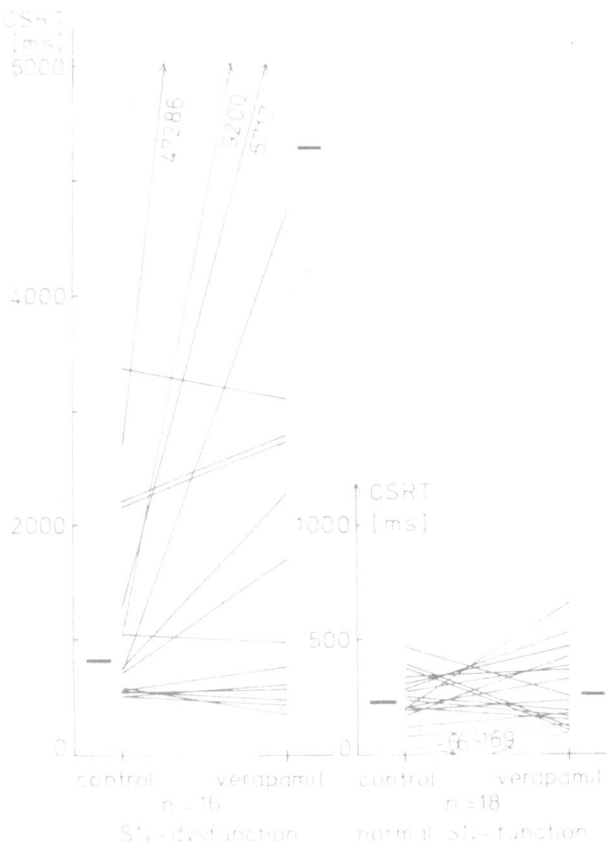

Figure 1. Sinus node recovery time corrected for heart rate (CSNRT) before and after verapamil administration (0.1 mg/kg iv) in patients with and without clinical signs of sinus node dysfunction.

In order to elucidate the mechanism of action of verapamil on sinus node function in man, the drug was tested in healthy volunteers before and after autonomic blockade (11). As expected, verapamil given iv without autonomic blockade led to a shortening of cardiac cycle length, i.e. to an increase in heart rate. During the next 15 min the cycle length increased without reaching the control values (Fig. 2). Simultaneously, there was a significant fall in mean systemic pressure. After autonomic blockade (propranolol 0.1 mg/kg, atropine 0.02 mg/kg iv) the cycle length shortened in comparison to the control situation. This rate represents the intrinsic heart rate, i.e. sinus node discharge without influence of the autonomic nervous system. This effect persisted

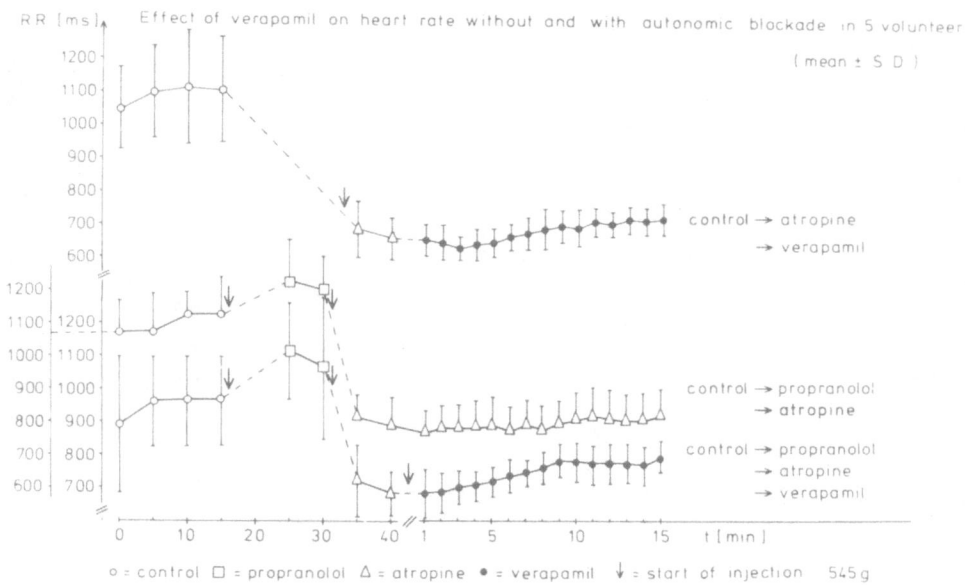

Figure 2. Effect of verapamil (0.1 mg/kg iv) on cycle length (R-R) before and after autonomic blockade in 5 volunteers.

for more than 15 min. On another day, verapamil was given iv after blocking the autonomic nervous system. In this situation, the additional application of verapamil caused a progressive increase in cycle length, i.e. a slowing of heart rate. Though changes were small, they were significant. The fall in systemic pressure was the same as after application of verapamil alone without autonomic blockade. The same effect of verapamil on the sinus node after autonomic blockade was demonstrated in experimental animals (1, 14, 79, 100). The results show that verapamil has a dual effect on the sinus node function. It exhibits a direct depressive effect on the sinus node which is unmasked after autonomic blockade. If the autonomic nervous system is unaffected, the concomitant fall in blood pressure induces an accelerating reflex mechanism which leads to an increase in heart rate. In addition to this indirect reflex mechanisms induced by verapamil via the baroreceptors, a direct catecholamine-releasing effect (18) and a vagolytic action (30) of Verapamil have been discussed. The results spread light on

the different effects of iv verapamil in patients with and without
sinus node dysfunction. In normals, the direct depressive effect
of verapamil on the sinus node is counteracted by the barorecep-
tor-induced cardioacceleration. In patients with SN-dysfunction,
the responsiveness of the sinus node to changes in autonomic tone
is reduced (19, 54). Therefore, the direct depressive effect of
the drug prevails that may lead to dangerous bradycardia and
asystole. On the other hand, iv verapamil may be useful in pro-
voking latent sinus node dysfunction. Whether the results also are
applicable to oral administration remains unsettled.

EFFECT ON THE A-V NODE

In the isolated preparation, all Ca-antagonists depress automaticity and conduction within the A-V node (44, 66, 74, 97). The
same effect is observed in the intact animal after iv application
(1, 30, 51, 55, 99). The effect is more pronounced if the drug is
given in the A-V nodal artery (40, 52, 60, 95). A possible explanation for this different action of Ca-antagonists on sinus and
A-V node is that the effect of the autonomic nervous system is
somewhat more pronounced on the sinus than on the A-V node. Therefore, the baroreceptor reflex predominantly influences the heart
rate (53). In contrast to the above mentioned results, nifedipine
has only small effects on the A-V node in experimental studies
(59, 60, 72, 74).

In man, many Ca-antagonists prolong conduction time and refractoriness of the A-V node. This has been demonstrated for verapamil
(31, 39, 63, 77, 82, 84, 86, 87), gallopalmil (D 600) (4, 87),
tiapamil (Ro 11-1781) (8, 32, 33, 87) and diltiazem (44, 68, 92).
Tab. 2 shows the effect of these four compounds on the A-V node in
patients with normal A-V conduction. In relation to the dose, D
600 has the most pronounced effect, tiapamil the weekest action on
the A-V node. In contrast to our results, some investigators (32)
found a significant decrease of the Wenckebach point after tiapamil in the same dose. Interestingly, the "pure" Ca-antagonist
nifedipine exerts no or only very small effect on the A-V node
when given in therapeutic doses (69, 81). The depressive effect of

Ca-antagonists on the A-V node can be counterbalanced by additional application of atropine or catecholamines (2, 33, 39, 45, 85).

Table 2. Effect of different Ca-antagonists on the A-V node (AVN). A-H = conduction time from the low right atrium to the bundle of His, FRP = functional, ERP = effective refractory period, SR = sinus rhythm, S-S paced cycle length, AV block = Wenckebach point during atrial pacing (cycle length).

	A-H S R	A-H S-S 600	FRP AVN	ERP AVN	AV block S-S
Verapamil 0.1 mg/kg iv	+13.2 %	+15.6 %	+11.0 %	+24.3 %	+14.0 %
D 600 0.03 mg/kg iv	+14.0 %	+25.0 %	+12.9 %	+31.2 %	+13.9 %
Tiapamil 1.0 mg/kg iv	+12.3 %	(+18.1 %)	-	-	(+ 8.9 %)
Diltiazem 0.15 mg/kg iv	(+5.6 %)	(+5.0 %)	-	(+13.1 %)	(+12.5 %)

EFFECTS ON OTHER CARDIAC STRUCTURES

Ca-antagonists have only little effect on action potential and refractoriness of the normal myocardium and the His-Purkinje system which becomes more pronounced only at high concentrations (16, 28, 50, 78, 90, 97, 100). Using suction electrodes in the dog's heart in situ, a change in the ratio of the duration of the monophasic action potential to the effective refractory period of the atrial muscle was observed (51). Spontaneous diastolic depolarization in Purkinje fibers has been observed to be depressed by verapamil (78), whereas other investigators noted a high resistence of pacemaker activity within the Purkinje system to verapamil (17, 24, 69, 99). However, nifedipine was reported to suppress abnormal automaticity in the partially depolarized Purkinje fiber (16, 17, 83, 94). Regenerative responses in the

spontaneously beating atrial muscle seem not to be influenced by
Ca-antagonists (66). Trigered activity in an atrial preparation
was abolished by verapamil in some studies (98), whereas other
investigators could not demonstrate this effect (99).

Electrophysiological studies in man were not able to show
significant effects of Ca-antagonists on atrial or ventricular
conduction and refractoriness (4, 31, 36, 39, 77, 84, 86, 87, 89,
92). In contrast, some investigators found a broadening of the
P wave in the surface ECG after verapamil (2, 5, 45). In addition,
the conductivity of the accessory pathway in patients with preexcitation syndrome is not influenced significantly by Ca-antagonists (34, 56, 64, 76, 91, 96). In some instances an acceleration
of conduction via the accessory pathway has been observed (64),
perhaps due to accelerating reflex mechanisms. The activity of
subsidiary pacemakers seems to be little influenced by Ca-antagonists (85, 92, 99). In higher doses, a depressive effect on latent
pacemakers was observed (26).

There are some studies in the isolated tissue indicating that
verapamil has some depressive effects on diseased myocardium that
may show slow channel conduction (18, 38, 71, 80). This may result
in an antiarrhythmic effect in these structures. In the ischemic
myocardium, verapamil was reported to reduce ventricular tachyarrhythmias, and to enhance fibrillation threshold (12, 29, 43,
75, 93). Paradoxically, verapamil seems to enhance impaired conduction in the ischemic myocardium, an effect which cannot be
explained by its slow channel blocking activity (22, 23). The results with nifedipine in this setting are controversial (17, 75).

WHAT ARE THE ELECTROPHYSIOLOGIC DIFFERENCES?
As mentioned in the introduction, the uniform concept of Ca-
antagonists has been questioned recently by some investigators (3,
15, 22, 28, 42, 48, 61, 62, 88). On the one hand, the way in which
different Ca-antagonists affect the kinetic of the slow channel
seems to be different. On the other, some Ca-antagonists have been
found to exert additional inhibitory effects on other ion channels.

Fleckenstein et al (28) distinguish three groups of so-called
Ca-antagonists: Group A (verapamil, D 600, nifedipine, diltiazem)
with outstanding specifity for the Ca-channel, group B (perhexiline, prenylamine, fendiline) with additional influences on the
Ca^{++}, Na^+, and Mg^{++} conductivities, and a third group (lidoflazine, tiapamil) which inhibit the fast Na-current equally or even
more intensively than the Ca-channel. The latter do not fulfil the
criteria for a specific slow channel blocker. In addition, concomitant effects on the (K^+) outward current have been assumed
(42). The effects of verapamil are a point of an intensive
discussion. In contrast to the results of Fleckenstein, Kaufmann
et al (3, 42) found that verapamil exerts some inhibitory effect
on the fast sodium channel. They speculate that the combination of
a slow channel blocker and a "local anaesthetic effect" resembles
the typical "class 4" action (42). "Pure" Ca-antagonists like
nifedipine are predominantly affecting the smooth muscle cells
causing a vasolidilatation (62). Fig. 3 tries to summarize these
data in a very speculative and oversimplificated manner.

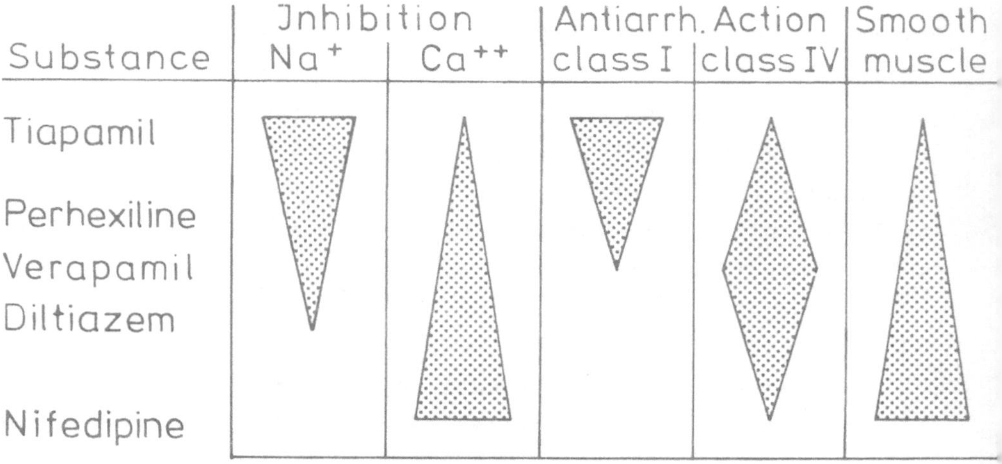

Substance	Inhibition		Antiarrh. Action		Smooth
	Na^+	Ca^{++}	class I	class IV	muscle
Tiapamil					
Perhexiline					
Verapamil					
Diltiazem					
Nifedipine					

Figure 3. Different effects of Ca-antagonists

CLINICAL IMPLICATIONS

From the reported electrophysiologic results some conclusion with regard to the therapy with Ca-antagonists can be drawn: Ca-antagonists in normal doses are not able to slow sinus rate. In very high doses this effect may be present. These drugs are therefore normally ineffective in sinus tachycardia, perhaps with the exception of true sinus node reentry tachycardia. In spite of this, Ca-antagonists should be used with caution in patients with sick sinus syndrome. Ca-antagonists, type verapamil are very useful in the acute treatment of tachycardias in which the A-V node is involved, i.e. A-V nodal tachycardias and reentry tachycardias in the preexcitation syndrome passing the A-V node. These drugs are able to slow ventricular rate in patients with atrial tachyarrhythmias, especially atrial flutter-fibrillation, if the impulse is conducted via the normal nodal pathway. (They are contraindicated if atrial fibrillation occurs in the WPW syndrome with antegrade conduction via the accessory pathway). Ca-antagonists of this type may lead to a higher degree A-V block in patients with A-V nodal conduction disturbances. This effect is not to be expected in patients with intraventricular (!) conduction defects. The reports on the efficacy of verapamil to suppress atrial or ventricular arrhythmias in patients with or without acute myocardial infarction are controversial.

In contrast to verapamil, nifedipine has no therapeutic value in supraventricular or ventricular arrhythmias. On the other hand, it does not induce A-V block in coronary patients with A-V nodal disease. In addition, the simultaneous application of nifedipine with beta blockers in patients with coronary heart disease may be less dangerous than the combination with verapamil. Therefore, the different electrophysiological effects of Ca-anta-gonists are of clinical relevance. These different effects should be studied very carefully before introducing a new calcium antagonistic drug.

REFERENCES

1. Angus JA, Richmond DR, Dhuma-Upakorn P, Kobbin LB, Goodman AH. Cardiovascular action of verapamil in the dog with particular reference to myocardial contractility and atrioventricular conduction. Cardiovasc Res 1976;10:623-632.
2. Bass O, Friedmann M. Ein Beitrag zum antiarrhythmischen Wirkungsmechanismus von Verapamil (Isoptin). Schweiz Med Wschr 1971;101:792-799.
3. Bayer R, Kalusche D, Kaufmann R, Mannhold R. Inotropic and electrophysiological actions of verapamil and D 600 in mammalian myocardium. III. Effects of the optical isomers on the transmembrane action potentials. Naunyn-Schmiedeberg's Arch Pharmacol 1975;290:81-97.
4. Beck OA, Witt E, Lehmann H-U, Hochrein H. Die Wirkung von Gallopamil (D 600) auf die intrakardiale Erregungsleitung und Sinusknotenautomatie beim Menschen. Z Kardiol 1978;67:522-526.
5. Belz GG, Bender F. 1974. Therapie der Herzrhythmusstörungen mit Verapamil. Stuttgart, Fischer, pp 8-13.
6. Bischoff KO, Hager W, Flohr E, Heredia D. Die Beeinflussung systolischer und elektrokardiographischer Zeitintervalle herzgesunder Patienten durch den Kalziumantagonisten Ro 11-1781. Z Kardiol 1978;67:268-272.
7. Blömer H, Wirtzfeld A, Delius W, Sebening H. 1977. Das Sinusknotensyndrom. Erlangen, Perimed, p 89.
8. Bödeker K, Bischoff KO, Menken U, Hager W. Hämodynamische und elektrophysiologische Wirkungen des neuen Calcium-Antagonisten Ro 11-1781. Z Kardiol 1980;69:790-796.
9. Breithardt G, Seipel L. 1976. The influence of drugs on sinoatrial conduction time in man; in Lüderitz: Cardiac pacing. Berlin, Springer, pp 58-72.
10. Breithardt G, Seipel L, Wiebringhaus E, Loogen F. Effects of verapamil on sinus node function in man. Europ J Cardiol 1978;8:379-394.
11. Breithardt G, Seipel L, Wiebringhaus E, Loogen F. The role of autonomic nervous system in the action of verapamil on the sinus node in man. Basic Res Cardiol 1978;73:637-647.
12. Broks WW, Verrier RL, Lown B. Protective effect of verapamil on ventricular vulnerability during coronary artery occlusion and reperfusion (Abstr.). Am J Cardiol 1978;41:426.
13. Carrasco HA, Fuenmayor A, Barboza JS, Gonzales G. Effect of verapamil on normal sinoatrial node function and on sick sinus syndrome. Am Heart J 1978;96:760-771.
14. Cavero I, Boudot JP, Lefevre-Borg F, Roach AG. 1979. Pharmacological evaluation of diltiazem and its desacetylated metabolite in several animal species. III. Mechanism of the cardiac acceleration evoked by diltiazem and desacetyldiltiazem in the conscious rabbit; in Bing: New drug therapy with a calcium antagonist. Amsterdam, Excerpta Medica, pp 81-88.
15. Chiba S, Kobayashi M, Furukawa Y. Effects of optical isomers of verapamil on SA nodal pacemaker activity and contractility of the isolated dog heart. Jap Heart J 1978;19:409-414.

16. Cranefield PF, Aronson RS, Wit AL. Effect of Verapamil on the normal action potential and on a calcium depent slow response of canine cardiac purkinje fibers. Circulation Res 1974;34: 204-213.
17. Dangman KH, Hoffman BF. Effects of nifedipine on electrical activity of cardiac cells. Am J Cardiol 1980;46:1059-1067.
18. Danilo P Jr, Hordof AJ, Reder RF, Rosen MR. Effects of verapamil on electrophysiologic properties of blood superfused cardiac purkinje fibers. J Pharmacol and Exper Therap 1980; 213:222-227.
19. Dighton DH. Sinus Bradycardia. Autonomic influences and clinical assessment. Brit Heart J 1974;36:791-797.
20. Dyrszka H, Wahn B. Klinisches Bild und Therapie einer Überdosis des Koronartherapeutikums Nifedipine (Adalat). Inn Med 1977;4:31-34.
21. Ehara T, Kaufmann R. The voltage- and time-dependent effects of (-)-verapamil on the slow inward current in isolated cat ventricular myocardium. J Pharmacol exper Ther 1978;207:49-55.
22. Elharrar V, Gaum WE, Zipes DP. Effect of drugs on conduction delay and incidence of ventricular arrhythmias induced by acute coronary occlusion in dogs. Am J Cardiol 1977;39: 544-549.
23. El-Sherif N, Lazzara R. Reentrant ventricular arrhythmias in the late myocardial infarction period. 7. Effect of verapamil and D-600 and the role of "slow channel". Circulation 1979; 60:605-615.
24. Endoh M, Yanagisawa T, Taira N. Effects of Calcium-Antagonistic Coronary Vasodilators. Nifedipine and Verapamil, on Ventricular Automaticity of the Dog. Naunyn-Schmiedeberg's Arch Pharmacol 1978;302:235-238.
25. Faire U de, Lundman T. Attempted suicide with verapamil. Europ J Cardiol 1977;6:195-198.
26. Feerst D, Talano J, Singer D, Lesch M. The effect of verapamil on latent pacemakers in the canine heart (Abstr.). Circulation Suppl 1978;58/II:183.
27. Fleckenstein A, Kammermeier H, Döring H, Freund HJ. Zum Wirkungsmechanismus neuartiger Koronardilatatoren mit gleichzeitig Sauerstoff-einsparenden Myokard-Effekten, Prenylamin und Iproveratril. Z Kreisl Forschg 1967;56:716-744.
28. Fleckenstein A, Späh F. 1981. Excitation-contraction uncoupling in the cardiac muscle; in Ebashi (ed.): Proc 8th intern Congr Pharmacol. London, Pergamon Press, p 23.
29. Fondacaro JD, Han J, Yoon MS. Effects of verapamil on ventricular rhythm during acute coronary occlusion. Am Heart J 1978;96:81-86.
30. Garvey HL. The mechanisms of action of verapamil on the sinus and AV nodes. Europ J Pharmacol 1969;8:159-166.
31. Gleichmann U, Seipel L, Loogen F. Der Einfluß von Antiarrhythmika auf die intrakardiale Erregungsleitung (His-Bündel Elektrographie) und Sinusknotenautomatie beim Menschen. Dtsch Med Wschr 1973;98:1487-1494.
32. Gmeiner R, Simma H, NG CK, Dienstl F, Knapp E. Die Wirkung von Ro 11-1781, einem Kalziumantagonisten, auf die atrioventrikuläre Überleitung. Z Kardiol 1977;66:238-241.

33. Gmeiner R, NG CK, Simma H, Gstöttner M. The effect of a new calcium antagonist (Ro 11-1781) on the cardiac conduction system in man. Europ J Cardiol 1979;9:77-86.
34. Gmeiner R, NG CK. Effect of tiapamil in the Wolff-Parkinson-White syndrome. J Cardiovasc Pharmacol 1981;3:237-250.
35. Grendahl H, Miller M, Sivertssen E. Registration of sinus node recovery time in patients with sinus rhythm and in patients with disrhythmias. Act Med Scand 1975;197:403-408.
36. Grohmann HW, Theisen K, Jahrmärker H. Einfach- und Doppel-stimulation des menschlichen Vorhofs. Untersuchungen zur Refraktärzeitbestimmung. Verh Dtsch Ges Kreislaufforschg 1971; 37:460-464.
37. Heng MK, Singh BN, Roche AHG, Norris RM, Mercer CJ. Effects of intravenous verapamil on cardiac arrhythmias and on the electrocardiogram. Am Heart J 1975;90:487-498.
38. Hordof AJ, Edie R, Malm JR, Hoffman BF, Rosen MR. Electrophy-siologic properties and response to pharmacologic agents of fibers from diseased human atria. Circulation 1976;54: 774-779.
39. Husaini MH, Kvasnicka J, Ryden L, Holmberg S. Action of vera-pamil on sinus node, atrioventricular und intraventricular conduction. Br Heart J 1973;35:734-737.
40. Iijima T, Taira N. Modification by manganese ions and vera-pamil of the responses of the atrioventricular node to norepinephrine. Europ J Pharmacol 1976;37:55-62.
41. Kaltenbach M, Hopf R, Keller M. Calciumantagonistische Thera-pie bei hypertrophisch-obstruktiver Kardiomyopathie. Dtsch Med Wschr 1976;101:1284-1287.
42. Kaufmann R, Bayer R. 1980. Combination of β-Blockers and calcium antagonists with regard to cardiac electrophysiology; in Roskomm, Graefe: Advances in β-Blocker therapy. Amsterdam, Excerpta Medica, pp 111-119.
43. Kaufmann AJ, Aramendia P. Prevention of ventricular fibrilla-tion induced by coronary ligation. J Pharmacol Exper Ther 1968;164:326-332.
44. Kawai C, Konishi T, Matsuyama E, Okazaki H. 1979. Effects of diltiazem on sinoatrial and atrioventricular nodes in com-parison with other calcium-antagonists; in Bing: New drug therapy with a calcium antagonist. Amsterdam, Excerpta Medica, pp 141-149.
45. Klempt HW, Bachour G, Reploh HD, Gradaus D, Brisse B, Bender F. Untersuchungen zum Wirkungsmechanismus von Verapamil. Verh Dtsch Ges inn Med 1972;78:1116-1120.
46. Kohlhardt M, Bauer B, Kraise H, Fleckenstein A. Differen-tiation of the transmembrane Na and Ca channels in mammalian cardiac fibers by use of specific inhibitors. Pfluegers Archiv 1972;335:309-322.
47. Kohlhardt M, Figulla HR, Tripathi O. The slow membrane channel as the predominant mediator of the excitation process of the sinoatrial pacemaker cell. Basic Res Cardiol 1976;71:17-26.
48. Kohlhardt M, Fleckenstein A. Inhibition of the slow inward current by nifedipine in mammalian ventricular myocardium. Naunyn Schmiedeberg's Arch Pharmacol 1977;298:267-272.

49. Kuhn H, Thelen U, Leuner C, Köhler E, Bluschke V. Langzeit-behandlung der hypertrophischen nicht obstruktiven Kar-diomyopathie (HNCM) mit Verapamil. Z Kardiol 1980;69:669-675.
50. Kupersmith J, Cohen R. Differing electrophysiologic effects of slow response inhibiting agents manganese and verapamil on ischemic, infarcted and normal tissue in situ. J Pharmacol exper Ther 1980;215:394-400.
51. Landmark K, Amlie JP. A study of the verapamil-induced changes in conductivity and refractoriness and monophasic action potentials of the dog heart in situ. Europ J Cardiol 1976;4: 419-427.
52. Lupi GA, Urthaler F, James TN. Effects of verapamil on auto-maticity and conduction with particular reference to tachyphy-laxis. Europ J Cardiol 1979;9:345-368.
53. Mancia G, Bonazzi O, Ferrari A, Gardumi M, Gregorini L, Perondi R, Pozzoni L. 1978. Baroreceptor control of atrio-ventricular conduction system in man; in Scharz, Brown, Malliani, Zanetti: Neural mechanisms in cardiac arrhythmias. New York, Raven-Presse, pp 339-343.
54. Mandel WJ, Hayakawa H, Allen HN, Danzig R, Kermaier AI. Assessment of sinus node function in patients with the sick sinus syndrome. Circulation 1972;46:761-769.
55. Mangiardi LM, Hariman RJ, McAllister RG, Bhargava V, Surawicz B, Shabetal R. Electrophysiologic and hemodynamic effects of Verapamil. Circulation 1978;57:366-372.
56. Matsuyama E, Konishi T, Okazaki H, Matsuda H, Kawai C. Effects of verapamil on accessory pathway properities and induction of circus movement tachycardia in patients with the Wolff-Parkinson-White syndrome. J Cardiovasc Pharmacol 1981;3: 11-24.
57. Melville KI, Shister HE, Huo S. Iproveratril: Experimental data on coronary dilatation and antiarrhythmic action. Canad Med Ass 1964;90:761-770.
58. Mertens HM, Mannebach H, Gleichmann U. 24stündiger elektrischer Herzstillstand nach intravenöser Gabe von 10 mg Verapamil. Z Kardiol 1980;69:414-416.
59. Motomura S, Taira N. Differential effects of organic slow inward current inhibitors, verapamil and nifedipine, on rate of atrioventricular rhythm and supraventricular tachycardia in the canine isolated, blood perfused AV node preparation. Naunyn-Schmiedeberg's Arch Pharmacol 1981;315:241-248.
60. Narimatsu A, Taira N. Effects on atrio-ventricular conduction of calcium-antagonistic coronary vasodilators, local anaesthe-tics and quinidine injected into the posterior and septal artery of the atrioventricular node preparation of the dog. Naunyn-Schmiedeberg's Arch Pharmacol 1976;294:169-177.
61. Nawrath H, Ten Eick RE, McDonald TF, Trautwein W. On the mechanism underlying the action of D-600 on slow inward current and tension in mammalian myocardium. Circulation Res 1977;40:408-414.
62. Nayler WG. Calcium antagonists. Europ Heart J 1980;1:225-237.
63. Neuss H, Schlepper M. Der Einfluß von Verapamil auf die atrio-ventrikuläre Überleitung. Lokalisation des Wirkungsortes mit His-Bündel Elektrogrammen. Verh Dtsch Ges Kreisl Forschg 1971;37:433-438.

64. Neuss H, Schlepper M. Influence of verious antiarrhythmic drugs (Aprinidine, Ajmaline, Verapamil, Oxprenolol, Orciprenaline) on functional properties of accessory A-V pathway. Act Cardiol Suppl 1974;18:279-288.
65. Obayashi K, Nagasawa K, Mandel WJ, Vyden JK. Cardiovascular effects of the new antiarrhythmic agent verapamil (Abstr.). Am J Cardiol 1975;35:161.
66. Okada T, Konishi T. Effects of verapamil on SA and AV nodal action potentials in the isolated rabbit heart. Jap Circulation J 1975;39:913-917.
67. Ono H, Himori N, Taira N. Chronotropic effects of coronary vasodilators as assessed in the isolated, blood-perfused sinoatrial node preparation of the dog. Tohoki J exp Med 1977; 121:383-390.
68. Oyama Y, Imai Y, Nakaya H, Kanda K, Satoh T. The effects of diltiazem hydrochloride on the cardiac conduction. A clinical study of His bundle electrogram. Jap Circulation J 1978;42: 1257-1264.
69. Padeletti L, Franchi F, Brat A, Dabizzi RP, Michelucci A. The cardiac electrophysiological effects of nifedipine. Intern J Clin Pharmacol Biopharm 1979;17:290-293.
70. Perkins CM. Serious verapamil poisoning: treatment with intravenous calcium gluconate. Brit Med J 1978;4:1127.
71. Peter T, Hamamoto H, McCullen A, Yamaguchi I, Mandel WJ. 1980. Verapamil effects in the setting of acute experimental myocardial ischemia; in Fleckenstein, Roskamm: Calcium-Antagonismus. Berlin, Springer, pp 75-85.
72. Raschack M. Differences in the cardiac actions of the Calcium antagonists Verapamil and Nifedipine. Arzneim Forschg 1976;26: 1330-1333.
73. Refsum H, Landmark K. The effect of a Calcium-antagonistic drug, nifedipine, on the mechanical and electrical activity of the isolated rat atrium. Act pharmacol toxical (Kbh) 1975;37: 369-376.
74. Refsum H, Glomstein A, Landmark K. The effect of nifedipine on the isolated rat heart. Act pharmacol toxicol (Kbh) 1976; 38:328-335.
75. Ribeiro LGT, DeBauche TL, Brandon TA, Maroko PR, Miller RR. Comparative effects of verapamil and nifedipine on reactive hyperemia and ventricular arrhythmias during coronary reperfusion. Europ Heart J 1980;1,suppl B:31-35.
76. Rinkenberger RL, Prystowsky EN, Heger JJ, Troup PJ, Jackman WM, Zipes DP. Effects of intravenous and chronic oral verapamil administration in patients with supraventricular tachyarrhythmias. Circulation 1980;62:996-1010.
77. Rizzon P, DiBiase M, Calabrese P, Brindicci G, Chiddo A. Electrophysiologic evaluation of intravenous verapamil in man. Europ J Cardiol 1977;6:179-194.
78. Rosen MR, Ilvento JP, Gelband H, Merker C. Effects of verapamil on electrophysiologic properties of canine cardiac purkinje fibers. J Pharmacol exper Ther 1974;189:414-422.
79. Ross G, Jorgensen CR. Cardiovascular actions of verapamil. J Pharmacol exper Ther 1967;158:504-509.

80. Rossner KL, Sachs HS. Electrophysiological study of syrian hamster hereditary cardiomyopathy. Cardiovasc Res 1978;12: 436-443.
81. Rowland E, Evans T, Krikler D. Effect of nifedipine on atrio-ventricular conduction as compared with verapamil. Intracardiac electrophysiological study. Br Heart J 1979;42:124-127.
82. Roy PR, Spurrel RAJ, Sowton E. The effect of verapamil on the cardiac conduction system in man. Postgrad Med J 1974;50: 270-275.
83. Saikawa T, Arita M. Effects of verapamil and its optical isomers on repetitive slow responses induced by electrical depolarization in canine ventricular myocardium. Jap Heart J 1980; 21:247-255.
84. Schlepper M, Neuss H. Changes of refractory periods in the A-V conduction system induced by antiarrhythmic drugs. A study using His bundle recordings. Act Cardiol (Brux) 1974;suppl 18: 269-277.
85. Seipel L, Breithardt G. 1980. Effects of Calcium-antagonists on automaticity and conduction in man; in Fleckenstein, Roskamm: Calcium-Antagonismus. Berlin, Springer, pp 87-96.
86. Seipel L, Both A, Breithardt G, Gleichmann U, Loogen F. Action of antiarrhythmic drugs on His bundle electrogram and sinus node function. Act Cardiol (Brux) 1974;suppl 18:251-267.
87. Seipel L, Breithardt G, Abendroth, R-R, Wiebringhaus E. Vergleichende klinisch-elektrophysiologische Untersuchungen verschiedener Ca-Antagonisten (Gallopamil (D 600), Dimeditia-pramin (Ro 11-1781), Verapamil). Z Kardiol 1980;69:551-555.
88. Shigenobu K, Schneider JA, Sperelakis N. Verapamil blockade of slow Na^+ and Ca^+ responses in myocardial cells. J Pharmacol exper Ther 1974;190:280-288.
89. Silvertssen E, Bay G, Grendahl H. The effect of propranolol and verapamil on atrial and atrioventricular refractory periods in man. Angiol 1975;26:605-618.
90. Singh BN, Vaughan Williams EM. A fourth class of antidysrhythmic action? Effect of verapamil on ouabain toxicity, on atrial and ventricular intracellular potentials, and on other features of cardiac function. Cardiovasc Res 1972;6:109-119.
91. Spurrell RAJ, Krikler DM, Sowton E. Effects of verapamil on electrophysiological properties of anomalous atrioventricular connexion in Wolff-Parkinson-White-syndrome. Br Heart J 1974; 36:256-264.
92. Sugimoto T, Ishikawa T, Kaseno K, Nakase S. Electrophysiological effects of diltiazem, a calcium antagonist, in patients with impaired sinus or atrioventricular node function. Angiol 1980;31:700-709.
93. Sugiyama S, Ozawa T, Suzuki S, Kato T. Effects of verapamil and propranolol on ventricular vulnerability after coronary reperfusion. J Electrocardiol 1980;13:49-54.
94. Tse WW, Han J. Effect of manganese chloride and verapamil on automaticity of digitalized purkinje fibers. Am J Cardiol 1975;36:50-55.
95. Urthaler F, James TN. Experimental studies on the pathogenesis of asystole after verapamil in the dog. Am J Cardiol 1979;44: 651-656.

96. Wellens HJJ. 1975. Effect of Drugs on Wolff-Parkinson-White syndrome; in Narula: His bundle electrography and clinical electrophysiology. Philadelphia, Davis Comp., pp 367-385.
97. Wit AL, Cranefield PF. Effect of Verapamil on the sinoatrial and atrioventricular nodes of the rabbit and the mechanism by which it arrests reentrant atrioventricular node tachycardia. Circulation Res 1974;35:413-425.
98. Wit AL, Fenoglio JJ, Hordorf AJ, Reemtsma K. Ultrastructure and transmembrane potentials of cardiac muscle in the human anterior mitral valve leaflet. Circulation 1979;59:1284-1292.
99. Yamaguchi I, Obayashi K, Mandel WJ. Electrophysiological effects of verapamil. Cardiovasc Res 1978;12:597-608.
100. Zipes DP, Fischer JC. Effects of agents which inhibit the slow channel on sinus node automaticity and atrioventricular conduction in the dog. Circulation Res 1974;34:184-192.

CLINICAL DIFFERENCES BETWEEN THE CALCIUM CHANNEL BLOCKING AGENTS*

ALFRED F. PARISI, M.D.**

The clinical differences between the different drugs which have been classified as calcium channel blocking agents are not as yet completely defined. The vast majority of literature which has appeared to date evaluates a single one of these drugs in comparison to placebo or less frequently in comparison to beta blockers. There are only a handful of studies which evaluate two or more of these new drugs in the same patient population. Assuming appropriate dose equivalency (which is not necessarily readily agreed upon), this latter type of study involves the least presumptions about clinical differences between these agents and thus potentially allows <u>direct</u> <u>comparison</u> of their relative efficacy and toxicity. However, the number of such studies is quite limited, the number of patients studied are small and dose equivalence between different agents is not as yet firmly established. Thus, most of the available information for comparing the different calcium channel blocking agents comes from independent studies of one or another of these agents. Such <u>indirect</u> <u>comparisons</u> can reasonably be inferred from studies of single agents when the clinical response appears to be a duplication and/or extension of pharmacologic effects observed in animals and when qualitatively different side effects are noted in the consensus of independent investigations. Table 1 lists the cardiovascular diseases and syndromes for which calcium channel blocking agents have been advocated. In this brief review I will indicate the clinical highlights of few emerging calcium channel blocking agents, emphasing the clinical differences that have been noted

---

   * Supported by the Medical Research Service of the U.S. Veterans Administration.
   **From the Department of Medicine, West Roxbury Veterans Administration Medical Center, Brigham and Women's Hospital and Harvard Medical School, Boston, Massachusetts.

when these agents have been used to treat cardiovascular disease and syndromes of major clinical importance.

Table 1. Conditions for which calcium channel blocking agents have been proposed as therapeutic agents.

Supraventricular tachycardia
Hypertension
Exertional angina
Vasospastic (variant) angina
Cardiomyopathy
Heart failure
Myocardial infarction
Cerebral vasospasm
Intestinal ischemia
Myocardial preservation (surgery)

I. CONTRASTING SPECTRUM OF CLINICAL APPLICATION

A. Supraventricular Tachyarrhythmias

Because of their differing effects on blood pressure and atrioventricular conduction, the spectrum of clinical application of the calcium channel blocking agents varies considerably. Of the currently popular calcium channel blocking agents verapamil has been available the longest, being introduced in Europe in 1962. To date, one of the most striking of these differences is the negative influence that verapamil has on atrioventricular conduction.

Kawai and colleagues recently reported a comparative study of verapamil, diltiazem and nifedipine on the sinoatrial and atrioventricular node function in 31 patients at cardiac catheterization (1). Electrophysiologic measurements were made before and after intravenous administration of each of these agents. Ten patients received diltiazem (10 to 20 mg), 13 patients received verapamil (10 mg) and 8 patients received nifedipine (1 mg). Nifedipine caused a significant increase in sinus rate (78 to 98 beats/minute) and shortened the sinus node recovery time (1331 to 1001 msec). Neither diltiazem nor verapamil influenced either of these measures of sinus node function significantly. In contrast both verapamil and diltiazem increased the AH interval, and prolonged the effective and functional refractory periods of the atrioventricular (AV) node, while nifedipine decreased these measures of AV node conduction and excitability. Verapamil had a more pronounced effect than diltiazem, increasing the AH interval 24 msec, the effective refractory period of the AV node 101 msec and the functional refractory period of the AV node 49 msec. None of the agents significantly altered His-Purkinje conduction (HV interval).

These pronounced effects of verapamil on AV nodal conduction underlie its efficacy in treating supraventricular tachydysrhythmias. Verapamil is most effective in treating AV nodal re-entrant supraventricular tachycardias, wherein more than 90% of patients convert to sinus rhythm within minutes of an intravenous bolus. Verapamil is also useful in treating atrial fibrillation and atrial flutter. After an intravenous administration, verapamil slows the ventricular response in approximately 90% of patients with atrial fibrillation, although less than 10% of these patients revert to sinus rhythm in this setting. In atrial flutter intravenous verapamil can be expected to slow the ventricular response in approximately 50% of patients; 30% will convert to sinus rhythm while 20% will convert to atrial fibrillation.

In a detailed clinical and electrophysiologic study of 28 patients with different forms of supraventricular tachycardia (SVT), Rikenberger et al showed that verapamil prolonged antegrade AV nodal conduction time, but did not affect retrograde AV nodal conduction time (2). Verapamil was successful in terminating SVT in all six patients with AV nodal re-entrant tachycardia. In six patients with SVT dependent on an accessory (WPW) pathway for retrograde conduction, verapamil terminated the rhythm in four patients and slowed it in two. In these patients the mechanism of dysrhythmia interruption was still slowing of antegrade AV nodal conduction. Verapamil did not affect the electrophysiologic properties of the accessory pathway. In three patients with automatic atrial tachycardias, verpamil produced AV node Wenckebach conduction but did not slow the rate of discharge of the ectopic atrial focus.

In the same study, oral verapamil was administered to 19 patients with somewhat less success for preventing dysrhythmias than occurred with the intravenous route for treating dysrhythmias. Within 30 days 10 of these patients discontinued the drug because of ineffectiveness or side effects. However, 7 patients did show evidence of long-term (mean 19 months) improvement with decreased frequency and shorter duration episodes of tachycardia.

B. Hypertension

Nifedipine was first introduced for clinical use in Japan in the mid 1970's. As compared to the other available calcium channel blocking agents, nifedipine has a considerably more pronounced arteriolar dilating effect. This property has made it a useful drug to treat hypertension.

Olivari, et al reported the effectiveness of nifedipine in 27 patients with moderately severe essential hypertension (diastolic pressure > 110) (3). After a ten day placebo-controlled run-in period during which blood pressures were closely monitored, patients were given nifedipine -- either 10 mg PO every six hours, or every twelve hours with placebo administration interposed at six hours. Nifedipine produced a 21% fall in systolic pressure and 19% fall in diastolic pressure within one hour; in patients receiving nifedipine twice daily, pressures rose to control levels by 12 hours from the preceding dose. Patients receiving nifedipine every 6 hours showed a sustained hypotensive effect to blood pressures approximately 20% less than control values. Blood pressure slowly rose to pretreatment levels by two days after nifedipine was withdrawn at the end of the trial.

Interestingly in individual patients the reduction in blood pressure related to the magnitude of the measured pretreatment peripheral arterial resistance. Those patients with the highest peripheral resistance had the greatest reduction in systolic and diastolic blood pressure. In a subsequent study the same group demonstrated that nifedipine could be effectively combined with methyldopa to lower blood pressure in a group of 23 patients with severe hypertension (diastolic pressure > 120 mm Hg) (4). The drug combination provided to be more potent than either agent alone, and produced a smoothing of intra-diem blood pressure fluctuations seen with nifedipine alone. Twenty-two of the twenty-three patients completed a 12-month follow-up study in which persistence of the efficacy of the drug combination was documented and beneficial effects on heart size, ECG and fundi were demonstrated.

Nifedipine has also been used in combination with beta blockade with propranolol to achieve an additive effect on blood pressure reduction. There is less extensive reported experience with other calcium channel blockers in hypertension. Some reports, however, have indicated that neither verapamil nor diltiazem produced a sustained hypotensive effect when administered chronically.

C. Exertional Angina Pectoris

Despite many years of experience with calcium channel blocking agents in treating patients with angina pectoris, it is only recently that studies

have emerged which adhere to well-designed scientific protocols. These
studies do not give a good insight into the comparative efficacy of different agents; however, from them one can glean minor differences in mechanism of action and differences in side effects and toxicity. The highlights of some of these studies which have shown statistically significant
results for drug efficacy are discussed below.

When verapamil was first used as an anti-anginal agent, it was employed
in low doses (40 to 80 mgs t.i.d.), and was not found to relieve angina
significantly more than placebo (5). Several subsequent investigations
which more fully explored its dose range, however, have found that larger
doses (80 to 120 mg t.i.d.) are effective not only in reducing anginal
attack rates and nitroglycerine consumption, but also in prolonging exercise tolerance (6-9). Sandler, et al found that 120 mgs t.i.d. had favorable effects on the amount and duration of ST segment depression which
occurs in the exercise electrocardiograms of patients with angina (6).
In a more recent study of treadmill exercise using computer-assisted
analysis of ST segment depression, verapamil as compared to a placebo,
slowed the rate of development of ST segment depression so that at comparable levels of exercise, ST segment depression was significantly reduced (9). However, at peak exercise, which occcurred later on verapamil
than on placebo, ST segment depression was unchanged as compared to placebo
therapy. In this study patients did not achieve a higher maximum double
product (heart rate x systolic blood pressure) indicating verapamil acted
by lowering myocardial oxygen requirements rather than increasing myocardial blood supply.

There has been considerable clinical experience with nifedipine in
treating chronic stable angina. Many early studies have reported that it
reduces angina frequency and nitroglycerine consumption (10). Most of
these early studies either did not involve well-designed protocols or
objective measures of efficacy. However, two recent randomized double-
blind crossover studies have confirmed the usefulness of nifedipine for
relief of anginal symptoms. Each also demonstrated that nifedipine
prolongs the duration of treadmill exercise. In ten patients, Moskowitz,
et al showed that nifedipine increased exercise duration to 523 sec from
a mean of 462 sec on placebo (11). Resting heart rate was slightly increased and resting systolic blood pressure, was 8 to 11 mm Hg lower after
nifedipine. At submaximal levles of exercise, the heart rate x blood

pressure product was lower on nifedipine than placebo; however, at end
(maximal) exercise, the double product was the same as achieved with
placebo therapy. Lynch, et al had similar results indicating that in
exercise-induced angina, nifedipine acts primarily by decreasing myocardial oxygen demands rather than improving myocardial blood supply (12).
As compared to placebo Lynch, et al also found fewer and less widespread
exercise-induced ST depression on nifedipine. In addition, fewer episodes
of ST segment depression were noted on 48 hr ambulatory electrocardiographic recordings. The latter group also compared the efficacy of nifedipine
(30 mg and 60 mg daily) to propranolol (240 mg and 480 mg daily) and the
combination of nifedipine plus propranolol. The drug combination proved
to be the most efficacious of the regimens examined. Very little has
been reported concerning the efficacy of combining other calcium channel
blockers with beta blockade.

Diltiazem has been widely used in Japan, particularly to treat variant
angina. Recently, several studies have appeared indicating that it has
promise for treating stable angina pectoris. Pool, et al found that doses
of 120, 180, and 240 mgs per day each improved treadmill performance in a
group of 15 patients studied in a double-blind, placebo-controlled crossover study (13). Thus, the time to onset of angina, onset of 1 mm ST
segment depression and total duration of exercise were prolonged.

Using a similar protocol, Hossack and Bruce showed that diltiazem
produced an increase in total exercise time, time to appearance of 1 mm
ST segment depression and time to onset angina which was most prominent
at the highest (240 mg) dose (14). Diltiazem slowed resting heart rate
by approximately 10% but did not alter the resting or maximum heart rate
blood pressure product. As is the case with nifedipine and verapamil,
the agent seems to be effective by lowering myocardial oxygen demands.
In both of these studies the effects of diltiazem on clinical measures
of angina (attack rates per week and nitroglycerine consumption) were
not reported, although Hossack and Bruce showed a tendency to less exercise-induced angina on treadmill testing during diltiazem therapy.

Two more recent reports using identical protocols to those above
found that the 120 and 180 mg dosages did not increase exercise time;
however, as compared to placebo, diltiazem in doses of 240 mg/day increased maximum exercise time and time to onset of angina (15, 16).
These early results are reminiscent of initial experience with verapamil

as an antianginal agent and suggest that more extensive evaluation of higher doses of diltiazem are needed to define its antianginal effectiveness more completely.

There is a very recent brief report of an acute study of 16 patients with stable angina, in which nifedipine and dilitiazem were compared directly (17). Each agent was given in a randomized double-blind protocol on alternate days prior to symptom-limited bicycle ergometry. As compared to control, both nifedipine and diltiazem significantly increased the exercise incurred workload. In the single doses used the beneficial effect of nifedipine (30 mg PO) was evident at 3 hours, but could not be detected in a second test 8 hours later. In contrast, diltiazem (180 mg PO) had a measurable effect in significantly increasing work performed up to 8 hours beyond its administration. Although both nifedipine and diltiazem are noted to have comparable serum half-lives (4 hours), assuming dose equivalency these results suggest a possible difference in biologic half-life. A longer biologic half-life could have advantages in dosing frequency and possibly in the emergence of symptoms after dose omissions. One recent study of diltiazem in patients with variant angina also suggests that its effects may be sustained beyond its measurable persistence in the body (18).

Lidoflazine is an antianginal agent developed and initially marketed in Belgium in 1969. Several well-designed trials have shown that it decreases anginal frequency, nitroglycerine consumption and prolongs exercise tolerance when compared to placebo (19). Unlike the other calcium blockers, its antianginal effects may not develop fully in the early weeks of therapy, but have been noted to achieve a maximum after 3 to 4 months of therapy. The agent does not alter resting or maximal heart rates, but blunts the rate response to submaximal levels of exercise. Thus, like the other calcium channel blockers, it appears to act by decreasing myocardial oxygen demands rather than by increasing myocardial blood supply.

In summary, when used to treat patients with exertional angina pectoris, in contrast to beta blockers, calcium channel blocking agents in currently reported clinical dosages do not have a pronounced negative chronotropic effect on the sinus node. Nifedipine, being most potent vasodilator, produces an increase sympathetic tone secondary to its hypotensive effect and is commonly associated with an increase in resting heart rate. In most patients this does not exceed 10 beats/minute. Verapamil and diltiazem do not produce a cardioacceleratory response, but rather a very mild degree of slowing. This effect is usually not as pronounced as beta blockade and in most studies is less than 10 beats/minute. Lidoflazine appears to have a minimum or no effect on resting heart rates in most patients.

Nifedipine lowers resting systolic blood pressure by 10 to 15 mm Hg in most normotensive patients who receive anti-anginal doses of the drug, while the remaining agents have a less pronounced or no hypotensive effect.

In patients with exertional angina, these calcium channel blockers have all been shown to prolong the duration of exercise before angina by lowering the heart rate x blood pressure product at submaximal levels of exercise; however, none of these agents increases the rate pressure product at symptom limited maximal exercise. Lidoflazine appears to act primarily by blunting the stress induced increment in heart rate with exercise while nifedipine appears to act mainly by blunting the exercise induced increase in systolic blood pressure.

D. Variant Angina Pectoris

Several recent reports have directly compared two or more calcium channel blocking agents in patients with variant angina. The group at the Montreal Heart Institute monitored efficacy of four different agents -- nifedipine, diltiazem, verapamil, and perhexiline -- by challenging patients with variant angina using graded doses of intravenous ergonovine (20). Nifedipine appeared to be more effective than the other agents in mitigating the ergonovine challenge. While these results might suggest some superiority in efficacy for nifedipine, it must be remembered that the model of an ergonovine challenge does not necessarily simulate the abnormal natural processes which provoke coronary spasm.

More recently Johnson, et al reported the results of a parallel, double-blind, double crossover protocol in which verapamil was compared to placebo (ten patients were studied) (21). At the end of four 2-month treatment periods, all patients were crossed over to nifedipine for an additional 2 months. They found that the number of chest pains per week, nitroglycerine consumption and the number of transient ST segment deviations on calibrated two channel ambulatory ECG monitoring, were similar during treatment with verapamil and nifedipine and less than with placebo (Table 2). Hospitalization for instability was required in two patients wile taking placebo and two while taking nifedipine, but in none while

Table 2. Comparative responses to therapy in variant angina.

	Placebo	Verapamil	Nifedipine
Anginal episodes/week	15.9	2.2	1.2
NTG tablets/week	18.3	3.2	2.4
ST deviations/week	40.1	6.5	9.8

All values are means. Excerpted from Johnson et al (21).

taking verapamil. The small number of patients involved hardly allows any conclusions regarding the relative efficacy of nifedipine and verapamil but casts some doubt about the appropriateness of conclusions drawn from the above cited study using ergonovine challenge. Despite this similar efficacy, nifedipine was less well tolerated -- its dosage had to be limited in six patients -- in two patients because of orthostatic hypotension, in one patient because of marked pedal edema and in three others because of gastrointestinal complaints. Another recent report also suggested that nifedipine was poorly tololerated when compared to verapamil (22). Gated blood pool scintigraphy at rest and during exercise showed that neither verapamil nor nifedipine significantly altered left ventricular volumes or ejection fraction.

The collective experience from eleven Japanese centers suggests that nifedipine, diltiazem and verapamil can all be used effectively in variant angina (23). 115 of 149 patients had complete elimination of attacks with nifedipine; 70 of 87 patients had complete elimination of attacks with diltiazem. Experience was considerably more limited with verapamil which was only used in 28 instances. While only 3 of these patients experienced complete elimintion of attacks, 21 had their attack rate cut by 50% or more.

II. SIDE EFFECTS AND TOXICITY

Several calcium channel blocking agents introduced earlier outside of the United States have had unacceptable side effects which will preclude their acceptance in this country. Specifically, prenylamine has caused Q-T prolongation and advanced ventricular arrhythmias; perhexiline has caused both dose dependent liver damage and peripheral neuropathy.

In general, the agents reviewed herein have been well-tolerated. Depending on the specific agent, a minority of patients have reported side

338

effects. In various studies one to five percent of patients need to discontinue medication for these reasons. Being vasodilators, headache, flushing and dizziness are the most common complaints experienced with calcium channel blockers. Side effects perculiar to individual agents include ankle edema, occurring in 8 of 16 patients on nifedipine reported by Lynch et al, (12) and constipation, responsive to laxatives, which occurred in 7 of 28 patients receiving verapamil (9). Table 3 lists side effects reported with the agents discussed in this review.

Table 3. Adverse effects attributed to calcium channel blocking agents.

NIFEDIPINE: Ankle edema, headache, dizziness, tinnitus, fatigue, nasal congestion, flushing, hypotension
VERAPAMIL: Constipation, headache, dizziness, nausea, sleepiness, palpitations, increased PR interval (higher degrees of AV block after intravenous dosages, often in patients receiving concomitant β blockers)
DILTIAZEM: Headaches, flushing, dizziness, nervousness, sleeplessness.
LIDOFLAZINE: Dizziness, headache, tired/painful legs, blurred vision

Side effects which appear peculiar to individual agents are underlined.

Studies of combinations of anti-anginal regimens which involve calcium channel blocking agents evaluating undesirable side effects and toxicity still need to be done. Sublingual nitroglycerine has been used in all the studies of calcium channel blockers cited herein and does not appear to be a problem; from this it cannot necessarily be inferred that large oral doses of nitrates and calcium channel blocking agents will be well tolerated. In particular, more studies need to be done with calcium channel blocking agents and beta blockers. Scant existing literature suggests this combination and can be exploited to treat hypertension and may make a more efficacious anti-anginal regimen. However, there is at least one report of an adverse interaction between nifedipine and beta blockade resulting in excessive blood pressure reduction in a hypertensive patient (24).

REFERENCES

1. Kawai C, Konishi T, Matsuyama E, Okazaki H. 1981. Comparative effects of three calcium antagonists, diltiazem, verapamil and nifedipine, on the sinoatrial and atrioventricular nodes. Circulation 63:1035.
2. Rinkenberger RL, Prystowsky EN, Heger JJ, Troup PJ, Jackman WM, Zipes DP. 1980. Effects of intravenous and chronic oral verapamil

administration in patients with supraventricular tachyarrhythmias. Circulation 62:996.

3. Olivari MT, Bartorelli C, Polese A, Fiorentini C, Moruzzi P, Guazzi M. 1979. Treatment of hypertension with nifedipine, a calcium antagonistic agent. Circulation 59:1056.

4. Guazzi MD, Fiorentini C, Olivari MT, Bartorelli A, Necchi G, Polese A. 1980. Short- and long-term efficacy of a calcium-antagonistic agent (Nifedipine) combined with methyldopa in the treatment of severe hypertension. Circulation 61:913.

5. Phear DN. 1968. Verapamil in angina: a double-blind trial. Br Med J 2:740-741.

6. Sandler G, Clayton GA, Thornicroft SG. 1968. Clinical evaluation of verapamil in angina pectoris. Br Med J 3:224-227.

7. Livesley B, Catley PF, Campbell RC, Oram S. 1973. Double-blind evaluation of verapamil, propranolol, and isosorbide dinitrate against a placebo in the treatment of angina pectoris. Br Med J 1:375-378.

8. Fagher B, Svenson SE, Persson S. 1977. Double-blind comparison of verapamil and propranolol in the treatment of angina pectoris. Postgrad Med J 53:61-65.

9. BalaSubramanian V, Paramasivan R, Lahiri A, Raftery EB. 1980. Verapamil in chronic stable angina. The Lancet, April 19.

10. Jatene AD, Lichtlen PR. 1976. The Third International Adalat Symposium. Excerpta Medica, Amsterdam.

11. Moskowitz RM, Piccini PA, Nacarelli GV, Zelis R. 1979. Nifedipine therapy for stable angina pectoris: preliminary results of effects on angina frequency and treadmill exercise response. Am J Cardiol 44:811-816.

12. Lynch P, Dargie H, Krikler S, Krikler D. 1980. Objective assessment of antianginal treatment: a double-blind comparison of propranolol, nifedipine, and their combination. Br Med J 184-187, July.

13. Pool PE, Seagren SC, Bonanno JA, Salel AF, Dennish GW. 1980. The treatment of exercise-inducible chronic stable angina with diltiazem. Chest 78:234-238.

14. Hossack KF, Bruce RA. 1981. Improved exercise performance in persons with stable angina pectoris receiving diltiazem. Am J Cardiol 47: 95-101.

15. Low RI, Takeda P, Lee G, Mason DT, Awan NA, DeMaria AN. 1981. Effect of diltiazem-induced calcium blockade upon exercise capacity in effort angina due to chronic coronary artery disease. Am Heart J 101:713.

16. Starling MR, Crawford MH, O'Rourke RA. 1981. Beneficial effects of diltiazem on exercise performance in patients with coronary artery disease and angina pectoris. Am J Cardiol 47:464 (abstract).

17. Broustet JP, Quern P, Pic A. 1981. Comparative effects of diltiazem, nifedipine and nitroglycerine in effort angina -- a double-blind study by symptom limited exercise test. Circulation 64:IV-150 (abstract).

18. Pepine CJ, Feldman RL, Whittle J, Curry C, Conti R. Effect of diltiazem in patients with variant angina: a randomized double-blind trial. Am Heart J 101:719.

19. Myocardial protection and exercise tolerance: the role of lidoflazine, a new anti-anginal agent. 1980. London, Royal Society of Medicine International Congress and Symposium Series No. 29, Academic Press Inc., Ltd.

20. Waters DD, Theroux P, Dauwe F, Crittin J, Affaki G, Mizgala HF. 1979. Ergonovine testing to assess the effects of calcium antagonist drugs in variant angina. Circulation 60:II-248 (abstract).

340

21. Johnson SM, Mauritson DR, Willerson JT, Hillis LD. 1981. Comparison of verapamil and nifedipine in the treatment of variant angina pectoris: preliminary observations in 10 patients. Am J Cardiol 47: 1295.
22. BalaSubramanian V, Bowles MJ, Davies AB, Khurmi NS, Raftery EB. 1981. Double-blind randomized comparison of verapamil and nidefipine in chronic stable angina. Circulation 64:IV-150 (abstract).
23. Henry PD. 1980. Comparative pharmacology of calcium antagonists: nifedipine, verapamil and diltiazem. Am J Cardiol 46:1047.
24. Opie LH, White DA. Adverse interaction between nifedipine and β-blockade. Br Med J 281:1462.

GENERAL GROUP DISCUSSION - Calcium Antagonists

Moderator: Dr. Robert O'Rourke

Dr. Lockhart: Has anyone had any experience with either nifedipine or verapamil being used with the class I antiarrhythmic drugs? Do you know of any interactions? Has anyone found any problems or have they attempted to even try it? The second question is that in Pisa recently there was a study in which they showed that beta blockers combined with nifedipine had an effect on cardiac output. They feel that cardiac output is maintained by sympathetic tone with the use of nifedipine and that you may be putting some patients into congestive failure or at least decreasing cardiac output by combining. Do you think this is realistic?

Dr. Seipel: I can't answer the first question because I have never tried to combine class I action with calcium antagonists. I have no experience, and I do not know any study in the literature concerning this point. The second point is speculative, but I think it is possible.

Dr. Rowland: All I can say is that from our own experience using the two drugs together, we have used verapamil and quinidine in large numbers of patients with AV reentrant tachycardia, the hypothesis being that by abolishing extrasystoles as well as having a depressant effect on the AV nodal function you can reduce the number of attacks of tachycardia. This is purely anecdotal. We think there is a slightly larger degree of success, but I haven't analyzed them sufficiently well enough to give you a scientific answer.

Dr. Epstein: We have some anecdotal experience relating to that particular question and have seen a couple of patients who unequivocally have had verapamil-quinidine interactions. We have seen, with repeated administration of the combination, postural hypotension which did not occur with either drug alone; and we saw one patient go into a frank pulmonary edema when he was quite stable taking verapamil alone and then when quinidine was added about after the 5th or 6th dose. I don't think it occurs often, but I think it would be just worthwhile for people to be aware of this and look out for it. It is a possible interaction.

Dr. O'Rourke: Were those patients with hypertrophic cardiomyopathy?

Dr. Epstein: Both of those patients had hypertrophic cardiomyopathy.

Dr. O'Rourke: Let me just comment on the problems with heart failure. There is no question if one looks at any of these drugs and looks at them in the intact pre-instrumented animal, they all depress myocardial performance if given in appropriate doses. You can see this manifested even more when you give it intracoronary and look at segmental wall motion in the area supplied by the coronary in which you injected that particular calcium blocking drug. It is also true that because of the vasodilatation that occurs systemically, and possibly a baroreceptor mediated effect, that in many situations in moderate doses, even intravenously, you do not produce severe depression of left ventricular performance. Dr. Sobel is going to talk later this afternoon, probably with much more sophisticated data, on the interactions and potential interactions of these drugs. In the animal studies it is interesting that when verapamil was looked at by Neumann and associates several years ago in the conscious dog, with beta blockade they showed marked potentiation of the depression of LV performance much greater than with nifedipine; but it was not accentuated in the animal that was beta blocked with a dose of propranolol that would prevent an isuprel bolus from stimulating the heart rate. So there are still some questions about interaction of these drugs in normal animals or man in various disease states whether you are looking at an attempt to try to improve diastolic properties of the ventricle or whether your patient has markedly depressed systolic function. It is interesting if one looks carefully at the number of studies that have been submitted for publication and some accepted that look at patients with coronary artery disease as the cause of the left ventricular dysfunction and you look at the ejection fraction by radionuclide techniques before and after giving the usual oral doses of these drugs in most situations, you do not see a marked depression of LV performance when they are given in doses that orally improve the symptoms of angina, improve the exercise performance, etc. I think it has yet to be completely resolved which patients might have major problems when the drugs that depress myocardial performance are used together.

Dr. Seipel: May I come back to the first point--combination for class I drugs and calcium antagonists. I have to correct myself. There is at least one study in German literature concerning this point in patients with atrial fibrillation. They also give quinidine to stop atrial fibrillation; and, in addition, they applied verapamil in order to slow the heart rate during atrial fibrillation. They stated that the combination of both drugs was much more effective in stopping atrial fibrillation and converting to sinus rhythm than both drugs alone. This study, as far as I remember, observed no serious side effects.

Dr. Guerrero: I believe that the comment on the quinidine and verapamil is right. In relation to the effects of verapamil on conduction, I think as Cranefield and Wit showed in the animal, the effect on the sinus node is mainly on the sick sinus node; and with normal sinus node there is no effect. A double-blind randomized study using placebo and nifedipine has shown that not only verapamil is superior to nifedipine for the treatment of stable angina pectoris, but 4 of 28

patients on nifedipine had to be discontinued from the study because of angina

pectoris. Now, as it has been our habit when we do these studies, we do Holter

tapes to look for changes in ST segment at other times then with effort. It has

been shown in these 4 patients one hour after the ingestion of nifedipine that they

did have tachycardia which induced the angina. Of course, in the literature it is

not unusual to find that these patients have angina induced by nifedipine. Most

likely, this is due to the tachycardia. So I believe that the tachycardia is

beneficial for the patient with angina. It is the bradycardia which is beneficial as

you all know having used propranolol for 20 years. Now as to Dr. Parisi's

statement on the tachphylaxis for nifedipine, I would like to refer him to a paper

in The American Journal of Cardiology in September where serial exercise testing

has been made which shows that verapamil's effects not only last but do improve

with time; and we have done well-controlled prospective studies in the U.S.A.

which, I believe, are much better than those done with nifedipine. We can tell you

that that effect lasts for a year, and there is no such a thing as tachyphylaxis with

verapamil. Now the tachycardia induced by nifedipine certainly is a problem when

you discontinue beta blockers, so I don't see how anyone can claim that the

combination is safe; because if a patient just forgets his beta blockers, he may

wind up in an unstable angina situation.

Dr. O'Rourke: Well, we thank you; and we'll give the other two drug companies

equal time in a few minutes. However, before that I would like to ask if any of

the members of the panel would like to respond in specific to any of the comments

that were just made.

Dr. Parisi: Well I think one of the problems that you have in this early stage of

the game is having a limited number of studies in highly-selected patients with different entry criteria in different studies. I think that time has to tell when a consensus is reached between these different small studies as to how one drug is really better than another or not. The equipotent dose is still a problem, and it is a problem for beta blockers which have been out for 20 years. So I think it is too early really to make statements about that. The tachyphylaxis had to do with the antihypertensive effects, not with antianginal effects that were mentioned; and there is literature that says verapamil is not a good long-term agent to treat hypertension. Perhaps, there is other data of which I am not aware; and I think that is what the tachyphylaxis referred to--not to other effects of verapamil.

Dr. Altman: I had a question for Dr. Kates. You just barely mentioned the possibility for stereo-selective first pass clearance, and I wonder whether there was any other precedent for that in the cardiovascular system and if you could comment on the degree.

Dr. Kates: There has been a study showing that there is a selective first pass hepatic clearance of the positive isomer with propranolol in this situation. I think there is a lot of precedent for stereo-selective handling of drugs in general. It is something that hasn't been addressed requires sophisticated chemical methodology or availability of optical isomers of drugs. Clearly quinidine and quinine have different effects. They are simply optical isomers. I think it is a whole area that needs to be investigated and probably a lot to be learned.

Dr. Watanabe: I have to make two comments. The first is concerned with terminology. I am happy to hear when Dr. Kates used a term calcium blockers rather than calcium antagonists or calcium internal blockers because as long as electrophysiology is concerned, especially in the sinus node and the AV node, the slowing of the current is mainly carried by slow sodium rather than slow calcium;

and, therefore, slow channel blockers are preferable to calcium channel blockers or calcium antagonists. There are two bits of evidence. The first one when we used the isolated perfused rabbit hearts when increased calcium concentration it actually depressed AV conduction, and also when I produced Wenkebach or 2:1 AV nodal conduction block with verapamil or diltiazem increased in the calcium concentration further aggravates the AV conduction block while an increase in the sodium concentration from 145 to 172 restores 1:1 conduction. A more recent experiment supports that most of the slow inward currents in the AV node are carried by slow sodium. My second point is regarding the increase in heart rate after verapamil. Sometimes you can see a faster heart rate after verapamil, and you indicated that this is mostly due to autonomic reflex. But again, using a similar preparation of very small AV node specimen, the size of which is about .2 mm where we can study automaticity and conduction and with lower concentrations of verapamil, you cannot see increased automaticity in the AV node. It is not entirely due to reflex action.

Dr. Seipel: These have in addition some vagolytic action as has been discussed for verapamil in the isolated preparation. I can't give any comment to that but it may be possible; but on the other hand, I remember a study injecting verapamil in the sinus node artery directly and the author observed a direct depressor effect in his animals, and he stated that there is only direct depressant effect of verapamil in these animals.

Dr. Watanabe: Well, of course, in those animals you cannot adhere to a given concentration; whereas, in these small specimens we can gradually increase the concentration and there you can demonstrate some acceleration of automaticity.

Dr. Taria: I would like to defend myself against the comments of Dr. Watanabe. I think that you are referring to the rabbit sinus node instead of the canine sinus node? We are now doing similar experiments on the canine atrioventricular nodal preparation and small concentrations of verapamil or diltiazem did not increase the rate of automaticity. I think there are differences in species here. You are working in the rabbit heart; I am working on the canine heart. I've been working on calcium antagonists for more than 10 years. Mr. Chairman, may I compliment the presentations given by the panelists. Dr. Watanable pointed out, regarding the two mechanisms as to why nifedipine does not depress the sinus node activity in the therapeutic dose? Why the other two calcium antagonists depress the sinus node activity or AV conduction. The misconception is prevailing, I think. If you see the preparations which are completely free from the influence of the central nervous system, nifedipine in a dilator dose, double the quantity of blood flow, but that does not affect the sinus node activity or AV conduction systems. So, in depressing sinus node or AV node activity you should see 9 times as much as the dose which increasing blood flow.

Dr. Bayer: May I add something to that. I agree that the 60's and the 70's were the time of calcium antagonists. We were working in the middle of the 60's at Fleckenstein's Institute on calcium antagonists and doing so until now. During this time we had to change the term calcium antagonists, and now in 1975 we find it given a new definition. It has given calcium antagonists a heterogeneous group of drugs which all reduce calcium available to induce or maintain several activities such as cardiac muscle contraction. Within these different drugs there is one group which we call slow channel inhibitors. That means that these drugs only inhibit the conductance of the slow channels and under some circumstances, as just was pointed out, the slow channel may carry calcium and sodium ions as well as calcium ions; but under normal conditions most of the current flowing through the slow channel is a calcium current. But within these different groups with the different drugs which are slow channel inhibitors, the action on the slow channel is different; and I am glad to hear that the action in the different modes of antiarrhythmic mode of action, the antianginal action, and so on are different as well. I just want to point out one very interesting difference between nifedipine and verapamil. Nifedipine does not act as depending on the resting membrane potential. That is very important. Verapamil acts very strongly negative inotropic, at least in isolated preparations. If the frequency is increased, the potency of verapamil increases tenfold to thirtyfold if the membrane potential becomes lower than -80 mV. At -40 mV there is no slow inward current anymore on the influence of verapamil. That means that all tissues having a slow resting potential, or a low maximum diastolic potential as the AV node or the sinus node, or injured myocardium are very sensitive to verapamil. That is the difference between nifedipine and verapamil. There is no use-dependence, as we call it. It is like this verapamil; if the muscle is stimulated repetitively or depolarized for a long time, verapamil is extensively bound to specific site of action within this low membrane channel. Nifedipine does not show such frequency and potential dependence.

Dr. Kates: I think your comments point out the heterogeneity of the slow channel classification. Where nifedipine is to the slow channel, tetraototoxin is to the fast channel; and the effects in no way are comparable to the verapamil-diltiazem effects which are frequency dependent on the kinetics in the slow channel. It is a difficulty we are having right now putting all these drugs in the same category. It is a very dissimilar compound.

Dr. Bayer: I would add that the action of nifedipine on the slow membrane channel is comparable to that of tetraototoxin on the fast channel and the action of verapamil on the slow channel is comparable to most local anesthetics on the fast channel that is use-dependent.

Dr. Ohrringer: There have been a number of reports in the literature regarding the use of calcium channel blockers in patients with congestive cardiomyopathies. I was wondering if anyone on the panel would care to address that and would care to comment on potential patient selection in the use of these drugs with patients with congestive cardiomyopathy.

Dr. O'Rourke: You are talking about the use of it as an unloading agent in individuals who have severe congestive cardiomyopathy with marked local dysfunction, ejection fractions in the range of 15 to 30%. The only experiments that we have with diltiazem that have been done in two patients in the experimental protocol during the cardiac catheterization laboratory have surprised us by how positive they have been, with a marked improvement with the unloading effect given intravenously in producing an increase in forward flow as well as decrease in filling pressures. I hate to make comments on two patients who have been done only on this protocol, but initially the data that we have in a design protocol to test that has been positive showing an important unloading effect similar to what might be seen with other agents that are being used as unloading agents. There obviously is a large amount of anecdotal data in the literature where individual patients have responded positively as far as fluid retention, congestion, etc. when given various of the three major slow channel calcium blocking. How that is going to hold up and which patients are candidates is going to require some very careful analysis. As we also know, in some countries propranolol has been used to improve diastolic properties in patients with severe congestive cardiomyopathy; and it is true that most of us would not ever give a beta blocking drug. That also has to be looked at.

<u>Dr. Guerrero:</u> In relation to that question, we did a study in 12 patients with ejection fractions below 40%. Two of those patients happened to have congestive cardiomyopathy. They did not deteriorate; and, maybe, there was a slight improvement. Overall, in that study there was no deterioration of myocardial infarction with about 3 or 4 times the therapeutic dose of verapamil given intravenously. I want to point out that it is very inaccurate to extrapolate from the <u>in vitro</u> preparation to the intact animal or intact man. We have approximately 60 patients studied in the U.S.A. with invasive and noninvasive methodology with all kinds of ejection fractions, and there is no replication of the so-called negative inotropic effects of verapamil; so let's kill another ghost right then and there. Furthermore, we have a study that I mentioned on patients with decreased myocardial function, and there were no negative inotropic effects. Further, we have 40 patients who were on the steady state treatment with beta blockers, and I mean at beta blocking levels. Of those patients again we gave about 3 times the dose of intravenous verapamil. There were no electrical or mechanical deleterious effects. Further, a study in 15 patients who were refractory to treatment with propranolol for unstable angina were administered verapamil orally in addition to propranolol which ranged from 160 to 1200 milligrams per day. There was a slight decrease of contractility which disappeared when propranolol was discontinued.

<u>Dr. Epstein:</u> May I just correct what I think is an important misconception. We did a study with verapamil in patients with coronary artery disease looking at ejection fraction at rest and with exercise by radionuclide techniques; and in fact, the drug does have negative inotropic potential when given chronically orally in clinical doses. There was a significant mean decrease in ejection fraction in the entire group of approximately 9 or 10 individuals. There was no individual who had a 10% fall in ejection fraction of 35% after a week's therapy, and three days

later that patient went into congestive heart failure. We have seen another patient going into congestive heart failure after some time on verapamil, and we have seen those with coronary patients. We have seen one patient with hypertrophic disease with no obstruction go into heart failure on nifedipine. So, I don't think this is a ghost that should be put to rest. I don't know how often it occurs. Probably not very often, but it is something we have to be aware of as clinicians. Certainly with verapamil, I'm not sure with nifedipine yet, maybe less so; but we have to be aware of it--it does occur.

Dr. O'Rourke: Let me comment to that in that I happen to agree completely with your comments, but I do also agree that it is probably a small percentage of patients where overt severe congestive heart failure is produced de novo. There are some patients who have coronary artery disease, with any of the beta blocking drugs going from rest to exercise measurements who no longer develop their global ischemia and who will actually have a slight improvement in their exercise ejection fraction because they do not develop the angina and myocardial ischemia that they would have developed had they not been on the antianginal agents. The same can be said for the beta blockers. On the other hand, there is no question that all of these drugs, usually in doses that may or may not be equivalent to what we will use orally, produce a degree of beta blockade if looked at very carefully by sensitive parameters looking at the effect on myocardial function with loading conditions controlled. How often that will be a problem in individual patient groups? It may be small, but it is not a ghost to be put to rest. I agree with your comment completely.

Dr. Chelly: As an anesthesiologist in cardiac surgery, I would like to know if, with regard to any exeriences concerning some patients chronically treated with the calcium blockers and operated on for cardiac surgery, there is some potential interaction between the anesthetic agent used for the cardiac surgery and the chronic treatment with calcium antagonists?

Dr. O'Rourke: I guess we can't answer that particular question. As you know, there has been a lot of work done where the calcium blocking agents have been used as additional cardioplegic solutions, particularly by Clark and associates, in preserving myocardium. Obviously, that does not relate to your question about interaction between anesthetics in patients on long-term calcium blocking agents in the treatment of their heart disease.

SUMMARY:

Dr. O'Rourke: I think it is impossible right now to give a summary on these particular topics. These are important agents. They do many things. They affect vascular smooth muscle, cardiac muscle, pacemaker sites, and I think a lot more information will be given. I happen to be one of those people to review those large numbers of abstracts.

HOW TO DEFINE CONTROLLED STUDIES IN CORONARY ARTERY SPASM

ROBERT A. O'ROURKE, M.D.

I. INTRODUCTION

In 1959, Prinzmetal and Associates (1) defined the syndrome of "variant angina" and proposed that the mechanism of chest discomfort in this group of patients was due to coronary artery spasm associated with "fixed coronary artery occlusive disease. Ensuing developments, including coronary angiography, long-term ECT recording, hemodynamic monitoring, myocardial radioisotope perfusion imaging and measurements of regional metabolism and coronary blood flow in man have substantiated the relationship between coronary artery spasm and the variant angina syndrome (2-11). Patient studies using these techniques have also implicated coronary artery spasm in the pathophysiology of many other ischemic syndromes besides variant angina pectoris (2,7,12-15). In addition, the provocation of coronary artery spasm by hyperventilation, by the intravenous administration of drugs by cold pressor testing has implicated a possible role of coronary spasm in ischemic heart disease in general (2, 16-22).

During the past decade a group of pharmacologic agents, known as the slow channel calcium blockers, have been used primarily outside the United States for the treatment of several forms of ischemic heart disease but primarily variant angina. These agents reduce the movement of calcium from the extracellular to the intracellular space and produce variable degrees of systemic arterial dilation, coronary artery dilation and reduced myocardial contractility (23-25). These drugs appear especially promising for treating patients with variant angina and multiple reports now indicate that they provide effective therapy of this entity as well as for patients with exercise-induced angina pectoris due to "fixed" occlusive coronary artery disease (24, 26-36). The purpose of this discussion will be to define variant angina, coronary artery spasm and its consequences and the various methods for detecting the presence of myocardial ischemia due to coronary spasm. Further information will be given concerning the techniques for establishing the diagnosis of coronary artery spasm and factors to consider when designing protocols to test drugs likely to be effective in treating patients with this disorder.

II. VARIANT ANGINA

The usual characteristics of patients with variant angina as classically described are listed in table 1.

Table 1. Characteristics of Variant Angina
1. Spontaneous episodes of chest pain at rest.
2. Reversible ECG ST segment elevation during pain.
3. Often, A-V block or ventricular arrhythmias with pain.
4. Results from coronary artery spasm.

In the initial descriptions by Prinzmetal and Conorkers (1), the patients had spontaneous attacks of angina, which usually occurred at rest and were associated with coincident electrocardiographic ST segment elevation, particularly in leads II, III and AVF. Physical examination and electrocardiograms during chest pain often demonstrated evidence of second or third degree atrioventricular block as well as the ST segment elevation, both ECT abnormalities disappearing when the chest pain resolved, usually in one or two minutes. In a smaller percentage of patients transient ventricular arrhythmias were associated with the other findings of variant angina.

More recently, it has been shown that chest pain due to coronary artery spasm may occur during exercise as well as at rest and that ST segment depression rather than elevation or no ECT changes at all often accompany chest pain due to mayocardial ischemia in patients with documented coronary artery spasm (2,37-43). Furthermore, it is now well-recognized that transient ST segment elevation at rest or with exercise may occur in patients with fixed coronary artery disease and no coronary artery spasm, particularly in those with increases in heart rate and/or blood pressure during emotional upset or exercise testing. These ST segment changes are most likely to occur in the same electrocardiographic leads that show evidence of a previous transmural myocardial infarction or in ECT leads corresponding to the site of major wall motion abnormalities (44-47).

III. CORONARY ARTERY SPASM

Coronary artery spasm may be defined as a transient, reversible, subtotal or total narrowing of a major epicardial coronary artery associated with objective evidence of myocardial ischemia. Coronary artery spasm has been documented to occur spontaneously in otherwise normal arteries or in arteries with additional "fixed" coronary artery narrowing due to atherosclerosis. The spasm of the coronary arteries that results in segmental or global myocardial ischemia may occur spontaneously or be produced by agents which increase coronary artery tone such as ergonovine maleate (see below) or circulating cathecholamines that stimulate coronary artery alpha adrenergic receptors. The later may be stimulated by use of cutaneous cold stimulation using a cold pressor test (22). Vigorous hyperventilation produces marked coronary artery vasoconstriction in certain patients with coronary artery spasm, presumably by diminishing hydrogen ion concentration (16). However, controversy exists as to whether this coronary artery constriction during hyperventilation is specific for coronary artery spasm and variant angina.

Theoretically, the use of beta blocking drugs could potentiate coronary artery spasm by promoting unopposed stimulation of coronary artery alpha-adrenergic receptors, resulting in more pronounced vasoconstriction (2). However, propranolol has produced salutary results in some patients with both severe occlusive coronary artery disease and an element of coronary artery spasm and the effects of beta-blocking drugs on coronary artery tone may vary depending on the presence or absence of local myocardial ischemia (2).

IV. CONSEQUENCES OF CORONARY ARTERY SPASM

It has been well demonstrated that the detrimental effects of naturally occurring coronary artery spasm are similar to those occurring in the experimental animal during an acute coronary artery occlusion (Table 2).

Table 2. Results of Coronary Artery Spasm

1. Angina pectoris or myocardial infarction.
2. ST segment elevation or depression.
3. Elevated left ventricular end-diastolic pressure.
4. Left ventricular systolic dysfunction.
5. Arrhythmias.
6. Myocardial perfusion defects.
7. Abnormal myocardial lactate metabolism.

ST segment elevation, wall motion abnormalities and elevation of left ventricular end-diastolic pressure usually occur prior to any elevation or depression in systemic arterial pressure and often without any major change in heart rate. In patients with either additional "fixed" coronary artery disease or normal artery coronary vessels, coronary artery spasm may produce typical angina pectoris, often at rest but also during exercise; and in some patients it results in acute myocardial infarction. In patients with coronary artery spasm, ST segment elevation indicating transmural myocardial ischemia or ST segment depression indicating subendocardial ischemia may occur. Arrhythmias are also common. As a result of coronary artery spasm, there is a sudden decrease in oxygen supply to contracting cardiac muscle resulting in important myocardial perfusion defects, and abnormal myocardial lactate metabolism has been demonstrated in the coronary venous efflux from areas of myocardial ischemia.

V. DETECTION OF MYOCARDIAL ISCHEMIA

There are multiple clinical non-invasive and invasive techniques now available for the detection of myocardial ischemia resulting from a disparity between myocardial oxygen supply and myocardial oxygen consumption. These methods are listed in Table 3.

Table 3. Identifying Myocardial Ischemia
1. Symptoms (angina pectoris).
2. ST segment changes (rest, exercise testing, ambulatory recording).
3. Rest and exercise 201-thallium scintigraphy.
4. Rest and exercise radionuclide angiography.
5. Hemodynamics during cardiac catheterization.
6. Ventricular cineangiography.

Angina pectoris, commonly occurring at rest, and often somewhat atypical is a hallmark of myocardial ischemia due to coronary artery spasm. However, angina at rest also occurs in patients with severe three vessel coronary atherosclerotic disease, particularly in those with an element of left ventricular decompensation as well. Angina frequently occurs at night in such patients due to augmented myocardial oxygen demands resulting from increased left ventricular volume in the supine position, dream states, and/or mild hypoxemia. ST segment changes may occur in patients

with myocardial ischemia who do not have definite symptoms of chest discomfort due to the ischemic myocardium. In patients with myocardial ischemia
due to coronary artery spasm, a twelve lead ECG often shows ST segment
elevation, particulary if recorded during an episode of pain. It is now
well known that ECG evidence of ST segment elevation or ST segment depression
during exercise testing may occur in patinets with coronary artery spasm
as well as in patients with fixed coronary artery lesions (37-43). In a
minority of patients, coronary artery with resulting myocardial ischemia
is almost always exercise-induced.

To assess patients with suspected coronary artery spasm during normal
activity, continuous ambulatory ECG recording using two ECG chest leads
is often useful. Such recordings will often show evidence of ST segment
elevation, depression or arrhythmias that correspond with the patient
symptoms of chest discomfort or frank angina. Additional episodes of ischemic
ST segments without chest pain may also be documented. To most effectively
determine such changes, it is prudent to place the ECG leads so that one
detects ST segment changes occurring over the anterolateral surface of the
heart and the other from the inferior left ventricular surface. Even
then, posterior wall ischemia may be missed.

In some patients with coronary artery spasm 201-thallium scintigraphy
may be very useful in establishing the correct diagnosis. Myocardial
perfusion scans during pain, whether at rest or during exercise, may show
decreased thallium uptake in the area of myocardial ischemia whereas later
redistribution scans, when no pain or ST segment elevation is present, are
completely normal.

Rest and exercise radionuclide angiography using technetium bound to
red blood cells or albumin is useful in patients with coronary artery
spasm as well as in patients with fixed coronary artery stenosis due to
atherosclerosis. This technique is particularly helpful in patients who
develop coronary artery spasm primarily during exercise. The presence of a
decrease rather than the normal 5% or greater increase in left ventricular
ejection fraction during exercise coupled with the presence of segmental
left ventricular wall motion abnormalities occurring during rest or exercise
pain may imply the correct diagnosis.

The hemodynamic measurements obtained during cardiac catheterization
often show important differences in patients with myocardial ischemia due
to fixed coronary artery lesions as compared to those with isolated coronary

artery spasm as the bases (2-4). In patients with fixed coronary artery disease, there is usually an increase in heart rate, systolic blood pressure, and left ventricular end-diastolic pressure at the onset of angina. In some instances, the hemodynamic changes actually precede the symptom of pain. In contrast, the heart rate is usually unchanged in patients with angina due to coronary spasm; the rise in left ventricular end-diastolic pressure occurs somewhat later; and there frequently is a marked decrease in the arterial blood pressure as sudden severe myocardial ischemia adversely affects left ventricular performance.

VI. DIAGNOSIS OF CORONARY ARTERY SPASM

The only way to establish the diagnosis of coronary artery spasm with certainty is by selective coronary arteriography. Although angina at ST segment elevations during chest pain and bradyarrhythmias during chest pain suggest the diagnosis of coronary artery spasm, these findings may occur in other situations. In patients with suspected coronary artery spasm but normal coronary arteriographic findings at rest or during spontaneous chest discomfort, provocative testing may be useful for detecting the presence of coronary artery spasm. The most frequently utilized test for this purpose is the intravenous injection of ergonovine maleate (17-21). In most patients with coronary artery spasm documented during spontaneous episodes of chest pain, intravenous ergonovine maleate has produced severe focal narrowing to complete occlusion of one or more coronary arteries when given in doses up to 0.4 mg. However, there is still some controversy as to the extent of narrowing necessary for a positive test and whether or not all patients with spontaneous documented spasm have a positive ergonovine coronary arteriographic response. Another provocative technique that has been utilized is the cold pressor test (22). In this method, the patient emerges his or her hand in a mixture of water and ice for one minute. Many patients with coronary artery disease demonstrate inappropriate coronary artery vasoconstrictor in response to this alpha adrenergic stimulas. In some patients, coronary artery spasm, often in addition to obstructive coronary artery disease, can be demonstrated arteriographically during the cold pressor test.

VII. MODIFYING FACTORS FOR CONSIDERATION

In considering the patient entrance criteria, the study design and the end points to be analyzed in evaluating a drug likely to improve symptoms in patients with coronary artery spasm, a number of modifying factors must be considered (Table 4).

Table 4. Factors to Consider When Designing Drug Trials
1. During spasm, ST segments may be elevated, depressed or unchanged.
2. ST segment elevation may occur transiently in patients without coronary artery spasm.
3. Many patients with spasm have episodic ischemic ST segment changes without pain.
4. Coronary artery spasm may be exercise-induced.
5. Many patients with spasm also have fixed atherosclerotic coronary disease.
6. The clinical course of variant angina is highly variable.
7. Ergonovine may induce symptoms of esophageal spasm with or without ECG changes.

First, in some patients coronary artery spasm may be exercise-induced. In such a situation, it might be useful to perform serial ECG exercise testing with 201-thallium scintigraphy on and off drug therapy to access the beneficial effects of the drug to be tested. Second, ST segment elevation, depression or no alterations at all may result during coronary artery spasm. This is not surprising considering the high incidence of right coronary artery involvement and the poor representation of the poster- ior surface of the left ventricular on the twelve lead electrocardiogram. Thus, there may be problems in individual patients in detecting symptomatic or asymptomatic myocardial ischemia by ECG in patients who are having definite episodes of coronary artery spasm. Third, ST segment elevation is not synonymous with coronary artery spasm and transient ST elevation may occur at rest or during exercise in patients with fixed coronary artery disease, particularly in those who had a prior myocardial infarction or have a left ventricular aneurysm (44-47). These factors should be considered when deciding on exclusion criteria for patients who have evidence of both fixed coronary artery disease and coronary artery spasm. Fourth, many patients with coronary artery spasm have episodes of ST segment elevation or depression representing myocardial ischemia at times when they have no angina. This fact must be recognized when designing the method for follow- ing patients during control periods and when they are receiving a drug intended to improve coronary artery spasm. The angina frequency could vary in one direction while the incidence of ST segment elevation or depression during continuous ambulatory recording could change in the opposite direction.

It must be emphasized that many patients with coronary artery spasm also have fixed coronary artery disease due to atherosclenosis. In these patients, myocardial ischemia may be due to coronary spasm or to the fixed coronary artery disease. Thus, it may be difficult to discern whether or not an improvement in symptoms is due to prevention of coronary artery spasm or whether it is due to an improvement in the disparity between myocardial oxygen supply and demand in the areas supplied by the severely narrowed coronary arteries.

Recently, it has been demonstrated that intravenous ergonovine maleate may induce symptoms and signs of esophageal spasm in patients who have no coronary artery disease. The symptoms resulting from spasm may mimic the chest discomfort of angina pectoris and non-specific ST-T wave changes may also occur. This information should be considered when deciding on the efficacy of a drug based upon a change in the incidence of atypical chest discomfort or episodes of non-specific ST-T wave changes.

Finally, the clinical course of patients with angina pectoris due to coronary artery spasm is highly variable. Several weeks with severe frequent episodes of variant angina may be followed by several weeks of almost no symptoms at all, the improvement occurring despite no medical therapy. Thus, a placebo controlled period with randomization is particularly necessary for accessing the effectiveness of a cardiovascular drug designed to diminish the frequency and severity of coronary artery spasm.

VIII. SELECTION OF PATIENTS FOR DRUG TRIALS

In order to obtain valid results from drug studies of patients with coronary artery spasm, the patient selection is extremely important. First, there should be no question concerning the diagnosis of coronary artery spasm. By far the best way to establish the diagnosis is selective coronary arteriography with provocative testing as necessary (see above). It is desirable to select patients who have frequent episodes of variant angina (at least five episodes per week). It is better to utilize patients who have associated ECG changes with ST segment depression, ST elevation and/or arrhythmias during the episodes of chest discomfort. In addition, to

obtain the best results, it is important to have definite, well-defined
exclusion criteria such as a history or ECG evidence of previous myocardial
infarction.

IX. CLINICAL DRUG TRIALS

Important factors in the proper design of a clinical drug trial for
patients with well-documented coronary artery spasm are included in
Table 5.

Table 5. Drug Protocol Design

1. Double-blind, randomized, placebo-controlled trials are desirable
   and possible.
2. All drugs except for short-acting nitrates for angina should be stopped.
3. If intractable angina with ECG evidence of ischemia occurs, patient
   can be advanced to next treatment with study still blinded.

Several large drug trials concerning the use of the slow channel calcium-
blocking drugs in patients with coronary artery spasm have been criticized
because of the lack of a controlled drug designed study (29). It should
be emphasized that a double-blind, randomized, placebo-controlled trial
of a drug likely to improve symptoms of myocardial ischemia in patients
with coronary artery spasm is both desirable and possible. Several recent
studies have utilized this approach with good results (33).

Randomization is an important factor in appropriate trial design because
it prevents bias in allocating patients to various interventions, insures
that study groups are comparable with respect to prognostic factors and
assures the validity of statistical tests of significance used to interpret
the results (48).

All drugs other than the short acting nitrates that are given as needed
for episodes of chest discomfort should be stopped. As indicated earlier,
it is even possible that some antianginal drugs, such as propanolol, may
predispose to coronary artery spasm.

Considerable concern has been expressed about the use of double-blind,
randomized controlled studies in patients with coronary artery spasm.
Acute myocardial infarction and sudden death have been reported to occur
in patients with this syndrome. However, if increasing angina with ECG
evidence of ischemia occurs during a double-blind randomized study, the
patient can be advanced to the next treatment (likely to be the active

medication) and the study is still blinded.

X. ASSESSMENT OF THERAPY

Various parameters (Table 6) have been utilized in patients with documented coronary artery spasm to document the effectiveness of specific drug therapy.

Table 6. Assessment of Therapy

1. Angina attack rate.
2. Number of short acting nitrates consummed.
3. Episodes of ST segment changes and/or arrhythmias on continuous ambulatory ECG recording.
4. ECG and hemodynamic response to exercise testing or intravenous ergonovine (in hospital).
5. Rest and exercise results of 201-thallium scintigraphy and radionuclide angiography.
6. Repeat coronary angiography before and with ergonovine provocation.
7. Appropriate statistical analysis.

The most commonly used method for assessing drug therapy is to compare the angina attack rate while the patient is receiving a placebo as compared to the number of episodes during one or incremental doses of the drug being tested. Also used is a pill count of the number of short acting nitrates consummed when the patient is on placebo therapy as compared to when he or she is receiving the drug designed to decrease coronary artery spasm. Another method that has been utilized to evaluate the results of drug therapy is of continuous ambulatory ECG recording on and off therapy with the number of episodes of ST segment evaluation or depression and/or the incidence of arrhythmias being compared during the two time intervals.

In those patients who have provacable coronary artery spasm with associated ECG changes, the ECG and hemodynamic changes (heart rate, blood pressure and heart rate, blood pressure product) during exercise testing may be assessed on and off medical therapy. Some investigators recommend the use of intravenous ergonovine in an attempt to induce coronary artery spasm with ECG heart rate and blood pressure monitoring in the Coronary Care Unit in order to demonstrate the efficacy of a drug known to improve coronary artery spasm. We believe that the intravenous administration of ergonovine outside of the cardiac catheterization laboratory is likely to be hazardous in some patients and do not recommend this approach.

In some patients, the rest and exercise results of 201-thallium scintigraphy and radionuclide angiography provide useful information, the former test showing decreased myocardial perfusion in areas of ischemia before but not during effective drug therapy and the latter demonstrating improved exercise performance of the left ventricular without major wall motion abnormalities on drug therapy as compared to a placebo study.

In several short term studies, coronary arteriography before and with ergonovine provocation has been utilized off and on medical therapy to show that a slow channel calcium blocking drug was effective in preventing ergonovine-induced spasm (34-37). In patients where this salutary effect has been demonstrated, initial long-term results with the specific drug employed have been excellent.

Finally, it must be stressed that an appropriate statistical analysis should be planned at the initiation of each specific protocol. With randomization, firm end-points and appropriate pre-planning, meaningful data can be obtained to assess accurately the efficacy of a drug; when not, the results are frequently negative even when the drug actually has a salutary effect.

REFERENCES

1. Prinzmetal, M., Kemnamer, R., Merliss, R., Wade, T., and Bor, N.: Angina pectoris. I. The variant form of angina pectoris. Am. J. Med. 27: 375, 1959.
2. Conti, C., Pepine, C., and Curry, J., Jr.: Coronary artery spasm: An important mechanism in the pathophysiology of ischemic heart disease. Curr. Probl. Cardiol. 4: 11, 1979.
3. Luchi, R., Chahine, R., and Raizner, A.: Coronary artery spasm. Ann. Intern. Med. 91: 441, 1979.
4. Hillis, L., and Braunwald, E.: Coronary-artery spasm. N. Engl. J. Med. Vol. 299 No. 13: 695, 1978.
5. Conti, C., and Curry, R., Jr.: Coronary artery spasm and myocardial ischemia. Mod. Concepts Cardiovasc. Dis. 49: 1, 1980.
6. Meller, J., Pichard, A., and Dack, S.: Coronary arterial spasm in Prinzmetal's angina: A proved hypothesis. Am. J. Cardiol. 37: 938, 1976.
7. Maseri, A., Severi, S., De Nes, M., L'Abbate, A., Chierchia, S., Marzilli, M., Ballestra, A., Parodi, O., Biagini, A., and Distante, A.: "Variant" angina: One aspect of a continuous spectrum of vasospastic myocardial ischemia. Am. J. Cardiol. 42: 1019, 1978.
8. Wiener, L., Kasparian, H., Duca, P., Walinsky, P., Gottlieb, R., Hanckel, F., and Brest, A.: Spectrum of coronary arterial spasm. Clinical, angiographic and myocardial metabolic experience in 29 cases. Am. J. Cardiol. 38: 945, 1976.

9. Feldman, R., Pepine, C., Whittle, J., Curry, R., and Conti, C.: Coronary hemodynamic findings during spontaneous angina in patients with variant angina. Circulation 64, No. 1, 1981.

10. Maseri, A., Parodi, O., Severi, S., and Pesola, A.: Transient transmural reduction of myocardial blood flow, demonstrated by thallium-201 scintigraphy, as a cause of variant angina. Circulation 54, No. 2, 1976.

11. Fuller, C., Raizner, A., Chahine, R., Nahormek, P., Ishimori, T., Verani, M., Nitishin, A., Mokotoff, D., and Luchi, R.: Exercise-induced coronary arterial spasm: Angiographic demonstration, documentation of ischemia by myocardial scintigraphy and results of pharmacologic intervention. Am. J. Cardiol. 46: 500, 1980.

12. Maseri, A., L'Abbate, A., Baroldi, G., Chierchia, S., Marzilli, M., Ballestra, A., Severi, S., Parodi, O., Biagini, A. Distante, A., and Pesola, A.: Coronary vasospasm as a possible cause of myocardial infarction. N. Engl. J. Med. Vol. 299, No. 23, 1978.

13. Braunwald, E.: (Editorial) Coronary spasm and acute myocardial infarction-New possibility for treatment and prevention. N. Engl. J. Med. Vol. 299, No. 23, 1978.

14. Buxton, A., Goldberg, S., Harken, A., Hirshfeld, J., Jr., and Kastor, A.: Coronary-artery spasm immediately after myocardial revascularization. N. Engl. J. Med. Vol. 304, No. 21, 1981.

15. Bharati, S., Dhingra, R., Lev, M., Towne, W., Rahimtoola, S., and Rosen, K.: Conduction system in a patient with Prinzmetal's angina and transient atrioventricular block. Am. J. Cardiol. 39: 120, 1977.

16. Yasue, H., Nagao, M., Omote, S., Takizawa, A., Miwa, K. and Tanaka, S.: Coronary arterial spasm and Prinzmetal's variant form of angina induced by hyperventilation and tris-buffer infusion. Circulation Vol. 58, No. 1, 1978.

17. Curry, R., Jr., Pepine, C., Sabom, M., Feldman, R., Christie, L., Varnell, J., and Conti, C.: Hemodynamic and myocardial metabolic effects of ergonovine in patients with chest pain. Circulation Vol. 58, No. 4, 1978.

18. Heupler, F., Jr., Proudfit, W., Razavi, M., Shirey, E., Greenstreet, R., and Sheldon, W.: Ergonovine maleate provocative test for coronary arterial spasm. Am. J. Cardiol. Vol. 41, No. 4, 1978.

19. Schroeder, J., Bolen, J., Quint, R., Clark, D., Hayden, W., Higgins, C., and Wexler, L.: Provocation of coronary spasm with ergonovine maleate. Am. J. Cardiol. Vol. 40, No. 4, 1977.

20. Helfant, R.: Coronary arterial spasm and provocative testing in ischemic heart disease. Am. J. Cardiol. 41: 787, 1978.

21. Schroeder, J., Bolen, J., Quint, R., Clark, D., Hayden, W., Higgins, C., and Wexler, L.: Provocation of coronary spasm with ergonovine maleate. Am. J. Cardiol. Vol. 40, No. 4, 1977.

22. Mudge, G., Goldberg, S., Gunther, S., Mann, T., and Grossman, W.: Comparison of metabolic and vasoconstrictor stimuli on coronary vascular resistance in man. Circulation, Vol. 59, No. 3, 1979.

23. Antman, E., Stone, P., Muller, J., and Braunwald, E.: Calcium channel blocking agents in the treatment of cardiovascular disorders. Part I. Basic and clinical electrophysiologic effects. Ann. Intern. Med. 93: 875, 1980.

24. Stone, P., Antman, E., Muller, J., and Braunwald, E.: Calcium channel blocking agents in the treatment of cardiovascular disorders. Part II. Hemodynamic effects and clinical applications. Ann. Intern. Med. 93: 886, 1980.

25. Walsh, R.A., Badke, F.R., and O'Rourke, R.A.: Differential effects of systemic and intracoronary calcium channel blocking agents on global and regional left ventricular function in conscious dogs. Am. Heart J. 102: 341, 1981.
26. Kimura, E. and Kishida, H.: Treatment of variant angina with drugs: A survey of 11 cardiology institutes in Japan. Circulation 63, No. 4, 1981.
27. Severi, S., Davies, G. Maseri, A., Marzullo, P., and L'Abbate, A.: Long-term prognosis of "variant" angina with medical treatment. Am. J. Cardiol. 46: 226, 1980.
28. Hosoda, S. and Kimura, E.: Efficacy of nifedipine in the variant form of angina pectoris. Proceedings International Nifedipine "Adalat Symposium" Tokyo Press Tokyo, 1975.
29. Antman, E., Muller, J., Goldberg, S., MacAlpin, R., Rubenfire, M., Tabatznik, B., Liang, C., Heupler, F., Achuff, S., Reichek, N., Geltman, E., Kerin, N.A., Neff, R.K., and Braunwald, E.: Nifedipine therapy for coronary-artery spasm: Collective clinical experience in 127 patients. N. Engl. J. Med. Vol. 302, No. 23, 1980.
30. Johnson, S.M., Mauritson, D.R., Willerson, J.T., and Hillis, L.D.: Comparison of verapamil and nifedipine in the treatment of variant angina pectoris: Preliminary observations in 10 patients. Am. J. Cardiol. 47: 1295, 1981.
31. Gunther, S., Green, L., Muller, J.E., Mudge, G.H., Jr., and Grossman, W.: Prevention by nifedipine of abnormal coronary vasoconstriction in patients with coronary artery disease. Circulation 63, No. 4, 1981.
32. Johnson, S.M., Mauritson, D.R., Corbett, J., Dehmer, G.J., Lewis, S.E., Willerson, J.T., and Hillis, L.D.: Effects of verapamil and nifedipine on left ventricular function at rest and during exercise in patients with Prinzmetal's variant angina pectoris. Am. J. Cardiol. 47: 1289, 1981.
33. Johnson, S.M., Jauritson, D.R., Willerson, J.T., and Hillis, L.D.: A controlled trial of verapamil for Prinzmetal's variant angina. N. Engl. J. Med. Vol. 304, No. 15, 1981.
34. Theroux, P., Waters, D.D., Affaki, G.S., Crittin, J., Bonan, R., and Mizgala, H.F.: Provocative testing with ergonovine to evaluate the efficacy of treatment with calcium antagonists in variant angina. Circulation 60, No. 3, 1979.
35. Waters, D.D., Theroux, P., Szlachcic, J., and Dauwe, F.: Provocative testing with ergonovine to assess the efficacy of treatment with nifedipine, diltiazem and verapamil in variant angina. Am. J. Cardiol. 48: 123, 1981.
36. Fiefenbrunn, A.J., Sobel, B.E., Gowda, S., McKnight, R.C., and Ludbrook, P.A.: Nifedipine blockade of ergonovine-induced coronary arterial spasm: Angiographic documentation. Am. J. Cardiol. 48: 184, 1981.
37. Chaitman, B.R., Waters, D.D., Theroux, P., and Hanson, J.S.: S-T segment elevation and coronary spasm in response to exercise. Am. J. Cardiol. 47: 1350, 1981.
38. Specchia, G., DeServi, S., Falcone, C., Bramucci, E., Angoli, L., Mussini, A., Marinoni, P., Montemartini, C., and Bobba, P.: Coronary arterial spasm as a cause of exercise-induced ST-segment elevation in patients with variant angina. Circulation, Vol. 59, No. 5, 1979.
39. Boden, W.E., Bough, E.W., Korr, K.S., Benham, I., Gheorghiade, M., Caputi, A., and Shulman, R.S.: Exercise-induced coronary spasm with S-T segment depression and normal coronary arteriography. Am. J. Cardiol. 48: 193, 1981.

40. DeServi, S., Specchia, G., Curti, M.T., Falcone, C., Gavazzi, A., Bramucci, E., Mussini, A., Angoli, L., Salerno, J., and Bobba, P.: Variable threshold of angina during exercise: A clinical manifestation of some patients with vasospastic angina. Am. J. Cardiol. 48: 188, 1981.

41. Lahiri, A.,Subramanian, B., Millar-Craig, M., Crawley, J., and Raftery, E.B.: Exercise-induced S-T segment elevation in variant angina. Am. J. Cardiol. 45: 887, 1980.

42. Yasue, H., Omote, S., Takizawa, A., Nagao, M., Miwa, K., and Tanaka, S.: Circadian variation of exercise capacity in patients with Prinzmetal's variant angina: Role of exercise-induced coronary arterial spasm. Circulation 59, No. 5, 1979.

43. Specchia, G., DeServi, S., Falcone, C., Angoli, L., Mussini, A., Bramucci, E., Marioni, G.P., Ardissino, D., Salerno, J. and Bobba, P.: Significance of exercise-induced ST-segment elevation in patients without myocardial infarction. Circulation 63, No. 1, 1981.

44. Chahine, R.A., Raizner, A.E., and Ishimori, T.: The clinical significance of exercise-induced ST-segment elevation. Circulation 54: 209, 1976.

45. Fortuin, N.J., and Friesinger, G.C.: Exercise-induced ST segment elevation. Clinical, electrocardiographic and arteriographic studies in twelve patients. Am. J. Med. 49: 459, 1970.

46. Bobba, P., Vecchio, C., DiGuglielmo, L., Salerno, J., Casari, A., and Montemartini, C.: Exercise-induced RS-T segment elevation. Electrocardiographic and angiographic observations. Cardiology 57: 162, 1972.

47. Longhurst, J.C., and Kraus, W.L.: Exercise-induced ST elevation in patients without myocardial infarction. Circulation 60: 616, 1979.

CALCIUM ENTRY BLOCKING AGENTS:
HOW TO DEFINE CONTROLLED STUDIES IN PATIENTS WITH ARRHYTHMIAS

Leonard S. Dreifus, M.D. and Eric L. Michelson, M.D.

There is an abundance of evidence now available indicating the importance of the slow channel in arrhythmogenesis.[1] The cells of the sino-atrial (SA) and atrio-ventricular (AV) node show no evidence of a fast component. Hence, in these fibers the entire action potential appears to result from a slow inward current.[1,2] Furthermore, electrophysiologic studies have demonstrated that the calcium "antagonistic" properties of some of the recently introduced coronary vasodilator agents might also offer important antiarrhythmic effects by inhibiting slow inward currents. While a number of drugs belonging to this class including diltiazem, nifedipine and verapamil will soon be available in the United States for a variety of clinical indications, only verapamil appears to exert important antiarrhythmic effects on the sinus node and atrio-ventricular node.[3] While earlier preclinical studies suggested that diltiazem might have important electrophysiologic effects by increasing the functional and effective refractory periods of the AV node and in particular, might worsen AV conduction in patients with underlying AV conduction disease, its clinical effects seem to be less pronounced than expected from studies in the isolated perfused electrophysiologic heart preparations.[3] Furthermore, calcium entry blockers show little or no direct effect in the management of ventricular arrhythmias.[4,5] Hence, the evaluation of drug treatment for calcium entry blockers will be discussed in the context of supraventricular arrhythmias, and especially one calcium entry blocker, verapamil, which has received extensive attention in the management of the supraventricular arrhythmias. However, those principles of protocol design that are also applicable to the study of ventricular arrhythmias will be noted.

The calcium entry blocking agents appear most effective in supraventricular tachycardias and reentry tachycardias involving the AV node, with or without an accessory pathway mechanism. Furthermore, since these agents have shown little or no effect on atrial refractory periods, it may be extremely important to establish the precise electrophysiologic mechanism for the supraventricular tachycardia to be studied. For instance, supraventricular tachycardias may respond differently depending on whether they are a result of sinus node reentry, intra- or interatrial reentry, such as reentry within Bachmann's bundle, or automatic atrial arrhythmias, as opposed to the mechanisms involving reentry within the AV node and/or perinodal AV tissues. Obviously, precise electrophysiologic studies cannot be attempted in all patients and consequently, the design of pharmacologic studies may not clearly define the effectiveness of an agent for a specific arrhythmia. Hence, attention to the specific classifications of the supraventricular arrhythmias, with some electrophysiologic proof when indicated would be ideal. The protocol designed to study the ventricular response in the presence of atrial flutter and atrial fibrillation must necessarily be different from acute studies to terminate supraventricular tachycardia, or chronic prophylactic studies to inhibit the number of atrial premature systoles or issues of paroxysmal supraventricular tachycardia.[6] Three specific strategies will be discussed:

1) Acute drug testing for:

    A) Supraventricular tachycardia

    B) Rapid ventricular rates in the presence of atrial flutter and fibrillation.

2) Prophylactic chronic administration to control atrial premature systoles and paroxysmal supraventricular tachycardias.

3) Chronic administration to control ventricular rates in the presence of atrial

flutter and fibrillation both at rest and exercise.

General Considerations

In addition to routine laboratory testing and electrocardiographic monitoring, hemodynamic studies are also required to fully evaluate new potential antiarrhythmic agents, including calcium channel blockers. In some specific instances of supraventricular tachycardias, the precise identification of the electrophysiologic mechanisms, e.g., atrio-ventricular nodal tachycardia vs. other atrial tachycardias are mandatory. In other instances, complex studies may be necessary involving drug combinations such as calcium entry blockers plus digitalis preparations or beta blocking agents. Since the calcium entry blocking agents have profound effects on the specialized tissues of the sinus and AV nodes, patients with evidence of preexisting disease should be excluded from these protocols. Furthermore, patients must be eliminated from any protocol in which significant negative inotropic effects would be deleterious to the patients' left ventricular function. Since digitalis preparations and beta blocking agents have significant interaction and additive effects with calcium entry blocking drugs, extreme care is required to prevent adverse hemodynamic or electrophysiologic complications.

I. Effect on acute supraventricular arrhythmias

A. Supraventricular tachycardia (AV nodal reentry)

Since supraventricular tachycardias are not usually life threatening, it is usually prudent to utilize placebo vs. active drug in a single or double blind protocol. When the drug is administered intravenously and its onset of action is within minutes, (e.g., verapamil) a single blind study utilizing placebo initially followed by the active preparation in single rising, appropriately timed doses is usually sufficient to identify the important properties of the antiarrhythmic agent (Fig.1). The expected endpoint is conversion to regular sinus rhythm.

Certain precautions are necessary during drug administration. An intravenous line should be in place prior to any intervention and continuous electrocardiographic monitoring initiated. Some investigators have advocated keeping the patient unaware of the exact time that an agent is being administered. Also, certain critical observations can be made during termination of the tachycardia regarding the arrhythmia mechanism. Careful obervation may reveal slowing of the tachycardia rate, inscription of a P wave without a following QRS indicating that the block occurred during the antegrade portion of the reentry loop, or change in P wave contour indicating a shift of the pacemaker. Observation of subsequent PR intervals following the establishment of sinus rhythm could indicate the relative influence of the agent on AV nodal conduction.

If the acute drug study is carried out in the catheterization laboratory in conjunction with electrophysiologic studies, other pertinent information can be obtained concerning sinus node function, atrial and atrio-nodal refractoriness, AH and HV intervals, as well as the location of the reentry circuit. Hence, a subset of patients should be studied in the catheterization laboratory during the electrical induction of the supraventricular tachycardia by programmed stimulation in order to gain further insight as to the electropharmacologic mechanisms of the antiarrhythmic agent. Utilizing a subset of patients with reentrant tachyarrhythmias reproducibly inducible with programmed stimulation of the atria, a double blind protocol can be used to determine the efficacy of an antiarrhythmic agent. Alternatively, a single blind modification can be utilized by administering a placebo initially followed by dose titration of the active drug (Figure 2).

II. Prophylactic therapy of atrial premature systoles and paroxsymal tachycardias.

The description of an adequate protocol to properly evaluate the antiarrhythmic efficacy of any antiarrhythmic drug in patients with either premature atrial systoles or paroxsyms of supraventricular tachycardia is extremely difficult. The unpredictable incidence and behavior of intermittent or transient events make it almost impossible to adequately determine antiarrhythmic drug efficacy in the presence of these arrhythmias. Atrial premature systoles, unlike their ventricular counterparts, are rarely seen in large numbers, and chronic drug protocols that are suitable for studying the efficacy of drugs in treating the ventricular arrhythmias are often unsatisfactory for atrial premature systoles. Using appropriate statistical methods and frequent 24 hour ambulatory ECG recordings it may be possible to study patients with as few as 100-300 atrial premature systoles per day, although patients with $\geq$ 30-60 premature beats per hour have been included in most studies of ventricular arrhythmias. A protocol for the study of premature beats is detailed in figure 3. This protocol is suitable for either atrial or ventricular arrhythmia studies.

On the other hand, frequent paroxysms of supraventricular tachycardia, for example, several episodes per month, as opposed to those that occur at extremely long intervals such as once or twice per year, may be suitable for the long term evaluation of antiarhythmic drugs with respect to tachyarrhythmia prophylaxis. Stringent selection of patients exhibiting at least one or two documented attacks per week are the most suitable candidates. As noted above, these patients can also be studied in the catheterization laboratory with programmed stimulation before and after the administration of either intravenous or orally administered antiarrhythmic agents (Fig. 2). It should be recognized that such studies may subject patients to long periods on the catheterization table and may also require the retention of a transvenous temporary cardiac pacemaker lead in the coronary sinus for several days. These studies are feasible and can be carried out in patients demonstrating predictably inducible supraventricular tachycardias. However, the influence of the autonomic nervous system on AV nodal function should not be underestimated. Therefore, the results of acute electrophysiologic drug dosing, although helpful, must be interpreted with some caution and must be correlated with the results of ambulatory, oral drug testing, also on protocol. This is true for both supraventricular and ventricular arrhythmias, but an especially important consideration in reentrant arrhytmias involving the AV node.

III. Effect of an antiarrhythmic drug on atrio-ventricular transmission in the presence of atrial flutter and fibrillaton.

Previous studies evaluating the effectiveness of beta blocking agents, digitalis and verapamil in the control of the ventricular rate in the presence of atrial fibrillation and flutter have led to a series of experimental protocols to evaluate the effect of an agent on AV transmission. Since all of these agents affect the N region of the AV node predominantly, and prolong the AV nodal functional and effective refractory periods, these agents can be studied either alone or in combination with each other.[1,7] In the case of atrial fibrillation, a reduction in the resting heart rate can be one end-point of therapy. However, during exercise testing an exaggerated increase in AV conduction can occur despite a slow ventricular rate at rest, particularly in patients on digitalis preparations. In comparison, in the case of either beta-blockers or verapamil, both resting and exercise heart rates are reduced following drug administration. Protocols have been designed both for patients in whom concomitant digoxin is to be prescribed and for those in whom digoxin is not otherwise indicated. Several protocols can be utilized in evaluating the response to an exercise challenge in the presence of atrial flutter and fibrillation.

In those patients in whom digoxin is indicated, optimal dosing of digoxin is required prior to randomization based on the resting heart rate, exercise heart rate and digoxin level. Thereafter, patients can be entered into an open, single blind titration phase. This would determine the dose of the drug necessary to optimally affect the ventricular rate in response to both resting and exercise periods. Only patients who achieve at least a 30 beat increase in heart rate with exercise and a 15% reduction in the exercise challenge test on drug would be accepted for randomization (Fig. 4). A more elaborate single and double blind protocol can be used to evaluate the combination of antiarrhythmic agents that are known to effect AV conduction alone and in combination, as seen in Fig. 4, by substituting another drug known to affect AV conduction, e.g., propranolol for the placebo. Hence, combined drug therapy can be evaluated in this manner although such a protocol is somewhat cumbersome. In addition, it is also feasible to add an arm to the protocol in which digoxin is weaned from digitalized patients once they are on the study drug to determine the efficacy of monotherapy. Furthermore, it may also be advisable to do adjunctive Holter monitoring at each stage of the protocol in this type of study design. In this way it is also possible to further evaluate both efficacy and possible adverse effects, such as excessive bradycardia.

In conclusion, the ability to evaluate the efficacy of calcium entry blocking agents in the presence of supraventricular arrhythmias is predicated upon the fact that these agents affect the slow response action potentials in the SA and AV node. In the case of reentrant tachycardias incorporating the AV node as part of the circuit, conduction block within the slow response cells of the AV node appears to terminate the reentry mechanism.[7] In a similar manner, agents affecting the slow response fibers within the N region of the AV node are also responsible for decreasing the ventricular response to atrial flutter and atrial fibrillation. Consequently, the evaluation of calcium entry blocking agents such as verapamil, diltiazem and nifedipine can be linked to the specific action of these agents on the slow response fibers within the SA node and the N region of the AV node.

REFERENCES

1. Cranefield PF: The conduction of the cardiac impulse. The slow response and cardiac arrhythmias. Mt. Kisco NY: Futura Publishing, 1975

2. Zipes DP, Fischer JC: Effect of agents which inhibit the slow channel on sinus node automaticity and atrioventricular conduction in the dog. Circ Res 34:184, 1974

3. Kawai C, Konishi T, Matsuyama E, Okazaki H: Comparative effects of three calcium antagonists, diltiazem, verapamil and nifedipine on the sinoatrial and atrioventricular odes: Experimental and clinical studies. Circulation 63:1035, 1981

4. Naito M, Michelson EL, Kmetzo JJ, Kaplinsky E, Dreifus LS: Failure of antiarrhythmic drugs to prevent experimental reperfusion ventricular fibrillation. Circulation 63:71, 1981

5. Naito M, Michelson EL, Kmetzo JJ, Kaplinsky E, Dreifus LS: Failure of antiarrhythmic drugs to effect epicardial delay during acute experimental coronary artery occlusion and reperfusion: Correlation with lack of antiarrhythmic efficacy. J Pharm Exp Therap 218:475, 1981

6. Kaplinsky E, Naggan L: Evaluation of drug treatment in supraventricular arrhythmias in the evaluation of new antiarrhythmic drugs. In: Morganroth J, Moore EN, Dreifus LS, Michelson EL,eds. The Evaluation of New Antiarrhythmic Drugs. The Hague: Martinus Nijhoff Publishers 1981:271

7. Mazgalev T, Dreifus LS, Bianchi J, Michelson EL: The mechanism of AV junctional reentry: Role of the atrionodal junction. Anat Rec 201:179, 1981

FIGURE 1

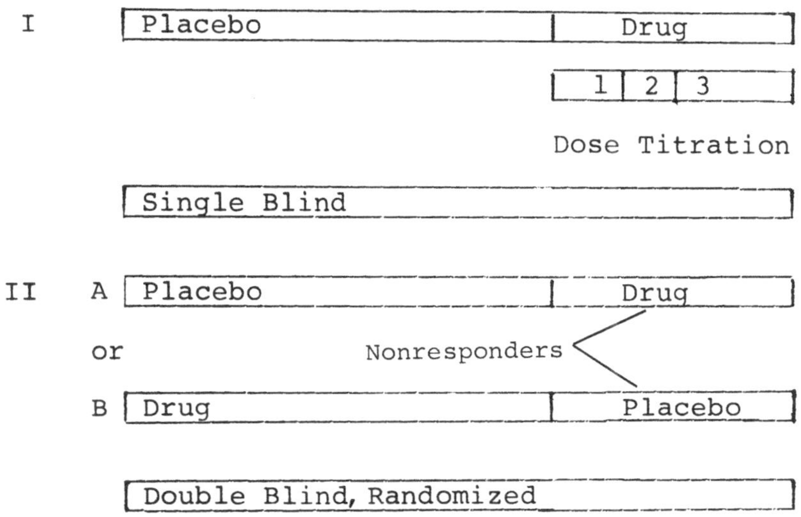

I
Placebo
Drug
1
2
3
Dose Titration
Single Blind
II
A
Placebo
Drug
or
Nonresponders
B
Drug
Placebo
Double Blind, Randomized

FIGURE 2

RANDOMIZATION
Dose Titration
Inducible Subset
1
2
3
Drug A
Prog Stim
Wean
Placebo
Prog Stim
Wean
1
2
3
Placebo
Prog Stim
Wean
Drug A
Prog Stim
Wean
Double Blind
Double Blind

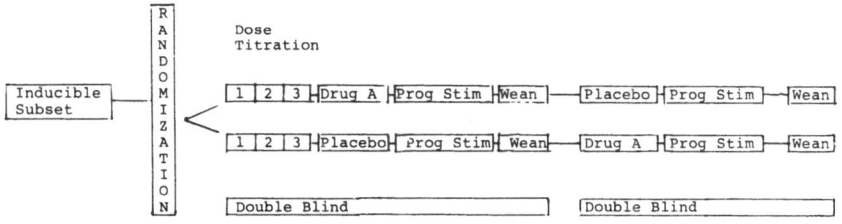

Prog Stim = programmed stimulation

FIGURE 3

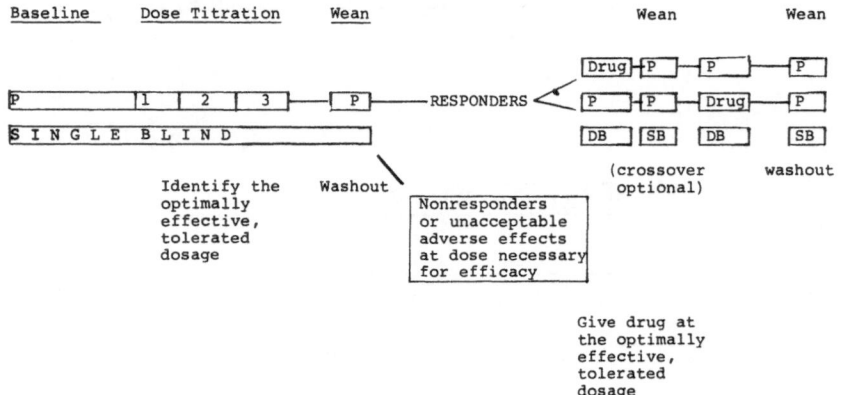

Baseline   Dose Titration   Wean   Wean   Wean

Identify the optimally effective, tolerated dosage

Washout

Nonresponders or unacceptable adverse effects at dose necessary for efficacy

(crossover optional)   washout

Give drug at the optimally effective, tolerated dosage

DB = double blind, randomized
P = placebo
SB = single blind

FIGURE 4

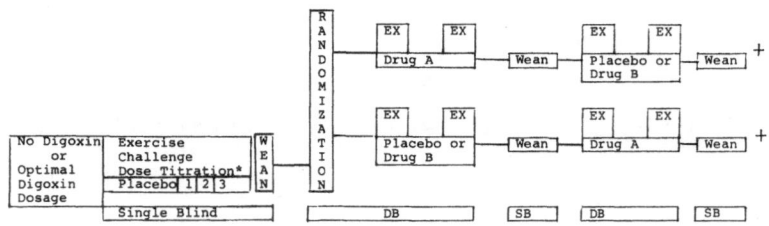

DB = double blind
SB = single blind
EX = exercise stress testing - usually Naughton protocol
* = optional - Holter monitoring for the 24 hours prior to each exercise stress test
      and throughout the study
+ = optional; if on digoxin, wean digoxin and evaluate drug vs placebo

EVALUATION OF BETA BLOCKERS AND CALCIUM ANTAGONISTS IN THE TREATMENT OF HYPERTROPHIC CARDIOMYOPATHY

STEPHEN E. EPSTEIN, M.D.

I. Problems in evaluating therapy for patients with hypertrophic cardiomyopathy

A. Great variability in symptoms -- day to day, week to week
1. Often experience symptoms at rest that are difficult to quantitate (fatigue, lightheadedness, chest pain, dyspnea)
2. Exercise end-point less reproducible than CAD patients

B. Great variability in pathophysiologic spectrum:
1. Obstructive vs nonobstructive
2. NSR vs AF
3. Decreased LV compliance vs. no or little change in compliance
4. Increase pulmonary capillary wedge pressure vs. no or small increase in pressure.

C. This variability in symptoms and pathophysiologic spectrum results in the need to study a fairly large number of patients in order to avoid a Type II error (failure to detect a significant effect when, in fact, such exists), since sample size increases exponentially in relation to increases in the coefficient of variation of end-point.

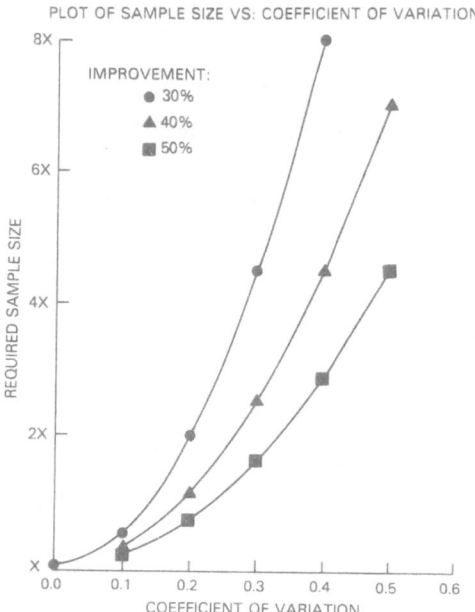

PLOT OF SAMPLE SIZE VS. COEFFICIENT OF VARIATION

Figure 2. Relation between sample size necessary
to detect a significant effect and spontaneous
variability of end point being tested. The three
curves represent relationship for progressively
more powerful interventions.

II. Broad patholophysiologic spectrum mean subgroups of patients might
respond differently to treatment. The problem that might arise is
how to identify subgroups of patients that might respond to therapy,
even though the majority of individuals might not.

A. Requires statistical models to establish the mean and spontaneous
variability of the end point being measured so that <u>individual</u>
deviation from the mean response to therapy can be identified.
This "searching" for subgroups" could lead to "significant" differences when, in fact, none existed. Hence, the subjects so
identified must constitute the patient cohort of a second study
designed to prospectively test a new hypothesis -- that the therapeutic intervention being tested benefits this specific subgroup
of patients.

III. Because of great variability in pathophysiologic spectrum and response to therapy, evaluation of therapy must be broad, encompassing several endpoints.

    A. Effects of drug on:
1. LV outflow tract obstruction
2. Pulmonary capillary wedge pressure
3. LV compliance
4. Patient's subjective appraisal
5. Exercise capacity
6. Traditional randomized double-blind crossover study
7. Survival

    B. However, clinical benefit cannot be detected merely by "favorable" responses to studies 1 through 4. Although such "favorable" responses are encouraging, they do not necessarily correlate with beneficial effect on symptoms, exercise capacity, or survival. Hence, true benefit can only be established by additional studies demonstrating favorable response to studies, 4, 5, 6, or 7.

DETERMINATION OF THE SAFETY OF CALCIUM ANTAGONISTS IN COMBINATION WITH
BETA-ADRENERGIC BLOCKING AGENTS -- THE CASE FOR CIRCUMSCRIBED CLINICAL TRIALS

Burton E. Sobel

Explicity, this topic is straight-forward. Implicitly however, it
reflects a source of tension between regulatory agencies and practitioners
of medicine regarding several issues. Before considerating specific
aspects of the clinical pharmacology involved, let us examine some of the
factors contributing to this tension, particularly with respect to these
two classes of agents.

In the Wall Street Journal on Monday, September 28, 1981, Dr. Hayes,
Commissioner of Food and Drugs, Department of Health and Human Services,
writes: "while the FDA already has improved and streamlined its drug
approval process, I am committed now to the most thorough review of the
intricate and complex system by which drugs are developed and evaluated.
On September 9, I announced the formation of a 21-member task force to
evaluate the entire process and recommend policy, regulatory, legislative,
and management changes. One issue being considered ... is whether drugs
... which are fairly safe but of unproven effectiveness, should be
provisionally approved by FDA while further studies are being completed.
The law now does not permit FDA such discretion." Undoubtedly, many
physicians object to laws that do not allow provisional acceptance
because of several considerations that will be discussed in this brief
essay. A companion letter by D. Creasey in the same issue of the Wall
Street Journal indicates that "such behavior (the bureaucratic propensity
for ignoring all sorts of possibilities for success just to avoid any
slight chance of failure and embarrassment) should be expected as a very
rational response by people working in a system which provides virtually
no rewards for a successful risk taking and promises political, congressional,
or media-induced punishment for failure." From even this single exchange
of views, it is evident that profound pressures have been exerted on
regulatory agencies regarding safety -- implicitly defined as avoidance

of potentially catastrophic outcomes from administration of drugs that could not be anticipated on the basis of the known mechanism of action of the agents or on the basis of data available from completed studies. Pressures on practitioners elicit a different bias, based on the desire to have potentially therapeutic agents available even when their efficacy has not yet been proven unequivocally.

Definitions of Efficacy:

With respect to agents in the two classes being considered in this discussion, efficacy of individual agents or combinations must be considered in terms of treatment of specific entities -- primarily hypertension, angina pectoris, and arrhythmia. For each, the most obvious explicit end-point of efficacy is not necessarily intimately linked to the implicitly desired end-points. For example, treatment of hypertension is directed explicitly toward lowering systemic arterial blood pressure. However, what is implicitly desired is reduction of vascular degeneration and injury, protection of target organs, and prolongation of life expectancy. Preliminary evidence suggests that calcium antagonists may be capable of reducing the extent of vascular injury sustained under at least some selected conditions predisposing toward vascular pathology. Thus, it is possible that calcium antagonists could protect the vasculature against injury whether or not they lowered blood pressure comparably to other drugs. Beta-adrenergic blocking agents inhibit release of renin, and high renin levels have been implicated by some as an independent variable contributing to vascular injury. Should this hypothesis prove to be true, protective effects on vasculature might be elicited by beta-adrenergic blocking agents whether or not they lowered peripheral arterial blood pressure comparably to other drugs.

Although the explicit goal of therapy of angina pectoris is the reduction of pain, we seek agents which will increase coronary flow, decrease ventricular oxygen requirements, improve ventricular performance by enhancing intrinsic ventricular function or by modifying systemic arterial or venous resistance and capacitance. Effects on these implicit end-points may be of considerably more importance with respect to long-term survival of treated patients than effects on the explicitly recognized end-point of pain per se.

Treatment of arrhythmia, particularly in patients with ischemic heart disease, is frequently directed explicitly toward reduction of the prevelance of premature ventricular complexes on ambulatory electrocardiograms or a related electrocardiographic end-point. What is desired implicitly however, is reduction of the propensity for ventricular fibrillation. In many circumstances, the two may be dissociated. Warning arrhythmias are not nearly as unequivocally associated with the likelihood of ventricular fibrillation in patients with acute coronary insufficiency as had been thought only a few years ago. Furthermore, it has become clear that suppression of PVCs with anti-arrhythmic agents is not tantamount to reduction of the propensity to ventricular fibrillation on the one hand, and that anti-fibrillatory agents may be remarkably ineffective in suppressing PVCs on the other.

From even these brief considerations about end-points, it is clear that definitive assessments of efficacy of a single drug is complex. The complexity is intensified when one seeks to establish efficacy of combinations of drugs or to compare their efficacy extrapolating from results obtained with a single agent or a different combination.

Drug Interactions and Efficacy:

When we consider beta-adrenergic blocking agents and calcium antagonists as anti-hypertensive agents, it is obvious that interactions between the two can led to synergistic effects on either explicit or implicit end-points. Since several calcium antagonists diminish peripheral vascular resistance and lower arterial blood pressure, they elicit increased release of renin from the kidney as a compensatory response. If the elevated plasma renin independently offset some of the protective effect on vascular pathology that would have been elicited by reduction of hypertension per se, concomitant use of a beta-adrenergic blocking agent with its inhibition of renal release of renin might be particularly helpful whether or not combination therapy lead to a larger decrement in systemic arterial blood pressure.

In a patient with angina pectoris treated with a calcium antagonist that lowered peripheral arterial resistance and arterial blood pressure, the physiological compensatory response might entail augmentation of heart rate which could offset the diminution in myocardial oxygen requirements implicitly sought. Administration of a beta-adrenergic

blocking agent concomitantly, with consequent inhibition of the acceleration of heart rate, might improve the balance between myocardial oxygen
supply and demand, augment coronary blood flow (because of the longer
cumulative diastolic perfusion interval), and improve ventricular
performance secondary to enhanced ventricular filling. On the other
hand, one can easily envision a situation in which the addition of a
beta-adrenergic blocking agent could led to modest CNS side-effects
ultimately resulting in the patient's diminished physical activity with
a consequent reduction of pain that was not reflective of cardiac
benefit.

Protective electrophysiological effects of calcium antagonists are
evident under some conditions (such as in treatment of reentrant
supraventricular tachycardia), but their influence on ventricular
arrhythmia is much less clear. Since the electrophysiological factors
responsible for ventricular fibrillation have not been delineated
definitively, and since it is not clear whether or not slow channel
action potentials contribute to high grade ventricular arrhythmia, it
is impossible to determine a priori whether calcium antagonists are
likely to preclude ventricular fibrillation induced by transitory
ischemia. Combination therapy with a beta-adrenergic blocking agent
might be expected to potentiate the inhibition of inward calcium flux,
based on some results in experimental animal preparations, and therefore
might potentiate anti-fibrillatory actions whether or not the combination
therapy influenced the frequency of PVCs detectable with ambulatory
electrocardiograms.

In addition to the complexities encountered when one evaluates the
efficacy of combination therapy in terms of explicit or implicit
end-points, the diversity of agents within each of the two classes must
be considered. For example, among calcium antagonists (Table 1) some
agents such as nifedipine exert their actions primarily or exclusively
on peripheral vasculature at conventional therapeutic doses. Such
agents function largely as vasodilators without substantial effects on
the heart itself under most circumstances. Conventional doses of other
agents, such as verapamil, exert substantial effects on the heart and
relatively modest effects on peripheral vasculature. Thus, even within
the overall group of calcium antagonists, anti-hypertensive, anti-anginal,
and anti-arrhythmic effects may result from diverse mechanisms. In the

first case, blood pressure may be reduced, angina diminished, and arrhythmia decreased primarily or exclusively because of reduction of peripheral vascular resistance and a consequent diminution of myocardial oxygen requirements, or because of enhancement of coronary perfusion due to inhibition of coronary vasospasm. In the second case, modest and potentially desirable decreases in contractility or diastolic stiffness of the ventricle may contribute to decreased systemic arterial blood pressure and diminished angina secondary to the decreased oxygen requirements. Direct effects on cardiac action potentials may influence cardiac rhythm.

Even among subclasses of calcium antagonists, marked diversity is evident. Available preparations of verapamil comprise two isomers with markedly different properties, one of which inhibits sodium channels in electrophysiologically excitable cells. Thus, the net effect of verapamil may differ depending on dose, prevailing blood level, and occupancy of several different types of receptors among other factors such as heart rate.

Diversity is evident when one considers beta-adrenergic blocking agents (Table 2) as well. Effects of some are attributable primarily or exclusively to $beta_1$ effects (the so called "cardioselective agents"), although receptor specificity tends to diminish for most agents when doses are increased. Other beta-adrenergic blocking agents have marked effects on vascular tone, and exert some of their clinical effects through this mechanism. Some of the agents are partial agonists, and effects of all of them will depend on the intrinsic sympathetic activity exhibited by the patient, and will therefore be somewhat variable. Diversity of this sort in addition to the diversity of pharmacokinetic properties makes it difficult to define the behavior of one agent based on results acquired in studies of another.

Statistical Considerations:

Factors underlying the enthusiasm for multi-center large scale double-blinded prospective clinical trials (which we shall refer to as global clinical trials), have been emphasized extensively throughout this symposium and merit the strongest possible consideration. Important conclusions regarding efficacy and safety can be established with global clinical trials, particularly when they are conducted according

to sophistificated criteria such as those developed by the National
Institutes of Health. The use of data monitoring boards to protect
patients against unexpected toxicity and to determine whether or not a
statistically significant result has been achieved permits blinding of
the investigators throughout the trial and facilitates objectivity in
its conduct. Statistical procedures have been developed to avoid
rejecting the null hypothesis inappropriately as a result of differences
occurring by chance during multiple evaluations of the data by such
boards, and to assure the effectiveness of the randomization process
and the comparability of baseline features of treated and control
groups. Unfortunately, however, global clinical trials are extraordinarily
expensive, making it incumbant upon policy makers to be extraordinarily
judicious in selecting appropriate agents or approaches for evaluation.
Even with the best of intentions, global clinical trials may be flawed
because of the lack of basic information available at their inception
or changes in perspective that evolve due to accretion of new information
while they are underway.

Such considerations apply to agents in both classes that we are
considering in this discussion. Beta-adrenergic blocking agents have
been used in clinical trials of ischemic heart disease, based initially
on the premise that they would be effective by improving the balance
between myocardial oxygen supply and demand. In fact, however, it
appears likely that beneficial effects of beta-adrenergic blocking
agents may be attributable to a reduction of the propensity toward
ventricular fibrillation in patients with coronary artery disease,
which may depend on properties of the drugs that were not even considered
when the trials were initiated. Since some (but not all) beta-adrenergic
blocking agents have direct membrane depressant effects, it is highly
likely that protective effects of one agent on sudden death may differ
from protective effects of another. Pharmacological differences among
the compounds make it particularly difficult to extrapolate results
obtained with one to results that might be anticipated with another.

Since the spectrum of agents available for clinical use will
continue to expand, it is essential, from a cost-effectiveness point of
view, that global clinical trials acquire as much information as
possible bearing on the mechanism of action of the agents studied in
specific settings as well as on the primary end-points. If for example,

beta-adrenergic blocking agents reduce the incidence of sudden cardiac death but do not change the frequency of premature ventricular complexes detectable by ambulatory monitoring, one would be hard pressed to use ambulatory monitoring as the sole or primary end-point in trials of other agents being tested for prophylaxis of sudden death because of their presumed anti-arrhythmic properties.

How Should Efficacy of Combinations be Evaluated?

Because of these considerations, it is necessary to construct circumscribed controlled clinical trials designed to acquire specific types of information needed for judicious selection of agents and approaches that ultimately may merit evaluation in global clinical trials. The primary focus of circumscribed trials should be to define the biological actions of the agents being evaluated with respect to fundamental physiological and pathophysiological phenomena. Circumscribed clinical trials can be completed with relatively small populations under conditions in which control can be particularly rigorous and the subjects can be rigidly stratified. The goals of such circumscribed trials are much more limited than those of global clinical trials. In the case of the agents we are considering in this discussion for example, circumscribed trials can define the extent to which specific calcium antagonists induce or exacerbate AV block in normal subjects, patients with ischemic heart disease without overt conduction system abnormalities, and patients with first degree AV block in the setting of coronary artery disease. Circumscribed trials can define the extent to which ventricular function is altered in patients stratified according to basal ventricular function, the severity and distribution of coronary artery disease, total peripheral arterial resistance, and ventricular filling pressure. Circumscribed clinical trials of beta-adrenergic blocking agents can define their electrophysiological properties in small subsets of patients studied definitively with invasive techniques and can also define the extent to which effects of the drug on ventricular performance and electrophysiology and dependent upon intrinsic sympathetic activity (ISA) by stratifying patients according to baseline ISA assessed rigorously. With information of this type available, additional circumscribed clinical trials could be undertaken so that interaction of agents of both types (beta-blockers and calcium antagonists)

can be studied in patients stratified according to those criteria found
to be important in determining the biological responses to each type of
agent alone, and predicated on an improved understanding of the mechanisms
involved in eliciting not only the explicit but also the implicit
therapeutic goals of therapy.

Safety:

Some of the tension between regulatory agencies and practitioners
results from different perceptions of what is meant by safety. No one
will argue that unexpected catastrophic events such as the grevious
consequences of widespread administration of Thalidomide before its
teratogenic effects were recognized must be avoided. Global clinical
trials provide one mechanism by which toxic effects can be recognized,
but clearly they can not supplant the need for vigorous, objective
monitoring and recording of potentially deleterious consequences of
administration of any agent to patients, whether such administration
occurs before or after the drug has been approved by a regulatory
agency. On the other hand, provisional utilization of an agent should
not depend on rigid adherence to the notion that it must have been
subjected to a prospective, double blinded, randomized patient-selection
global clinical trial, since toxicity can be evaluated by monitoring
whether or not the agent is being studied in such a trial. Unfortunately,
safety is a relative matter. The patient who is being threatened by a
high risk of sudden cardiac death may well elect to take a modest risk
of skin rash, paresthesias, flushing, CNS depression, or other predictable
possible effects of calcium antagonists or beta-adrenergic blocking
agents even before the unequivocal benefit of either or both in combination
as a prophylactic measure for sudden cardiac death is established.
Paradoxically, such patients do not provide the ideal substrate for
evaluation of possible late or catastrophic types of toxicity since
they are likely to be treated with multiple agents, to suffer from
consequences of severe underlying disease, and to fail to survive for
the protracted intervals necessary to more definitively exclude such
late, possible idiosyncratic, and certainly unexpected toxicity.

The Nature of Toxic Reactions:

Most "toxic" reactions of drugs are consequences of their pharmacological action. For example, calcium antagonists which cause vasodilitation may lead to postural hypotension, reflex tachycardia, peripheral edema (due to hydrostatic consequences of the altered peripheral vascular resistance), and cutaneous flushing. These and related phenomena may be accentuated when other agents with vasodilator properties are administered concomitantly. On the other hand, such effects may be blunted by concomitant adminsitration of agents with different pharmacological properties such as beta-adrenergic blocking agents that obviously may inhibit the acceleration of heart rate that might be induced by peripheral vasodilation alone. In addition to the intrinsic pharmacological properties of drugs, the physiology that governs their action will obviously determine the incidence and possible severity of adverse effects of this type. For example, if absorption or protein binding of a drug is modified so that more of the agent is available in free form for binding to receptors than would be the case otherwise, knowledge of dose or blood level will not accurately predict the biological effect of the drug in a given setting, nor provide insurance against adverse effects. Even if the free concentration of the agent at the receptor site could be delineated definitively, it would be difficult to predict the intensity of the biological response and hence the likelihood of adverse reactions which are in fact extensions of the agent's intrinsic pharmacological properties because of compensatory changes in receptor number and affinity that may occur in response to specific levels of agonists. Matters become particularly complex when agents are used in combination. For example, administration of cimetidine to a patient taking propranolol may modify the plasma propranolol level because of alterations induced by cimetidine on hepatic blood flow and because of the extensive metabolism of propranolol in the liver. However, changes in beta-receptor number resulting as a response to the increased free propranolol level due to this alteration may compensate for the otherwise augmented biological response that would have occurred.

How Can We Best Utilize These and Related Considerations in Developing Criteria for Defining Safety?

Again, one attractive approach is development and implementation of circumscribed clinical trials designed to characterise the dependence of biological response on intrinsic properties of the agent, specific physiological processes, and basic mechanisms invovled in drug action. In the case of an agent with a flat dose response curve, such as penicillin, marked changes in serum levels will not be a major safety concern because toxicity is not directly related to the prevailing blood level. Conversely, an agent like streptomycin which has a steep dose response curve with respect to toxic effects, must be administered within a framework of considerable information regarding factors that may modify prevailing blood levels by as little as 30%, since such factors may change a benign dose into one that is toxic.

A Proposed Strategy:

Several different types of studies are needed to assess the efficacy and safety of individual agents and combinations of calcium antagonists and beta-adrenergic blocking drugs.

Safety:

Potential toxicity of single agents should obviously be evaluated first in experimental animals prior to human testing, but with awareness that species differences may be profound and that the doses administered to animals may be largely irrelevant to the ultimately employed clinical dose particularly if massive doses are used in screening studies performed with animals. For evaluating safety in patients, persistent monitoring is required -- not only in the context of pre-approval circumscribed or global clinical trials since such trials do not guarantee detection of all possible toxic effects. Thus, continuing post-marketing surveilance is particularly important for detection of catastrophic types of toxicity that are not predictable based on the known pharmacological actions of drugs used alone or in combination and that may occur only infrequently.

Adverse effects of drugs attributable to their intrinsic properties and mechanism of actions are best assessed with circumscribed clinical trials of single agents alone first and subsequently combinations deemed to be therapeutically attractive. Information from such circumscribed trials coupled with knowledge of pharmacokinetics, interactions of drugs with receptors, the relative advantages of the agent in a specific setting in comparison to the relative risk of adverse reactions of this type, and the mechanisms of actions of individual drugs and combinations is essential for the practitioner who must decide whether or not to use an agent or combination of agents in treating an individual patient.

Efficacy:

Much of the tension between regulatory agencies and practitioners would disolve if the agencies recognized the need for and relied more fully on the individual practitioner's ability to make judgements based on results of circumscribed clinical trials and provided him with more freedom to do so, while protecting the safety of the population at large by vigorous monitoring for detection of major, potentially catastrophic toxicity that is unpredictable in terms of the known pharmacological properties of agents employed. Circumscribed clinical trials are particularly well suited for defining mechanisms of action of individual agents, beneficial interactions of combinations designed to achieve implicit as well as explicit therapeutic goals, and interactions of combinations designed to ameliorate adverse reactions attributable to the pharmacological properties of each drug alone. Circumscribed clinical trials can provide definitive, focused information regarding efficacy, difficult if not impossible to acquire from global trials. A global trial might detect a finite incidence of first degree A-V block in patients treated with an arbitrarily selected combination of a calcium antagonist and a beta-blocker. However, circumscribed clinical trials with rigidly stratified subsets of patients, sequential studies in the same subjects, and invasive electrophysiological measurements can much more definitively answer questions such as: What is the dose response curve for each drug alone and the combination with respect to affecting A-V conduction in normal subjects stratified according to age or gender, patients with pre-existing conduction system disease of specified type and severity, coronary artery disease with or without overt conduction system abnormalities, patients with pre-excitation, patients with bundle branch block, patients with hypokalemia (such as might result from concomitant treatment with a diuretic) among others.

Answers to these and similar questions are needed to provide the basis for judgements concerning the liklihood of benefit of the drug or the combination in individual patients. Information from circumscribed clinical trials should be employed by regulatory agencies as an aid to provisional approval of drugs. It should be employed in judicious selection of use of such agents by practitioners, whose judgemental responsibilities unfortunately have often been usurped by agencies concerned not only with surveillance for assessing safety but also with defining efficacy largely or exclusively in terms of global clinical trials. Finally, information from circumscribed clinical trials is essential for appropriate selection of agents suitable for ultimate evaluation in global clinical trials and determination of when such trials should be undertaken.

TABLE 1

Calcium Antagonists

Property	Agent		
	Verapamil	Diltiazem	Nifedipine
Coronary and peripheral vasodilation	++	++	+++
Depression of myocardial contractility	++	++	+
Depression of AV conduction	+++	++	0
Noncompetitive sympathetic antagonism	+	++	0
Local anesthetic effect	++	++	0
Oral dose	80-160 mg q 8 hr	60-80 mg q 8 hr	10-20 mg q 8 hr
Plasma half-life	5 hr	4 hr	4 hr
Side effects	Cardiac	Cardiac	Peripheral

TABLE 2

Beta-Receptor Blocking Agents

Drug	Cardio-selectivity (low doses)	ISMA[1]	Membrane depression	Lipid solubility	Potency[2]	Average dose (mg) q.d.	Plasma T1/2 (hr)	Therapeutic plasma level (ng/ml)
Acebutolol	+	+	+	++	0.3	600-1200	8	200-2000
Alprenolol	0	++	+	+++	0.3	400	2-3	50-100
Atenolol	+	0	0	+	1	100	6-9	200-500
Metoprolol	+	0	1	++	1	150-300	3-4	50-100
Nadolol	0	0	0	+	2-4	80-240	17-24	50-150
Oxprenolol	0	++	+	++	0.5-1	120-400	2	80-100
Pindolol	0	+++	+	++	6	7.5-22.5	3-4	50-150
Practolol	+	++	0	+	0.3	400	6-8	1500-5000
Propranolol	0	0	++	+++	1	120-400	3.5-6	50-100
Sotalol	0	0	0	+	0.3	240-480	5-13	500-4000
Timolol	0	1	0	++	6	15-45	4-5	5-10

[1]ISMA refers to intrinsic sympathomimetic activity.
[2]Expressed as potency vs 1-propranolol.

GENERAL GROUP DISCUSSION - How to Define Controlled Studies In:

Moderator: Dr. Leonard S. Dreifus

Dr. Meinertz: I would like to ask the panel if the calcium antagonists have any effect on ventricular arrhythmias.

Dr. Michelson: It is my impression that the effect of calcium blocking agents on the ventricular arrhythmias has not been studied very well. Furthermore, the actions of these agents have not been studied in enough drugs. Our preliminary evidence in this country does not appear to offer very promising results. They may be effective in patients who have a very specific etiology for the arrhythmia such as a vasospastic etiology. However, from the animal models and clinical evidence, it appears that the calcium blocking agents are not very promising in the presence of ventricular arrhythmias induced by ischemia. There has been some exciting work done in Dr. Sobel's department that suggests that the calcium entrance blocking agents may have a role in relationship to reperfusion arrhythmias. However, in the models that we have, and even in those animals in which we can elicit inducible sustained ventricular tachycardia, diltiazem and verapamil have not been found to be efficacious.

Dr Sobel: I would agree with Dr. Michelson, that from a clinical point of view, we have studied acute myocardial infarction induced ventricular arrhythmias, in one trial and there was no substantial change in the frequency of ectopic ventricular beats with therapeutic doses of nifedipine. However, this does not directly address the effectiveness of verapamil in this particular setting. It is my impression that others share the view that Dr. Michelson expresses. As far as the reperfusion arrhythmia story is concerned, Peter Corr has studied reperfusion arrhythmias using a cat preparation because it resembles the human heart in many ways. There is a truly dramatic suppression of reperfusion ventricular arrhythmias in this preparation. Both verapamil and nifedipine appear effective in these instances. However, in these animal models there appears to be vasospastic component. Furthermore, there is also a suppression of these arrhythmias by alpha adrenergic blockade and we are excited as to whether there appears to be a common mechanism of action.

Dr. Michelson: To reiterate what was demonstrated on some slides this afternoon, there appears to be a tremendous species differences, and particularly the cat, since this animal is so alpha sensitive, so that one has to be very careful in dog studies under similar circumstances. However, we do not know the action of these agents in man as there is not sufficient evidence available at this time.

Dr. Epstein: We have conducted similar studies in the dog. In these studies, we were not able to show protection with verapamil, nifedipine, or diltiazem. Conceivably, there is a species problem.

Dr. Abrams: I do not think in the discussions over the last several days that I have heard an expression or seen evidence of comparative efficacy of the beta blockers and calcium channel blockers in so-called common angina. A parallel question to this one is in the so-called common angina where there is evidence of a spastic element. How does one evaluate these agents in the presence of a spastic component?

Dr. Dreifus: I was interested in this question myself, Dr. Abrams. I am particularly concerned how we evaluate the beta blocking and calcium entry blocking agents in various subsets of patients. For instances, those with predominant vasospastic components as opposed to those with predominantly fixed obstruction. Perhaps the subsets should be clearly identified by both noninvasive as well as invasive techniques including cardiac catheterization. Perhaps even the knowledge of the family history, lipid patterns, stress induced vs. rest induced angina should be utilized to derive the various subsets for study.

Dr. Temple: The issue appears quite complex following the discussions that I have listened to this afternoon. Clearly, there appears to be two classes of patients, those with effort induced angina and those with rest angina. Admittedly, this may be partially due to vasospastic components but most likely it is due to fixed lesions. There is some published information, particularly that by Dr. Krikler. He studied nifedipine and propranolol alone and in combination as well as against placebo. In that setting, the combination of nifedipine and propranolol was best. Propranolol was next and nifedipine was third and placebo was last. There are a couple of other studies but I doubt that they have been published as yet. In Dr. Epstein's study he picked propranolol nonresponders. In this study verapamil in high doses was better than propranolol. However, the issue cannot be considered settled as yet. In another study, verapamil appeared to do somewhat better than nifedipine. However, I am not sure whether the dosages were comparable. There are relatively few comparisons and remarkably there are no adequate comparisons utilizing long acting nitrates. There are no publications to my knowledge in effort angina and there is only one, but not published, in vasospastic angina. Dr. Carl Pipine is carrying out a cross-over study of nifedipine vs. isosorbide. Interestingly, that study is being carried in what was thought of to be nitrate nonresponders, and the results so far seem to indicate that there was no difference in effectiveness between these two agents. To get to the other question, it may be sufficient to have a group of patients that is 90% effort angina and/or 90% vasospastic angina.

Dr. O'Rourke: There are several articles currently for editorial consideration in patients who have had coronary angiography as part of their entrance criteria. Beta-blocking agents are being compared to calcium blocking agents. In a study by Dr. Kelly from Australia, the comparison of propranolol vs. verapamil was considered. In addition to this, there are studies from Dr. Bramah Singh in Los Angeles. In addition, there are a large number of studies which are about to be published comparing verapamil to beta blocking agents. Although the results are variable, the majority of these studies indicate that both agents are effective as compared to placebo. However, there is not a clear decision at this moment as to whether one or the other is more efficacious.

Dr. Epstein: As you know, in our study we chose patients specifically that did not respond to propranolol. In these patients they did however, respond to verapamil. I think it is important that you can have a propranolol nonresponder and yet have an agent which will be effective. What we conclude, is that in some patients, a beta blocker is better than a calcium antagonist, while in others, the opposite may be true. This may identify patients in which the mechanism for precipitating angina pectoris is different.

Dr. Dreifus: Dr. Meinertz, do you know of any studies in which patients with supraventricular arrhythmias have been studied in subsets as to their precise electrophysiologic mechanism?

Dr. Meinertz: To my knowledge there are no really controlled studies. This has been in spite of the huge numbers of studies and case reports that are available.

Dr. Dreifus: What would you consider as minimal criteria to study the safety factor of these agents? I would like you to consider both the type of patient and the dosages of these agents. Perhaps you would even like to elaborate on the dose titrations and loading dosages of these agents.

Dr. Sobel: Obviously, this is a very difficult question to answer. For instance let us take verapamil. Furthermore, let's just look at these agents for use for supraventricular tachycardias. It is obvious that the efficacy of the drug in reverting supraventricular tachycardias is much greater than for its prophylaxis. There are many possible reasons as to why this may be true. Consider the fact that a patient with a supraventricular tachycardia may have a major adrenergic response to the arrhythmia itself. In this instance, the drug may be effective merely against the adrenergic response. Furthermore, receptor saturation could be achieved with a single intravenous dose. This could accomplish what it is intended to with oral administration. In light of the hepatic removal and metabolism of these agents there could be a compensatory mechanism for these receptors under other circumstances. However, it may not be possible to achieve a satisfactory response with oral or prophylactic administration. Hence, I cannot come up with a specific list of dose titrations. I would propose that we define, for example, what is the effect of a specific dose in normal subjects or what is the effect of a single dose in normal subjects on the major properties of AV function, sinus node function as well as other parameters of cardiac electrophysiology. Furthermore, we would like to know what is the effect of a comparable dose range on these parameters in people with SA or AV nodal disease. We may wish to evaluate the effect of these agents in patients such as with single, double or triple vessel coronary disease and use these conclusions as guides based on what we have learned initially and to see what happens in terms of experience with continuing surveillance to be certain that these guides are appropriate. I am sorry to be so vague, but I think by nature some of these questions have to have vague answers.

Dr. Morganroth: Dr. Temple, could you address this issue. I think this is really a troublesome problem in terms of hot new drugs which make it difficult at times for the clinicians to interact with pharmaceutical companies and likewise for pharmaceutical companies to interact with the FDA. For instance, if you take a drug which belongs to a new class and they read about this in the Wall Street Journal, New York Times or in one of the peer review journals. Let me take nifedipine for an example. Pfizer may receive thousands of calls from clinicians wishing to utilize these agents such nifedipine in their own patients with spasm. This often becomes a difficult problem because the companies must respond to this ethically. Do you have any advice to the industry and subsequently to clinicians how these problems can be handled?

<u>Dr. Temple:</u> It turns out, fortunately, or unfortunately, that most of the hot drugs that people want are in the cardiovascular area because cardiovascular disease embraces most of the problems leading to death. The means there will never be a time that any agent with promise won't be desired by the clinicians. Hence, there will never be a time when clinicians will not be demanding access to hot new effective drugs. There are then two questions. First, how can you keep that excitement from prejudicing the drug evaluation. Occasionally, the excitement is ill-founded and this should not prevent the in-depth precise orderly process to study the effectiveness and safety of these new drugs. Furthermore, it is not very helpful when a rather large but poorly controlled trial is presented and there is no immediate plan to carry out a precisely controlled trial. I do not want to be difficult, but it is my opinion that qualified physicians should be encouraged to participate in controlled studies. However, there may be patients that these clinicians and investigators do not feel can be treated in such trials. I would have no objection to the use of these new agents when it seems appropriate. These are probably patients who should not be introduced to a placebo. Secondly, my answer concerns the encouragement of the investigators to keep and accurate records. For instance, they should not give the drugs away to their friends and adhere precisely to the guidelines which have been set forth for the clinical trial of these agents. Hence, a maximal use of the data can be achieved even though the patient is not in a controlled study category. Dr Sobel mentioned earlier that the only way to identify catastrophic events is to have the drug administered to a large number of individuals. In the case of nifedipine, we have had a rather well controlled exposure to at least 5000 or 6000 people and this drug has been administered to these patients under the so-called emergency IND. In my mind this is at least as valid an experience as any post-marketing surveillance study. The optimal technique for this type of exposure is to be able to identify every single patient that has received this agent and finally, attempt to ascertain the

fate of every one of these individuals. Even though it is not a controlled study you will certainly be able to identify the worse cases and problems. In this instance, all you have to assume is that everything that happened is due to the drug and then you can assume what the worse possible effects of the drug can produce. In the case of nifedipine there may not be as many controlled studies as we would like, but the experience is rather impressive. The information that we receive would indicate that nothing too bad does happen to these people on drug.

Dr. Wenger: Dr. Dreifus, I would like to ask you specifically that in your study of patients with atrial fibrillation on drugs you suggested exercise evaluation of heart rate response and I was struck by the failure of the patients to respond with heart rate on verapamil, how much exercise are you recommending and what kind of heart rate would you expect a patient to achieve?

Dr. Dreifus: I am not so sure that only suppression of heart rate with exercise is what you want to achieve in a drug trial. The case that I showed was not to represent precise numbers per se. We use a criteria before randomization of at least the ability to increase the heart rate by 30 beats per minute with exercise. In order to determine the effectiveness of an agent, we would insist on at least a 15% reduction in heart rate from the control level at the same level of exercise after drug is administered. We use a modified stress test in order to achieve this rate of graded exercise for three minutes. Obviously, a strict protocol such as the Bruce or Balke could be used. However, we are not attempting to achieve maximal heart rates, but to utilize only a controlled period of exercise, say for 3 minutes which is just enough to increase the heart rate sufficiently in the presence of atrial fibrillation so that any significant reduction of more than 15% from the control level would be considered an effect due to the drug that we administered.

<u>Dr. Michelson:</u> Dr. Dreifus, I think Dr. Wenger's point is a little different. One criteria that you could use is to determine how far they can exercise in a protocol, that is, could they exercise for a longer period of time with less symptoms and that could be considered an end point and a favorable response. However, patients with atrial fibrillation usually show an inappropriate increase in the ventricular rate with exercise. In these patients it may even take toxic doses of digitalis to adequately control the ventricular rate. Hence, in these exercise protocols you are interested in the accelerated response very early in the protocol. That may even be within the first minute of a very low level protocol such as a Naughton or modified Balke test.

SYMPOSIUM ON THE EVALUATION OF

NEW BETA BLOCKER AND CALCIUM ANTAGONIST DRUGS

Gunnar Aberg, Ph.D.
Director, Cardiovascular Pharmacology
Ciba-Geigy Corporation

William B. Abrams, M.D.
Executive Director, Clinical Pharmacology
Merck Sharp & Dohme Research Labs

Fred Alexander, M.D.
Clinical Research
Smith Kline & French Research Labs

Douglas Allin
Clinical Research Associate
American Critical Care

Cynthia B. Altman, M.D.
Associate Director, Clinical Investigation
Smith Kline Corporation

Keiko B. Aogaichi, M.D.
Research Physician
Hoffman-LaRoche Inc.

Jeffrey Anderson, M.D.
Assistant Professor of Internal Medicine
University of Utah

Sherrin Baky
Senior Clinical Research Associate
Syntex, Inc.

Carla Ballard
Cardiovascular Product Manager
SmithKline Corporation

James A. Bannon, Pharm D.
Clinical Research Associate
Philadelphia Association for Clinical Trials

Allan H. Barker, M.D.
Associate Clinical Professor of Medicine
University of Utah

Walter M. Barker, Ph.D.
Assistant Director, Clinical Research
Abbott Laboratories

John Barlow, M.D.
Director, Clinical Investigation
Merrell Dow Pharmaceutical Inc.

Priv. Doz. Dr. R. Bayer
Universitat Dusseldorf
West Germany

Mirza A. Beg, M.D.
Group Director, Medical Affairs
Smith Kline & French Laboratories

Bruce Berger, M.D.
Assistant Director, Clinical Pharmacology
Revlon Health Care Group

Dr. Hartmut Bethge
Prof. Dr. Med.
E. Merck, West Germany

James Biddison, M.D.
Greater Baltimore Medical Center

Phillip H. Bookman, M.D.
Director, Clinical Investigation
McNeil Pharmaceutical

Martin Borggrefe, M.D.
Universitat Dusseldorf
West Germany

R. Michael Borland, M.D.
Assistant Director, CV/Pulmonary Section
Ciba-Geigy Corp.

Gunter Breithardt, M.D.
Universitat Dusseldorf
West Germany

David M. Capuzzi, M.D., Ph.D.
Director
Lankenau Medical Research Center

Joan Carter
President
Cardio Data Systems

Frank Caruso, M.D.
Director, Clinical Pharmacology
Revlon Health Care Group

Jacques Chelly, M.D.
Associate Professor of Pharmacology
University of Paris, France

P. Y. Chi, Ph.D.
Assistant Director, Biostatistics
Ciba Geigy Corporation

James Coakley
Product Manager, Cardiovasculars
Miles Pharmaceuticals

James L. Cockrell, Jr.
Physiologist
VA Medical Center, Washington, D.C.

Jay N. Cohn, M.D.
Professor of Medicine
University of Minnesota

David L. Copen, M.D.
Associate Clinical Professor of Medicine
Yale University

Stanley Cortell, M.D.
Professor of Clinical Medicine
Columbia University

Rebecca B. Costello, M.S.
Research Associate
VA Medical Center

George H. D'Addamio
Manager, Clinical Trials
Smith Kline & French Laboratories

Richard R. Dean, Ph.D.
Head, Department of CV Pharmacology
Abbott Laboratories

Philip L. Dern, M.D.
Medical Officer, Cardio-Renal Drugs
Food and Drug Administration

Robert DiBianco, M.D.
Assistant Chief Cardiology
VA Medical Center, Washington, D.C.

Leonard S. Dreifus, M.D.
Professor of Medicine and Physiology
Jefferson Medical College

Stewart J. Ehrreich, Ph.D.
Deputy Director
Food and Drug Administration

Charles A. Ellis, Jr., M.D.
President Medical Staff
Lawrence General Hospital, Lawrence MA

Toby R. Engel, M.D
Professor of Medicine
Medical College of Pennsylvania

Stephen E. Epstein, M.D.
Chief, Cardiology Branch
National Heart, Lung & Blood Institute

John L. Fischetti, M.D.
Associate Director, Marketed Products
ICI Americas Inc.

Dr. J. D. Fitzgerald
Head of Research Dept II
Imperial Chemical Industries Ltd, England

James E. Foley, Ph.D.
Associate Clinical Pharmacology Director
E. R. Squibb & Sons, Inc.

Lawrence Friedman, M.D.
Medical Officer, Clinical Trials Branch
National Heart, Lung & Blood Institute

Curt D. Furberg, M.D.
Chief, Clinical Trials Branch
National Heart Lung & Blood Institute

Ronald R. Gauch, Ph.D.
Vice President - Regulatory Affairs
Ciba-Geigy Pharmaceutical Co.

John A. Gillespie, M.D.
Assistant Professor of Medicine
University of Rochester

Robert Glaser
Product Manager
Merck Sharp & Dohme Research Laboratories

Sidney Goldstein, M.D.
Clinical Professor of Medicine
University of Michigan

Hector J. Gomez, M.D., Ph.D.
Director of Clinical Pharmacology International
Merck Sharp & Dohme

Leonard M. Gonasun, M.D.
Associate Director Clinical Research
Sandoz, Inc.

Stanley Gottlieb, M.D.
Senior Clinical Research Fellow
McNeil Pharmaceutical

Lawrence S. C. Griffith, M.D.
Associate Professor of Medicine and Pharmacology
Johns Hopkins Hospital

Juan R. Guerrero, M.D.
Director, Medical Research
Knoll Pharmaceuticals

Dr. F. Hagemeijer
Sint Franciscus Gasthuis
The Netherlands

Dr. Klaus-Jurgen Hahn
Prof. Dr. Med.
Knoll AG, West Germany

Harold F. Hailman, M.D.
Assistant Vice President, Director Scientific Liason
Hoffman-LaRoche Inc.

Donald C. Harrison, M.D.
Chief of Cardiology
Stanford University

Arthur H. Hayes, Jr., M.D.
Commissioner
Food and Drug Administration

Harry M. Helfrich, M.D.
Associate Director, Clinical Operations
Smith Kline & French Laboratories

Judith A. Hemberger, Ph.D.
Clinical Research Team Leader
Marion Laboratories, Inc.

John Hermanovich, Jr., M.D.
Assistant Professor of Medicine
Hershey Medical Center

Ake Hjalmarson, M.D.
Associate Professor of Medicine
Sahlgren Hospital, Sweden

M. J. Hoffman, M.D.
Clinical Associate Professor of Medicine
University of Rochester

Geoffrey Holmes
Clinical Associate
Merck Sharp & Dohme Research Laboratories

William L. Holmes, Ph.D.
Chairman, Department of Research
Lankenau Medical Research Center

Saichi Hosoda, M.D.
Professor of Medicine
Jichi Medical School, Japan

John E. Jefferis, M.D.
Vice President, Medical Director
Pfizer Pharmaceuticals

Bengt W. Johansson, M.D.
Associate Professor
General Hospital, Sweden

Norman M. Kaplan, M.D.
Professor of Medicine
University of Texas

Nadim Kassem, M.D.
Senior Director, Internal Medicine
Schering Corporation

Robert E. Kates, Ph.D.
Assistant Professor
Stanford Medical Center

Francis J. Kenney, M.D.
Director, Clinical Research
Norwich-Eaton Pharmaceuticals

Edward B. Kirsten, Ph.D.
Director, Clinical Pharmacology
Knoll Pharmaceuticals

Harris Koffer, Pharm.D.
Clinical Research Associate
Philadelphia Association for Clinical Tria

John B. Kostis, M.D.
Chief, Cardiology
Middlesex General Hospital

Donald C. Kvam, Ph.D.
Manager, Clinical Pharmacology
Riker Laboratories, Inc.

Ezra Lamdin, M.D.
Director, Medical Affairs
ICI Americas Inc.

David P. Lauler, M.D.
Chairman, Department of Medicine
Lawrence & Memorial Hospitals

Norman W. Lavy, M.D.
Vice President, Drug Regulatory Affairs
E. R. Squibb & Sons, Inc.

Ian K. Lee, M.D.
Director, Pharmaceutical Clinical Development
Mead Johnson Company

Barrie Levitt, M.D.
Clinical Professor of Medicine in Cardiology
Albert Einstein College of Medicine, New York

Bengt Ljung, M.D.
AB Hassle
Sweden

Earle Lockhart, M.D.
Associate Director, Cardiovascular
Clinical Research
Bristol-Myers Company
Robert Loring
Vice President and General Manager
Cardio Data Systems

Dr. Serge Lubin
Director of Therapeutic Research in Cardiology
Sanofi Research, France

Bo Lundgren, Ph.D.
AB Hassle
Sweden

George E. Maha, M.D.
Executive Director, Clinical Research-Domestic
Merck Sharp & Dohme Research Laboratories

Sara A. Mahler, M.D.
Associate Medical Director
Endo Laboratories

Valerie McCall
Research Supervisor
Cardio Data Systems

Prof. Dr. Thomas Meinertz
University of Mainz
West Germany

Eric L. Michelson, M.D.
Director, Clinical Research Unit
Lankenau Medical Research Center

Howard Miller, M.D.
Director of Medical Research
Sandoz, Inc.

Hideo Mitamura, M.D.
Research Associate
Lankenau Medical Research Center

E. Neil Moore, D.V.M., Ph.D.
Professor of Physiology in Medicine
University of Pennsylvania

Joel Morganroth, M.D.
Chief, Cardiac Research and Education
Lankenau Medical Research Center

T. Nakagawa
Tanabe
Japan

M. Nakamura
Tanabe
Japan

Edward S. Neiss, M.D., Ph.D.
Vice President, Research
Revlon Health Care Group

Jeffrey Nickel, Ph.D.
Merck International Division

Ole-Jorgen Ohm, M.D.
Research Associate
Lankenau Medical Research Center

S. Bertil Olsson, M.D.
Associate Professor
Sahlgrenska Hospital, Sweden

Robert O'Rourke, M.D.
Chief of Cardiology
University of Texas

Carl E. Orringer, M.D.
Acting Head, Section of Cardiology
Ochsner Clinic

Alfred F. Parisi, M.D.
Chief, Cardiology Section
West Roxbury VA Medical Center

Manley A. Paulos, Ph.D.
Assistant Director Clinical Research
American Critical Care

Gerd Petrik
Helopharm W. Petrik & Co. KG
West Germany

T. P. Pruss, Ph.D.
Division Director, Biological
Research and Development
Revlon Health Care Group

Joseph Reiser, Ph.D.
Associate Professor of Medicine and Physiology
Hahnemann Medical College

Robert Reynolds, Ph.D.
Group Leader, Cardiovascular Pharmacology
American Critical Care

Samuel Ringel, Ph.D.
Assistant Director, Clinical Pharmacology
Revlon Health Care Group

Robert E. Robinson, M.D.
Director, Clinical Research/Internal Medicine
Merrell Dow Pharmaceuticals Inc.

Thomas Robinson, M.D.
Pfizer Laboratories

Barry A. Rofman, M.D.
Director of Clinical Research
Merck Sharp & Dohme

Edward Rowland, M.D.
Senior Research Fellow
Royal Postgraduate Medical School

Alberto Rosenberg, M.D.
Director, Investigational Drugs
ICI Americas Inc.

Magdi Sami, M.D.
Assistant Professor
McGill University, Quebec

Timothy Saxton
Clinical Research Associate
Endo Laboratories

James A. Schoenberger, M.D.
Professor of Medicine
Rush-Presbyterian St. Luke's Medical Center

John J. Schrogie, M.D.
Executive Director
Philadelphia Association for Clinical Trials

Alexander Scriabine, M.D.
Director
Miles Institute for Preclinical Pharmacology

Ludger Seipel, M.D.
Director of Cardiology
University of Tubingen, West Germany

Dr. Theodore Selby
Associate Medical Director
Smith Kline Corporation

S. Ben Sen, M.D.
Director, Cardiovascular/
Pulmonary Section
Ciba-Geigy Corporation

David Seymour, M.D.
L.E.R.S.
France

Arthur Simon, M.D.
Director, CV Clinical Research
Bristol-Myers Company
International Division

Steven Singh, M.D.
Washington, D.C.

Burton E. Sobel, M.D.
Cardiologist-in-Chief
Barnes Hospital, St. Louis

Peter Somani, M.D., Ph.D.
Professor of Pharmacology & Medicine
Medical College of Ohio

Joseph F. Spear, Ph.D.
Professor of Physiology
University of Pennsylvania

Hubert C. Stanton, Ph.D.
Director Biologic Research
Mead Johnson & Co.

W. J. Stein, M.D.
New York

Alfred Steinman, M.D.
Director Clinical Research
American Critical Care

Eberhard Stengele, M.D., Ph.D.
Godecke AG
West Germany

Kurt Stoepel, M.D.
Bayer AG
West Germany

Norio Taira, M.D.
Professor of Pharmacology
Tohoku University, Japan

Davis L. Temple, Ph.D.
Director, Chemical Research
Mead Johnson & Co.

Robert Temple, M.D.
Director, Division of Cardio-Renal Drugs
Food and Drug Administration

J. Gerald Toole, M.D.
Associate Director, Clinical Therapeutics
Warner-Lambert Company

Phoebe Tribble
Manager, Cardiovascular Clinical Research
Bristol-Myers Company

P. Turlapaty, Ph.D.
Clinical Investigation Associate
Ives Laboratories

Svetislav K. Vanov, M.D., Ph.D.
Director of Medical Research
Miles Pharmaceuticals

Yoshio Watanabe, M.D.
Professor of Medicine
Fujita Gakuen University, Japan

Jerome Weinstein, M.D.
Director, Clinical Research
Hoechst-Roussel Pharmaceuticals, Inc.

Thomas L. Wenger, M.D.
Sr. Clinical Research Scientist
Burroughs Wellcome Co.

Lars Werko, M.D., F.R.C.P.
Executive Vice President
AB Astra, Sweden

Richard R. Wilson, M.D.
Director, CV/Renal Clinical Research
G. D. Searle & Co.

Robert A. Wolbach, M.D., Ph.D.
Associate Director Clinical Research
Abbott Laboratories

Alastair J. J. Wood, M.D.
Associate Professor of Pharmacology
Vanderbilt University

Raymond L. Woosley, M.D., Ph.D.
Associate Professor of
Medicine and Pharmacology
Vanderbilt University Medical Center